T0302228

Medically Unexplained Symptoms, Somatisation and Bodily Distress

Developing Better Clinical Services

Medically Unexplained Symptoms, Somatisation and Bodily Distress

Developing Better Clinical Services

Edited by

Francis Creed
Professor of Psychological Medicine, School of Community-Based Medicine, University of Manchester, Manchester, UK

Peter Henningsen
Professor of Psychosomatic Medicine, Technical University Munich, Munich, Germany

Per Fink
Professor of Functional Disorders, Research Clinic for Functional Disorders and Psychosomatics,
Aarhus University Hospital, Aarhus, Denmark

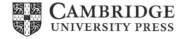

CAMBRIDGE
UNIVERSITY PRESS

CAMBRIDGE
UNIVERSITY PRESS

University Printing House, Cambridge CB2 8BS, United Kingdom

Cambridge University Press is part of the University of Cambridge.

It furthers the University's mission by disseminating knowledge in the pursuit of education, learning and research at the highest international levels of excellence.

www.cambridge.org
Information on this title: www.cambridge.org/9780521762236

© Cambridge University Press 2011

First published 2011

A catalogue record for this publication is available from the British Library

Library of Congress Cataloguing in Publication data
Medically unexplained symptoms, somatisation, and bodily distress : developing better clinical services / [edited by] Francis Creed, Peter Henningsen, Per Fink.
   p. ; cm.
Includes bibliographical references and index.
ISBN 978-0-521-76223-6 (hardback)
1. Somatoform disorders.   2. Medicine, Psychosomatic.   3. Neuroses.   I. Creed,
Francis.   II. Henningsen, Peter, M.D. III. Fink, Per.
[DNLM: 1. Neurotic Disorders.   2. Somatoform Disorders   3. Psychophysiologic Disorders.
WM 170]
RC552.S66M43 2011
616.85'24–dc22
2011011503

ISBN 978-0-521-76223-6 Hardback

Contents

Preface

It is very common that patients present to their doctor with bodily symptoms, such as headaches, fatigue, back, chest and other pains, which cannot be explained by a recognised physical disease. All medical specialists and GPs see large numbers of such patients and these symptoms are the fifth most common reason for patients visiting doctors in the USA. Some doctors and many patients express despair about our lack of knowledge regarding the origin of these symptoms and how best to treat them.

This book addresses several aspects of this problem. The most important is the continued suffering endured by patients who have persistent symptoms without appropriate treatment. Another is the high cost associated with these symptoms because of frequent doctor visits, expensive investigations and the associated disability, which leads to time missed from work. They form one of the most expensive categories of healthcare expenditure in Europe. This book makes the case for shifting some of this expenditure away from numerous investigations for organic disease and towards effective treatment of bodily distress.

Another problem addressed by this book is that of classification and nomenclature. Throughout the book the authors make it clear that the problem of numerous bodily symptoms is one which encompasses both body and mind. As such, it is served poorly by our healthcare system which is sharply divided into 'mental' and 'physical' domains. Since the traditional labels 'medically unexplained symptoms' or 'somatisation' are so unhelpful, we propose the term 'bodily distress' as a more useful name for these disorders, which need to be recognised in their own right if patients are to receive appropriate treatment.

This book is timely because the major diagnostic systems in psychiatry (the American 'Diagnostic and Statistical Manual' and the World Health Organisation's 'International Classification of Diseases') are currently being revised and it is important to present up-to-date information about diagnosis and nomenclature.

The international authors who have contributed to this book provide a detailed review of the epidemiology of bodily distress and the current evidence concerning the efficacy of treatment. On this basis, we make evidence-based recommendations for improving the management of bodily distress syndromes. This involves helping doctors to acquire the necessary skills to manage these problems appropriately and enabling them to find adequate time to do so. We must seek to overcome the negative attitudes towards psychological illnesses in our society and modify the way that patients, doctors and social agencies approach these problems. There are a few examples of new service provision and good practice, which we have highlighted.

Contributors

Arthur Barsky
Director of Psychiatric Research, Brigham and Women's Hospital, Boston, MA, USA

Chris Burton
Centre for Population Health Sciences, University of Edinburgh, Edinburgh, UK

Richard Byng
University of Plymouth, Plymouth, UK

Francis Creed
School of Community-Based Medicine, University of Manchester, Manchester, UK

Jef de Bie
Liaison Psychiatrist, Liege, Belgium

Christian Fazekas
Medical Psychology and Psychotherapy Department, Medical University Graz, Graz, Austria

Per Fink
Research Clinic for Functional Disorders and Psychosomatics, Aarhus University Hospital, Aarhus, Denmark

Kurt Fritzsche
Department of Psychosomatic Medicine and Psychotherapy, University Medical Center Freiburg, Freiburg, Germany

Alka Gudi
Newham Centre for Mental Health, East London NHS Foundation Trust, London, UK

Else Guthrie
School of Community-Based Medicine, University of Manchester, Manchester, UK

Constanze Hausteiner-Wiehle
Technical University Munich, Munich, Germany

Peter Henningsen
Technical University Munich, Munich, Germany

Peter Hindley
Department of Child Psychiatry, St George's Hospital Medical School, London, UK

Kurt Kroenke
Department of Medicine, Indiana University, Indianapolis, IN, USA

Astrid Larisch
University of Marburg, Marburg, Germany

Sing Lee
Hong Kong Mood Disorders Center, Prince of Wales Hospital, Shatin, Hong Kong

Kari Ann Leiknes
Department of Psychiatry, Norwegian Knowledge Centre for the Health Services, Oslo, Norway

Charlotte Ulrikka Rask
Aarhus University Hospital, Aarhus, Denmark

Winfried Rief
University of Marburg, Marburg, Germany

Gudrun Schneider
Department of Psychosomatics and Psychotherapy, University Hospital Münster, Münster, Germany

Andreas Schröder
Aarhus University Hospital, Aarhus,
Denmark

Michael Sharpe
Psychological Medicine Research,
Royal Edinburgh Hospital, Edinburgh, UK

Wolfgang Söllner
Department of Psychosomatic Medicine
and Psychotherapy, General Hospital
Nuremberg, Nuremberg, Germany

Athula Sumathipala
Institute of Psychiatry,
King's College London, London, UK and
Institute for Research and Development,
Colombo, Sri Lanka

Christina van der Feltz
Netherlands Institute of Mental Health,
Utrecht, The Netherlands

Emma Weisblatt
Laboratory for Research into Autism;
Department of Experimental Psychology,
University of Cambridge, Cambridge, UK

Peter White
Centre for Psychiatry, Wolfson Institute
of Preventative Medicine, Queen Mary
University of London, St Bartholomew's
Hospital, London, UK

Chapter

1

Epidemiology: prevalence, causes and consequences

Francis Creed, Arthur Barsky and Kari Ann Leiknes

Introduction

The epidemiology of medically unexplained symptoms will be considered under the following headings: prevalence, causes and consequences. For the first and last of these headings the data will be considered in three categories: medically unexplained symptoms, somatoform disorders and functional somatic syndromes (see Chapter 2). These 'diagnostic' labels describe different groups of patients but they also overlap considerably. The term 'medically unexplained symptoms' is a broad one; somatoform disorders and functional somatic syndromes are subgroups within it. These subgroups are represented diagrammatically in Figure 1.1 and are described below.

Prevalence

For each of the three groups, medically unexplained symptoms, somatoform disorders and functional somatic syndromes, the nature of the group will be described briefly and then the prevalence of these will be described in cross-sectional studies in primary, secondary care and population-based studies. Then each section will include data from longitudinal studies that show the outcome of medically unexplained symptoms.

Medically unexplained symptoms

The term 'medically unexplained symptoms' has been used widely and there is a considerable amount of data concerning the prevalence and outcome of these symptoms. The findings from secondary care will be considered first as this is where the concept was developed. It arose because many patients attending secondary care clinics had symptoms that, after appropriate (and sometimes very extensive) investigation, could not be explained by organic pathology or well-recognised physiological dysfunction [1;11]. In this way the term 'medically unexplained symptoms' describes a group of patients by what they do not have. The next section examines how often this occurs.

Prevalence of medically unexplained symptoms in secondary care

Secondary care studies in the Netherlands, UK and Germany have shown that medically unexplained symptoms are the presenting problem for 35–53% of new outpatients at specialist medical clinics (Table 1.1). The most common symptoms are: headache; back, joint, abdominal, chest and limb pains; fatigue; dizziness; bloating; palpitations; hot or cold sweats;

Medically Unexplained Symptoms, Somatisation and Bodily Distress, ed. Francis Creed, Peter Henningsen and Per Fink. Published by Cambridge University Press. © Cambridge University Press 2011.

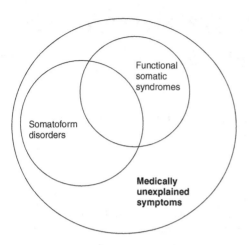

Figure 1.1 Diagram to show how the term 'medically unexplained symptoms' embraces a wide group of patients, and that somatoform disorders and functional somatic syndromes are smaller subgroups within the wider group.

Table 1.1 Proportion of patients attending secondary care clinics whose presenting complaint is diagnosed as 'medically unexplained'

Study	Type of clinic	Number of patients included in the study	Per cent diagnosed with 'medically unexplained symptoms'
Van Hemert *et al.*, 1993 [2]	General medical	191	52
Hamilton *et al.*, 1996 [3]	Gastroenterology, neurology and cardiology	324	35
Nimnuan *et al.*, 2001 [4]	Seven different specialties	550	52
Fiddler *et al.*, 2004 [5]	Gastroenterology, neurology and cardiology	295	39
Kooiman *et al.*, 2004 [6]	General medical	321	53
Targosz *et al.*, 2001 [7]	Neurology	57	30
Carson *et al.*, 2000 [8]	Neurology	300	30
Stone *et al.*, 2009 [9]	Neurology	3781	30
Mangwana *et al.*, 2009 [10]	General medical	200	50

nausea; trembling or shaking; and numbness or tingling sensations [11;12] In seven clinics in one UK hospital, the proportion of patients with medically unexplained symptoms varied between 24% in the chest clinic to 64% in the neurology clinic (mean 52%) [4].

The high prevalence of medically unexplained symptoms in neurology clinics has led to numerous studies and a summary of data from seven neurology clinics showed prevalence rates between 26% and 45% (median 30%) [9]. In the largest survey, the most common categories of diagnosis were: (i) headache disorders (26%); (ii) an organic

Table 1.2 Proportion of patients attending primary care whose presenting complaint is diagnosed as 'medically unexplained'

	Clinics	Number of patients	Per cent diagnosed with 'medically unexplained symptoms'
Mumford et al., 1991 [14]	Primary care patients consulting with illness (i.e. excluding 'routine' visits	554	7–12.6
Peveler et al., 1997 [15]	Booked consultations	170	19
Kirmayer and Robbins, 1991 [16]	Primary care attenders	685	23.6
Palsson, 1988 [17]	Sweden		16
Kisely et al., 1997 [18]	Weighted sample of primary care attenders	5447	15.4 Had 5+ medically unexplained symptoms
Duddu et al., 2008 [19]	119	119	33

neurological disease was present but the presenting symptoms were not explained by it (26%); and (iii) conversion symptoms (motor, sensory or non-epileptic attacks) (18%) [13]. The second category is important as it indicates that medically unexplained symptoms commonly occur in people who have physical illness but the presenting symptoms cannot be explained by that physical illness. Examples include non-epileptic attacks, which occur in people who also have epilepsy, and non-cardiac chest pain in people with heart disease.

Prevalence of medically unexplained symptoms in primary care

In primary care, the general practitioner (GP) will usually make a clinical judgement that a symptom is not explained by organic disease, without necessarily using special investigations. Such symptoms generally form between 10% and 33% of presenting complaints in primary care (Table 1.2). A systematic review concluded that medically unexplained symptoms constitute the primary reason for consulting the GP in 15–19% of patients [20].

The proportion of all patients whose symptoms are classified as 'medically unexplained' varies greatly between GPs and this variation cannot be attributed to variation in the GPs' patient populations; instead it reflects GPs' tendency to use this categorisation [21]. There is, however, a relevant diagnostic category in the *International Classification of Diseases* (ICD), under which many of these patients may be classified: 'Signs, symptom and ill-defined conditions' (ICD code 780–789). In the UK, this accounts for the one of the largest diagnostic categories of hospital outpatients and the fourth largest category in primary care. In USA, it is the fifth most frequent reason for visiting a doctor (60 million per annum) – see Table 1.3 [22].

Table 1.3 Number of visits to the doctor in USA by diagnostic group (2005) [22]

Diseases of	Million visits per annum	Per cent of total
Respiratory system	110	11.5
Nervous system	86	8.9
Circulatory system	81	8.5
Musculoskeletal	80	8.4
Symptoms, signs; ill-defined conditions	**60**	**6.3**
Endocrine, nutritional and metabolic	56	5.9
Mental disorders	47	4.9

Prevalence of medically unexplained symptoms in population-based studies

Surveys in the general population show that pain is the most common medically unexplained symptom – headache and back, joint, abdominal and limb pain being the most common; fatigue, dizziness, bloating, food intolerance and sexual difficulties are also common [23;24]. These symptoms are reported by over a fifth of the population but only a small proportion report that they are severe [24].

Outcome of medically unexplained symptoms

Prospective studies are concerned usually with one of two outcomes: Does an organic disease come to light that explains the symptom(s)? Do the symptoms persist over time?

With regard to the first question, follow-up studies have been performed to assess whether medically unexplained symptoms turn out to have a medical cause after a period of time. In fact, this rarely occurs even though it is uppermost in some doctors' minds and contributes to their decision to perform repeated investigations. In a German one-year follow-up study, five out of 284 patients classified as having medically unexplained physical symptoms later turned out to have a physical illness that could explain their symptoms [6]. In the largest neurology survey, only four out of 1030 patients (0.4%) had acquired an organic disease diagnosis that was unexpected at initial assessment and could plausibly be the cause of the patient's original symptoms [9].

With regard to the second question, population-based studies suggest that most medically unexplained symptoms wane over time; fewer than half persist over one year [24;25;26;27] and two-thirds recede over a longer period [28]. The long Norwegian study reported that painful medically unexplained symptoms may persistent over many years in approximately 8% of the general population, mostly women [28].

Although up to a fifth of new symptoms presented to GPs are medically unexplained [15;29], only 10% of these (i.e. 2.5% of all patients attending the GP) had persistent symptoms that led to repeated consultation – the rest consulted for a single episode only [30]. In secondary care clinics symptoms tend to be more severe and persistent than those seen in primary care. Over a one-year follow-up period, approximately two-thirds of patients report improvement in medically unexplained symptoms but about 40% report some continued symptoms causing ill health [6;31]. The proportion may be higher in neurology clinics [9].

Therefore, we can conclude that medically unexplained symptoms are very common both in the general population and in primary and secondary care, but at least in the first two settings most are transient. These may not require medical intervention other than reassurance about their frequency in healthy people and a check that they do not indicate physical disease. In secondary care the symptoms tend to be more persistent and may have more severe consequences (see below). In both primary and secondary care, doctors need to use appropriate strategies in managing patients with these symptoms. The rest of this section is concerned with medically unexplained symptoms that persist over six months or more.

Somatoform disorders

This term includes several disorders where a high number of medically unexplained symptoms is the main feature. It is a diagnostic category in both the *Diagnostic and Statistical Manual of Mental Disorders* (DSM)-IV and ICD-10 classification systems [32;33], where it also includes several other diagnoses (see below). This book is concerned with the first two main categories (a and b below) but there have been several modifications, two of which (c and d) are also included here. In this chapter we used 'somatoform disorder' as an umbrella term to include the following disorders:

(a) '*somatisation disorder*', defined by numerous bodily symptoms that are disabling and/ or lead to medical help-seeking [32]; there are slight differences in the way the two diagnostic systems define this disorder but both require multiple somatic symptoms spread throughout the body (Table 1.4)

(b) '*undifferentiated somatoform disorder*', which requires presence of one or more unexplained physical symptoms causing clinically significant distress or impairment for six months [32]

(c) '*abridged somatisation disorder*', which is defined by the somatoform symptom index (SSI) either as four medically unexplained symptoms in men and six in women (SSI-4/6) or by three medically unexplained in men and five in women (SSI-3/5) [34;35]

(d) '*multisomatoform disorder*', which requires presence of three current medically unexplained symptoms, one of which must have been present for two years [36].

This large number of diagnoses reflects the fact that 'somatisation disorder' as originally defined, had a very high number of medically unexplained symptoms, which meant that this disorder was very rare in population-based studies [37]. The other diagnoses have been developed as they have a lower threshold and are more relevant in primary care and population settings.

The remaining major group of disorders concerns high health anxiety (hypochondriasis), which also has rather a high threshold. Persistent disease conviction (the worry that one has a serious illness) occurs in approximately 6.5% of the population but the additional criteria of seeking medical help and refusal to accept appropriate medical reassurance reduces the prevalence of the diagnosis in population-based samples to less than 1% [37;38;39].

The diagnostic category 'somatoform disorders' includes also the diagnoses of pain disorder (pain not fully explained by organic disease and associated with psychological factors) and conversion disorder, which refers to sensory or motor symptoms for which no medical explanation can be found, but which are disabling and lead to medical help-seeking [32;33]. Pain disorder is not considered separately from the somatoform disorders as the epidemiology is similar; many people have multiple pains [40]. Conversion disorder

Table 1.4 Selected somatoform disorders in DSM-IV and ICD-10 [32; 33]

DSM-IV		ICD-10	F45
Somatisation disorder:	300.81	Somatisation disorder:	F45.0
– a history of many medically unexplained symptoms before age 30		– at least two-year history of medically unexplained symptoms	
– resulting in treatment sought or psychosocial impairment		– resulting in repeated (three or more) primary care or specialist consultations	
– a total of eight or more medically unexplained symptoms from across the four groups: • at least four pain • two gastrointestinal • one sexual • one pseudoneurological		– a total of six or more medically unexplained symptoms, from at least two separate organ groups (gastrointestinal, cardiovascular, genitourinary, skin and pain)	
Undifferentiated somatoform disorder	300.81	Undifferentiated somatoform disorder	F45.1
Hypochondriasis	300.7	Hypochondriacal disorders	F45.2
Pain disorder associated with psychological factors	307.80	Persistent somatoform pain disorder	F45.4
		Somatoform autonomic dysfunction	F45.3
Body dysmorphic disorder	300.7	Hypochondriacal – dysmorphophobia	F45.2
		Neurasthenia	F48.1

is not considered in detail in this book as it is rare in clinical practice and has not been studied widely [41;42]. Body dysmorphic disorder is a condition characterised by a distressing and disabling preoccupation with an imagined or slight defect in appearance [43;44;45]. It differs considerably from the very common disorders which are the main concern of this book.

ICD-10 includes neurasthenia (chronic fatigue), as one of the somatoform disorders. This is considered here as chronic fatigue syndrome under the heading of functional somatic syndromes. ICD-10 also includes somatoform autonomic dysfunction, which refers to symptoms of autonomic arousal with preoccupation and distress relating to a particular organ [33].

Prevalence of somatoform disorders in primary and secondary care

The prevalence of somatoform disorders in primary care studies is shown in Table 1.5. The third column of Table 1.5 shows the prevalence of somatoform disorders as a whole, i.e. somatisation disorder, undifferentiated somatoform disorder, somatoform disorder, not otherwise specified, pain disorder, hypochondriasis, conversion and abridged somatisation (SSI-4/6) and multisomatoform disorder. It can be seen in the last column that the diagnoses undifferentiated somatoform disorder, somatoform disorder, not otherwise specified, abridged somatisation (SSI 4/6) and multisomatoform disorder are much more frequent than the other disorders, reflecting their lower threshold.

Most of the studies have used a standardised research interview to assess diagnosis. The most commonly used interviews are the Schedule for Clinical Assessment in Neuropsychiatry (SCAN)[55], the Primary Care Evaluation of Mental Disorders (PRIME-MD) [56], and, in population-based studies, the Composite International Diagnostic Interview (CIDI) [57]. During these interviews respondents are asked about each of many bodily symptoms and, for each symptom reported, whether a doctor has declared that it is 'medically unexplained' and that it causes distress or impairment. A few studies, however, have simply used a self-administered questionnaire (e.g. the Personal Health Questionnaire (PHQ-15)) to ask respondents to tick on a checklist those bodily symptoms that they have experienced recently and found bothersome. This approach counts all bodily symptoms, regardless of whether they are medically explained or unexplained. It cannot lead to a formal diagnosis but it has been found that a high score on such a questionnaire is associated with impaired functioning and high healthcare use even after adjusting for concurrent psychiatric and physical disorders [53;54;58]. Patients scoring in the top 10–20% on this questionnaire were given a provisional diagnosis of 'probable somatisation' [53] and are represented in the bottom three rows of Table 1.5.

The use of different measures and different samples leads to considerable variation in the prevalence rates reported in Table 1.5, but most studies provide an overall prevalence in the range of 8–20%. The median for abridged somatisation SSI-4/6 is 16% which concurs with a systematic review [37] (Table 1.6).

One systematic review examined the prevalence of somatisation and hypochondriasis in primary care using abridged forms of both diagnoses (Table 1.6) [37]. It can be seen that the median prevalence figure for abridged somatisation was 16% in primary care and this concurs with a further systematic review which found that between 16% and 22% of patients had abridged somatisation [20]. The median prevalence rate for hypochondriasis is approximately 10% of patients attending primary care.

Very few primary care studies reporting prevalence of somatoform disorders provide clear data regarding concurrent physical illnesses. One study reported that 42% of patients with somatoform disorders had diseases of the circulatory system, 29% of the musculoskeletal/connective, 20% respiratory, and 18% endocrine, nutritional and metabolic diseases [49]. Another showed that 58% of patients with medically unexplained symptoms had two or more chronic diseases, most commonly chronic chest and cardiovascular diseases [59]. Of the last two studies in Table 1.5, one reported that the mean number of physical disorders was approximately 1 in the patients with high somatic symptoms score [54]. The other reported that 41% had at least one serious concurrent medical illness [53]. This shows clearly that somatoform disorders coexist with recognised physical diseases.

There have been fewer studies of somatoform disorders in secondary care. In patients newly referred to a neurology clinic, the most frequent current diagnoses were somatoform disorders (33.8%; 95% confidence interval (CI) 25.9–42.7%) [12]. In two-thirds of these patients the somatoform disorder occurred in addition to a clear organic neurological disorder, emphasising the frequency with which somatoform and organic disorders can co-occur. A study of medical inpatients, most of whom would have had serious physical illness, found 1.5% had somatisation disorder and 10% had undifferentiated somatoform disorder,

Table 1.5 Prevalence of somatoform disorders in primary care

Study	Sample (N) and measure[a]	Proportion with any somatoform disorder,[b] % (95% CI) or median % and range (R)	Prevalence (rate %) of individual somatoform disorders (see text) and further data concerning incidence or persistence
Fink et al., 1999 [46]	Denmark (18–60 yrs) (SCAN 2.1) N = 199	Any somatoform disorder: 22.3% (16.4–28.1%) for ICD-10 57.5% (50.5–64.5%) for DSM-IV	Prevalence: (DSM-IV): 30.3% (23.8–36.9) if somatoform disorder, NOS excluded 12.6% (7.9–17.4) if somatoform disorder, NOS and undifferentiated somatoform disorder excluded
de Waal et al., 2004 [47]	The Netherlands (25–80 yrs) (SCAN 2.1) N = 473	Any somatoform disorder: 16.1% (12.8–19.4%)	Somatisation disorder: 0.5% (0.0–0.9) Undifferentiated somatoform disorder : 13.0% (9.8–16.2) Pain disorder: 1.6% (0.7–2.4) Hypochondriasis: 1.1% (0.4–1.8) Conversion disorder: 0.2% (0–0.6)
Toft et al., 2005 [48]	Denmark (18–65 yrs) (SCAN) (Present state rate) N = 701	Any somatoform disorder (using ICD-10) Total: 35.9% (30.4–41.9%) F: 38.3% (31.5–45.6%) M: 31.7% (22.6–42.4%)	Diagnoses by ICD -10: F44.4–48.0 Somatisation: 10.1% (7.5–13.5) Undifferentiated somatoform disorder: 1.7% (0.7–4.0) Hypochondriasis : 2.4% (1.1–5.2) Seasonal affective disorder: 4.3% (2.8–6.7) Pain disorder: 4.4% (2.7–6.9)
Hanel et al., 2009 [49]	Germany (18–65 yrs) N = 1751	18.4%	Somatoform disorders/ functional disorder diagnoses by 75 GPs

Table 1.5 (cont.)

Study	Sample (N) and measure[a]	Proportion with any somatoform disorder,[b] % (95% CI) or median % and range (R)	Prevalence (rate %) of individual somatoform disorders (see text) and further data concerning incidence or persistence
Kroenke et al., 1997 [36]	USA (18–91yrs) (PRIME-MD) (PHQ-15) N = 1000	Any somatoform disorder 14%	Multisomatoform disorder: 8.2% Somatoform disorder, NOS: 4.2% Hypochondriasis: 2.2%
Jackson et al., 2008 [50]	USA (Follow-up 5 yrs) (PRIME-MD) (PHQ-15) N = 500 (baseline)		Multisomatoform disorder: 8% (at baseline) Stability: 22% (7/32) had multisomatoform disorder at five-year follow-up)
Ustun and Sartorius, 1995 [51]	6 European sites PSE/SCAN/ CIDI/SCID		Somatisation disorder: median = 1.7% (range: 0.4–3.0) Hypochondriasis: median = 0.5% (range: 0.1–1.0) Neurasthenia: median = 9.3% (range: 4.6–10.5)
Lowe et al., 2008 [52]	Germany (18–95 yrs) (PRIME-MD) (PHQ-15) N = 2091	9.5% (PHQ-15 score ≥15)	
Barsky et al., 2005 [53]	USA (PHQ-15) N = 1546	20.5% (PHQ-15 high score)	
Kroenke et al., 2002 [54]	USA (PHQ-15) N = 3000	10% (PHQ-15 score ≥15)	

[a] Adults >18 years, unless otherwise specified.
[b] Total and M and F.
M, male; F, female; CI, confidence interval; NOS, not otherwise specified; DSM, *Diagnostic and Statistical Manual of Mental Disorders*; ICD, International Classification of Diseases; SCAN, Schedule for Clinical Assessment in Neuropsychiatry; PRIME-MD, Primary Care Evaluation of Mental Disorders; PHQ, Patient Health Questionnaire; CIDI/SCID, Composite International Diagnostic Interview/Structured Clinical Interview for DSM.

Table 1.6 Summary of findings regarding prevalence of abridged somatisation and abridged definition of hypochondriasis [37]

	Abridged somatisation	Abridged hypochondriasis
Population-based	Median = 14% (range: 4.4–19%) Four studies	Median = approx. 7% (range: 1.3–10.7%) Four studies
Primary care attenders	Median = 16.6% (range: 7.3–35%) Six studies	Median = 10.7% (range: 2.2–14%) Eight studies

using DSM-IV criteria [60]. In a larger study of patients with serious physical illnesses the prevalence of somatoform disorders (15.3%) was significantly higher than in a population-based sample of healthy controls (5.7%) [61].

Prevalence of somatoform disorders in population studies

The prevalence of somatoform disorders in population-based studies is summarized in Table 1.7. Once again, there is considerable variation in the prevalence rates reflecting the use of different measurement instruments. One systematic review of population-based studies included only somatoform disorders diagnosed using the standardised CIDI. In seven studies, with a total of 18 894 respondents, the 12-months prevalence ranged from 1.1% to 11% (median = 6.3; 95% CI 2.1–7.8) [62]. The authors of this study estimated that the number of residents aged 18–65 years in the European Union (EU) (total 301 million) affected by somatoform disorders within the previous 12 months was 18.9 million (95% CI 12.7–21.2).

Outcome of somatoform disorders

There have been remarkably few prospective studies of somatoform disorders [27;37;74]. From the results of two systematic reviews it appears that half of patients with abridged somatisation reported remission of the disorder over one year and in half the symptoms persist [27;74]. The same is true of patients with hypochondriasis [27].

Symptoms are more persistent in those studies which have selected patients with particularly severe or chronic symptoms [74]. In adolescents, where symptoms tend to be of recent onset, symptoms of somatoform disorders persisted in approximately one-third of participants over a 15-month follow-up period [62]. In another study of adolescents, approximately 45% of those with undifferentiated somatoform disorder continued to have the disorder one year later, but the proportion was larger (two-thirds to three-quarters) in those with pain disorder or abridged somatisation disorder [64;65].

Functional somatic syndromes

The term functional somatic syndromes covers the individual, well-recognised medical syndromes such as irritable bowel syndrome, fibromyalgia (chronic widespread pain), chronic fatigue syndrome, temporomandibular joint pain and multiple chemical sensitivity. These diagnoses are made frequently in clinical practice but their cause is unclear so they are generally regarded as 'medically unexplained' syndromes. Each syndrome has clear diagnostic features that have been refined by expert committees[75;76;77]. These detailed diagnostic

Table 1.7 Prevalence of somatoform disorders in population-based samples

Population-based study	Sample (N)[a]	Proportion with any somatoform disorder,[b] % (95% CI) or % (SE)	Prevalence (rate %) of individual somatoform disorders (see text) and further data concerning incidence or persistence
Essau et al., 2007 [62;63]	Germany Adolescents (12–17 yrs) (lifetime rate) (M-CIDI) N = 523	Total: 12.2% F: 18.2% M: 5%	Undifferentiated somatoform disorder : 11.0% Pain disorder: 1.6% Conversion disorder: 1.5%
Lieb et al., 2002 [64;65]	Germany Adolescents (14–34 yrs) (lifetime rate) (M-CIDI) N = 3021	Total: 12.5% (11.0–14.0%) F: 17.6% (15.3–20.1%) M: 7.2% (5.8–8.9%)	Undifferentiated somatoform disorder : 9.0% (7.8–10.3) Pain disorder: 1.7% (1.2–2.4) Abridged somatisation (SSI-4/6): 1.7% (1.2–2.3)
Leiknes et al., 2007 [66]	Norway (18–66+ yrs) (6-month rate) Current (M-CIDI) N = 1247	Total: 24.6% (22.2–27.0%) Any severe somatoform disorder (with impairment) Total: 10.2% (8.5–11.9%) F: 14.4% (11.6–17.1%) M: 5.9% (4.0–7.7%)	Somatoform disorder, NOS: 19.2% (17.0–21.4) Multisomatoform disorder: 14.1% (12.2–16.0)
Jacobi et al., 2004 [67]	Germany (18–65 yrs) (12-month rate) (M-CIDI) N = 4181	Total: 11.0% (0.6) F: 15.0 (0.8) M: 7.1 (0.6)	Abridged somatisation (SSI-4/6): 4.3% (0.3) Pain disorder: 8.1% (0.5)
Wittchen et al., 2005 [68;69]	Four European countries (Czech Republic, Italy, Norway, Germany) and seven studies combined (18–65 yrs) (12-month rate) (CIDI and M-CIDI) N = 18 894	Total: 11% (10.1–12.1%) F: 15.0% (13.4–16.7%) M: 7.1% (6.1–8.4%)	

Table 1.7 (*cont.*)

Population-based study	Sample (N)[a]	Proportion with any somatoform disorder,[b] % (95% CI) or % (SE)	Prevalence (rate %) of individual somatoform disorders (see text) and further data concerning incidence or persistence
Kringlen *et al.*, 2006 [70]	Norway (18–65 yrs) (12-month rate) (CIDI 1.1) N = 1080	Total: 2.2% (0.4) F: 1.5% (0.5) M: 3.0% (0.7)	Not available
Kringlen *et al.*, 2001 [71]	Norway (18–65 yrs) (12-month rate) (CIDI 1.1) N = 2066	Total: 2.1% (0.3) F: 3.7% (0.6) M: 1.2% (1.3)	No information about included disorder subtypes
Sandanger *et al.*, 1999 [72]	Norway (18–65+ yrs) (2-week rate) (CIDI 1.0) N = 617	Total: 5.9% (3.5–8.2%) F: 7.1% (3.7–10.4%) M: 4.5% (1.2–7.8%)	Somatoform disorder by ICD-10: F44-F45.4 Incidence: 6.5 (2.0–30.4) per 1000 per annum
Rief *et al.*, 2001 [73]	Germany (14–92 yrs) (SOMS-7) N = 2050		(Self-rated by SOMS) Somatisation (300.81): 0.3% (F: 0.5; M: 0.1) SSI-3/5: 23.6% (F:18.5 M: 30.1) Hypochondriasis: 7.0% (M: 5.7 F: 8.0)

[a] Adults >18 years, unless otherwise specified.
[b] Total and M and F.
M, male; F, female; CI, confidence interval; NOS, not otherwise specified; CIDI, Composite International Diagnostic Interview; M-CIDI, Munich-Composite International Diagnostic Interview; SOMS, Screening for Somatoform Symptoms; SSI, somatoform symptoms index.

criteria are symptom-based as there is no known organic cause and no specific abnormality that can be detected by suitable investigation.

Prevalence of functional somatic syndromes in primary and secondary care

These syndromes are found frequently in both primary and secondary care. Findings will be presented here for three syndromes, irritable bowel, chronic fatigue syndrome and fibromyalgia (also known as chronic widespread pain). These are typical of the functional somatic syndromes and have been most thoroughly studied. Although the prevalence is presented for individual syndromes, it must be recognised that these syndromes overlap a great deal [78;79;80].

Irritable bowel syndrome and functional dyspepsia are known collectively as 'functional gastrointestinal disorders'. Such disorders account for 4–5% of all consultations with a GP and 41% of patients attending a gastroenterology clinic [81;82]. Chronic fatigue is a main presenting feature in approximately 7% of primary care attenders [83;84]. Chronic fatigue syndrome, on the other hand, is much less frequently recorded as a diagnosis in primary care, partly because of the reluctance of many doctors to use this diagnosis. Approximately a third of patients presenting in primary care with disabling fatigue of six or more months duration have chronic fatigue syndrome [85].

Approximately 2% of patients on a GP list present persistently with fibromyalgia [86]; many more will present with less persistent symptoms but these are inconsistently reported, rather like chronic fatigue syndrome. A quarter of patients in a rheumatology clinic have fibromyalgia and this diagnosis accounted for 14.5% of all medical outpatients in one study [87]. In another report, 15% of hospitalised patients in an internal medicine ward had fibromyalgia [88].

The UK-based study by Nimnuan and colleagues in seven clinics at a tertiary care hospital found that there was a predominance of the 'expected' syndrome for each clinic [4]. For example, in the gastroenterology clinic, irritable bowel syndrome was found in 25% of patients but tension headaches, aching muscles and joints and cardiac chest pain were also common. Similarly, in the rheumatology, clinic fibromyalgia was very common, but this was also seen commonly in respiratory, gastroenterology and gynaecology clinics. Non-cardiac chest pain is not only a very common symptom presenting to cardiac clinics and emergency departments but it is also commonly seen in most other specialist clinics [87].

This UK study demonstrates how the organisation of secondary medical care into specialty clinics can increase the chance that patients with multiple bodily symptoms are seen in many different clinics [4;87]. In most healthcare systems, specialist doctors work in discrete clinics and a patient who presents with, for example, abdominal pain and diarrhoea is likely to be investigated for these symptoms. If the investigations prove to be negative, and the patient also has chest pains, they are likely to be referred to a cardiologist for investigations of the chest pain. The appropriate investigations will be performed and, if no medical illness is found to explain the chest pains, the patient is at risk of being referred to a chest physician if they also have breathing difficulties and/or a neurologist for headaches. In this way high healthcare costs accrue but the patient may receive little help with their symptoms.

Prevalence of functional somatic syndromes in population-based samples

Systematic reviews of the prevalence of irritable bowel syndrome in population-based samples have indicated that the prevalence varies considerably with the definition of the syndrome. A recent systematic review found four studies that used the Rome definition in satisfactory population-based samples (n = 32 638). The pooled prevalence was 7% (95% CI 6–8%) [82].

There are differences in the prevalence of chronic fatigue syndrome according to the definition used. One recent large study estimated a prevalence of 2.5%, which concurs with a previous UK primary care study [89;90], although previous estimates have been lower because several definitions exclude all comorbid conditions, including psychological morbidity. The proportion of the population with disabling, unexplained fatigue is approximately 10% [90;91].

The prevalence of fibromyalgia varies with the method of ascertainment. Estimates in North America have varied between 2% and 3.3% for fibromyalgia according to the

American College of Rheumatology (ACR) criteria [92;93;94]. Higher estimates (4.5–12%) have emerged from population-based studies of chronic widespread pain, which does not included the allodynia of fibromyalgia [95;96;97;98]. The Declaration of the European Parliament (P6_TA(2009)0014) states that fibromyalgia affects 14 million persons in the EU and 1–3% of the general population worldwide.

Outcome of functional somatic syndromes

Follow-up studies of the functional somatic symptoms have shown that very few people with these diagnoses are found later to have organic disease that caused their symptoms [82;99;100]. In a series of follow-up studies of irritable bowel syndrome, less than 3% were later diagnosed with organic gastrointestinal disease [101]. A systematic review of follow-up studies of chronic fatigue syndrome found that only three out of more than 2000 patients died, but up to 10% developed physical illness that could have been responsible for the original fatigue [102]. Fibromyalgia has been associated with the later onset of cancer but the reason for this association is not clear; lack of exercise and use of analgesics have been suggested [103;104]. It has also been associated with an increased risk of suicide [105;106].

With regard to the course of the disorder, over half of patients with irritable bowel syndrome continue to have symptoms some years later and it is regarded as a chronic and recurrent disorder [82;101]. Established cases of chronic fatigue syndrome have a poor outlook as less than 10% improve greatly, though the majority of children with the condition do so [102]. With less severe cases of disabling chronic fatigue, such as that seen in primary care, the outlook is better with at least 40% showing improvement over one year [102]; in one population-based study the proportion was even higher [107]. The situation is very similar with fibromyalgia; in one clinic study only 15% of patients improved over 4 years, but in a population-based cohort nearly half were free of chronic widespread pain (defined as ACR criteria for fibromyalgia) one year later [108].

Relationship between functional somatic syndromes and somatisation

The previous two subsections have reviewed somatoform disorders and functional somatic symptoms. Because both are based on 'medically unexplained' symptoms it has been assumed by some that these are synonymous. In one sense this is true as undifferentiated somatoform disorder involves one or more persistent medically unexplained symptoms that leads to impairment. Each of the functional somatic syndromes fits this description. When we consider multiple somatic symptoms, however, the picture is rather different. Only a proportion of people with a functional somatic syndrome have multiple somatic symptoms.

Numerous somatic symptoms are closely associated with irritable bowel syndrome in population-based studies [109;110]. In fact, only a third have raised somatisation scores and the proportion is similar in primary care patients with irritable bowel syndrome [111]. Among patients attending specialist clinics with severe and persistent irritable bowel syndrome, up to a half have multiple medically unexplained somatic symptoms, or a raised somatic symptom score [112;113]. Systematic reviews have shown that approximately one half of irritable bowel syndrome patients have concurrent psychiatric disorders, including somatisation, and approximately half also have other functional somatic symptoms [114;115]. Similar findings have been reported in fibromyalgia and temporomandibular joint pain [116;117;118]. In population-based samples of people with disabling low back pain, chronic widespread pain, orofacial pain and chronic fatigue the proportion with numerous somatic symptoms is between 26% and 36% [80;119].

Gastroenterologists recognise that some patients with irritable bowel syndrome have 'extra-gastrointestinal' symptoms of irritable bowel syndrome, namely headaches, fatigue, muscular and joint pains, etc. [120;121]; these are common somatic symptoms and also the symptoms of chronic fatigue syndrome and fibromyalgia. It has been recognised recently that some people with irritable bowel syndrome have only the gastrointestinal symptoms of this disorder ('uncomplicated' or 'single' irritable bowel syndrome), whereas others have numerous 'extra-gastrointestinal' symptoms ('complicated' or irritable bowel syndrome with multiple symptoms) [122;123]. The same is true of other functional somatic syndromes [124;125].

Conclusion

This section has indicated that medically unexplained symptoms are common in the general population and present frequently to doctors. It is only those symptoms which are persistent and lead to impairment or distress that are diagnosed as 'somatoform disorders'. Such disorders are common, occurring in approximately 6% of the population, 16% of primary care attenders and up to 33% of patients in secondary care clinics.

Functional somatic syndromes are also common but only some patients with these syndromes also have numerous somatic symptoms. Patients with symptoms of functional somatic symptoms alone are now described as having 'uncomplicated, single functional somatic syndromes' whereas those who have numerous somatic symptoms, in addition to those of the functional syndrome, are referred to as having 'complicated' functional somatic syndromes [124]. Alternatively, in the new 'bodily distress disorder' classification, approximately half of patients with functional somatic syndromes are classified as severe, multiorgan type of bodily distress syndrome, as opposed to single-organ type, which is much more common generally [12;126]. We shall see in a later section that this is very important when it comes to impairment and costs.

Evidence-based aetiological factors

Much of the evidence regarding the aetiological factors associated with medically unexplained symptoms, somatoform disorders and functional somatic syndromes comes from cross-sectional studies. This means that they are correlates rather than true aetiological factors, which can only be determined in prospective studies. This section will briefly review these findings and add the few data that have been collected in prospective studies. The latter have mostly concerned the functional somatic syndromes rather than somatoform disorders. Finally the data concerning prediction of persistent medically unexplained symptoms, somatoform disorders and functional somatic syndromes will be added as these are important in identifying people who are at highest risk of disability and high healthcare costs.

Correlates of medically unexplained symptoms and somatoform disorders

It is widely accepted that somatisation is associated with female sex, fewer years of education, low socioeconomic status, other psychiatric disorders (especially anxiety and depressive disorders) and recent stressful life events [37;127;128;129]. It is unclear why numerous somatic symptoms occurs more often in females and the reasons suggested include: sex differences in prevalence of depression and anxiety, in pain threshold and awareness/reporting of bodily symptoms, in experience of childhood abuse; and the socialisation of women to be less stoical than men [130]. Many of these findings relate to studies of the more severe forms of somatisation. Abridged somatisation is less clearly related to a female predominance and there is no evidence of a sex difference in the prevalence of hypochondriasis, although the association with anxiety and depression is clear [37].

Some people are predisposed to develop somatoform disorders. There is some evidence of a genetic predisposition to develop numerous somatic symptoms. It is unclear whether this is independent of a predisposition to develop psychiatric disorders in general but several studies suggest this is so [121;131;132]. Early childhood experiences that are associated with somatoform disorders include a parent with poor health or high neuroticism, persistent abdominal pain as a child and childhood abuse [5;129;133;134]. The personality trait of neuroticism has been identified as an independent correlate of medically unexplained symptoms [135;136;137]. Prior experience of physical illness may predispose individuals to somatoform disorders.

Correlates thought to be important in the onset of somatoform disorders include a physical or psychiatric illness and/or a stressful life event (either direct involvement in a traumatic event or serious illness or death of a close relative) [138;139]. Four prospective studies have shown that the following are associated with new onsets of somatoform disorders: female gender, lower social class, prior psychiatric disorder (especially anxiety and depression), physical illness, a negative view of one's health, and reported traumatic sexual and physical threat events [26;64;140;141].

Since medically unexplained symptoms are universal, studies have tried to explain why in some people they become established and lead to consultations with doctors, whereas most other people either ignore such symptoms or do not act upon them. These features are mostly cognitive – and depend on people's response to bodily symptoms – and complex and beyond the scope of the present chapter, but they include sensitisation to pain, heightened attention to bodily sensations, increased worry about symptoms and illness (health anxiety), attributing bodily symptoms to a possible medical illness rather than recognising them as a normal phenomenon or psychological stress [127;142;143]. These features are generally though to predict persistence of symptoms, which is considered in the next section.

Predictors of persistence of medically unexplained symptoms or somatoform disorders

As mentioned above, there are too few prospective studies of somatoform disorders. The study that examined patients attending primary care with *persistent* medically unexplained symptoms, as opposed to all medically unexplained symptoms, found that this group was significantly older and more likely to be female, unemployed, from non-Western background, with fewer years of education and to have consulted for a psychological disorder than patients attending with a medical diagnosis [30].

One of the few prospective studies found that, over a 10-year period, persistent somatoform pain disorder was more likely to be reported by women; depression at the first assessment was the only other predictor [28]. A one-year prospective study did not find that depression was a predictor; older age, poor self-evaluation of health and impaired work role were predictors [26]. In a prospective study of adolescents the factors associated with persistent somatoform disorders were female gender, concurrent depressive or other psychiatric disorder, parental psychiatric disorders and negative life events [65;140].

Medically unexplained symptoms are more likely to be persistent if they are numerous and there is high health anxiety and/or continued depression [6;27;144]. The psychological variables listed in the last paragraph of the previous section are considered to be predictors of persistent somatoform disorders. One study suggested that chronic physical disease, negative affectivity and selective attention/somatic attribution are independently associated with number of persistent medically unexplained symptoms [59]. Among patients attending a neurology clinic with rather more severe medically unexplained symptoms, persistence over a year occurred in two-thirds and this was associated with a patient's belief that they would not improve, a failure to attribute the symptoms to a psychological cause and the receipt of illness-related financial benefits [13].

Correlates of functional somatic syndromes

All of the functional somatic syndromes are more common in women than men. All are associated with younger age, lower socioeconomic status, anxiety, depression, and stressful life events. The similarity of associated features has led to the suggestion that they might be part of the same disorder [78;145]. In a meta-analysis, Henningsen and Zimmerman showed that a significantly greater proportion of patients attending medical clinics with functional somatic syndromes (irritable bowel syndrome, functional dyspepsia, chronic widespread pain and chronic fatigue syndrome) have well-documented anxiety or depressive disorders than patients with comparable organic diseases or healthy controls [146].

The functional somatic syndromes are also associated with physical illness. In population-based studies there is a clear association between chronic fatigue and physical illness, even after adjustment for potentially confounding variables [147;148]. The association occurs with a wide range of physical illnesses including cardiovascular, chest disease, cancer and sleep disorders [107;149], as well as a wide range of medications taken for physical illness.

Studies of onset of functional somatic syndromes have shown that post-infectious irritable bowel syndrome is associated both with prior gastrointestinal infection and with anxiety, depression, neuroticism, recent stressful life events and health anxiety [150;151]. One of the most interesting aspect of this work has been the repeated finding that it is psychological factors, such as anxiety, stress, somatisation, and negative illness beliefs, which explain the onset of post-infectious irritable bowel syndrome among those who have experienced the infection [150;152;153]. There is some evidence that the nature of the triggering infection is associated with the type of functional somatic syndrome; chronic fatigue is most likely to follow infectious mononucleosis [153;154;155].

Inactivity in childhood and inactivity after infection have been found to increase the risk of chronic fatigue syndrome in adults [156], but one recent study suggested that overactivity in childhood and obesity in adulthood were associated with later onset of chronic fatigue in the absence of concurrent psychiatric disorder [157]. In the presence of concurrent psychiatric disorder the risk factors differed somewhat; they included negative life events and family history of psychiatric disorder [157].

Predictors of onset and persistence of functional somatic syndromes

Prospective clinical studies have shown that risk factors for persistent functional somatic syndromes include: demographic features (female sex, older age, fewer years of education, lower socioeconomic status, unemployment), a reported history of sexual abuse/other childhood adversity, multiple symptoms, concurrent chronic physical illness or psychiatric disorder (depression, anxiety, dysthymia, panic), social stress, and reinforcing social factors such as illness benefits [102;127;129;145;158] Many of the perpetuating factors for the functional somatic syndromes are psychological. Persistent worry about having a serious illness, hypervigilance to bodily symptoms and the tendency to 'catastrophise' in relation to pain, a strong conviction of an underlying physical disease and an expectation that the illness will have marked adverse consequences, are all recognised in this context [102;127;129;143;145;156].

For patients with irritable bowel syndrome, successful contact with a gastroenterologist that is followed by improvement in symptoms of irritable bowel syndrome is associated with reduced anxiety, reduced fears of cancer or other serious illness, greater likelihood of attributing symptoms to stress and less catastrophising in relation to bodily symptoms [159]. This confirms the importance of these factors in persistent irritable bowel syndrome.

Consequences of persistent medically unexplained symptoms/somatisation

Impairment of function

This section will demonstrate the extent to which medically unexplained symptoms, somatoform disorders and functional somatic syndromes are associated with impairment of function. The first part will examine the relationship between severity of medically unexplained symptoms and somatoform disorders and degree of impairment. It will show also that medically unexplained symptoms and somatoform disorders may be associated with a degree of disability that is comparable with that associated with major physical diseases and psychiatric disorders such as depression. Lastly we shall see that when medically unexplained symptoms or somatoform disorders occur concurrent with physical illness and anxiety/ depression the effect on impairment appears to be additive.

This section cites studies which have used most frequently the measure of health status developed for the Medical Outcomes Study (Short Form 36 [SF-36] or derivatives, such as SF-20) [160]. This is a self-administered questionnaire that assesses perceived disability in several areas, which can be grouped together as two summary scores. The physical component summary score includes physical limitations, such as going up stairs or carrying shopping, role limitation (illness affects daily life) attributed to physical illness and to bodily pain and general health. The mental component summary score refers to mental ill health and how its affects daily life, vitality and social functioning. These subjective reports will be supplemented by objective records of days off sick where appropriate.

Medically unexplained symptoms and somatoform disorders

Impairment of health status increases with number or severity of medically unexplained symptoms

There is a spectrum of severity of medically unexplained symptoms which is correlated with degree of impairment. An increasing number of medically unexplained symptoms is associated with increasing levels of disability indicating a dose–response relationship [161]. The

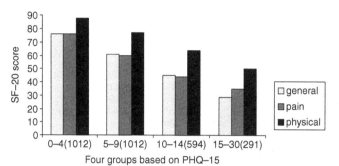

Figure 1.2 Health status (Short Form (SF)-20) for general, pain and physical scores by four groups of patients based on somatisation score [54]. (Low SF-20 score represents impairment.) Number of participants in each group given in parentheses. PHQ, Patient Health Questionnaire.

same is true of health anxiety [162]. This holds true when *all* bodily symptoms are recorded using a self-report questionnaire (e.g. PHQ-15) instead of measuring only medically unexplained symptoms.

Figure 1.2 shows a sample of 2917 primary care patients divided into four groups according to the number of somatic symptoms rated as bothersome on the PHQ-15 questionnaire (0–4, 5–9, 10–14 and 15–30 symptoms) [54]. It can be seen that general, painful and physical dimensions of health status all show greater impairment as number of bodily symptoms increases after adjustment for age, sex, years of education and number of physical illnesses. The 10% with the greatest number of somatic symptoms (scores 15–30) have greatly impaired health status. The same relationship of increasing disability with increasing number of somatic symptoms has been recorded in attenders at UK secondary care gastroenterology, neurology and cardiology clinics [31]. This study showed also that the correlation between number of bodily symptoms and health status (R = −0.57) was almost identical for patients whose symptoms were medically explained or unexplained.

The data presented above relate to self-rated disability. The same relationship has been observed between the number of somatic symptoms and number of days 'off sick'. After adjustment for age, sex, years of education and number of physical illnesses, people who report numerous somatic symptoms (top 10% scores on PHQ-15) have twice as many days off sick as those with moderate score (10 to 14) [47].

One study compared patients with medically unexplained symptoms, patients with somatoform disorders and healthy controls [163]. On the SF-36 physical component score, the first two groups showed marked impairment compared with the last. On the mental component summary score, however, only patients with somatoform disorder showed impairment. Thus people with medically unexplained symptoms which are not sufficiently severe to fulfil the criteria for somatoform disorder did not show impairment on the mental health dimension.

The impairment of health status associated with medically unexplained symptoms is comparable with that of depressive disorders or general medical disorders

Primary care

In primary care, one study showed that patients with medically unexplained symptoms were impaired in seven of eight dimensions of functioning compared with the general population [164]. Patients with depressive disorder were impaired in five dimensions. The pattern of impairment differed (Figure 1.3). Medically unexplained symptoms were associated

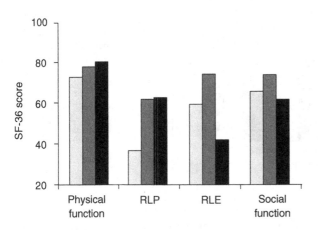

Figure 1.3 Short Form (SF)-36 scores for patients with medically unexplained symptoms (light grey), general population (dark grey) and people with major depressive disorder (black). High scores represent good health status; and low scores indicate impairment [164]. RLP, role impairment physical; RLE, role impairment emotional.

with impairment especially in physical functioning (illness affects walking upstairs, carrying shopping, etc.) and role limitation physical (the physical effect of the illness on daily life). Depressive disorder showed greatest impairment on role limitation emotional (the emotional effect of the illness on daily life) and social functioning. Thus the impairment associated with medically unexplained symptoms is comparable with that of depressive disorder alone although the areas of functioning affected are different.

Secondary care

Among patients attending specialist gastroenterology, neurology and cardiology clinics, the SF-36 physical component scores in patients with medically unexplained symptoms were comparable with those in patients whose symptoms were explained by demonstrable organic disease [31]. For the mental component score (MCS), however, the patients with medically unexplained symptoms had a significantly lower (more impaired) score than the patients with symptoms explained by organic disease (39.3 (standard error of mean (1.1) and 44.8 (0.9) respectively; $p<0.001$) Six months later this pattern was maintained.

Impairment of function when somatoform disorder occurs with concurrent anxiety and depression

It is often thought that somatoform disorder is a form of anxiety or depressive disorder. This is not so. As we have just seen, the pattern of impairment is different for patients with anxiety and depressive disorders compared with somatoform disorders. It is important to recognise, however, the additional impairment in patients with somatoform disorder who also have anxiety and depression. When somatoform disorder is accompanied by anxiety or depression, the impairment of physical functioning and of physical aspects of role functioning are greater than when either occurs alone [47]. When somatoform disorder is accompanied by both depressive and anxiety disorders, the degree of impairment is almost five times that of somatoform disorder alone [49].

Much of the impairment in primary care patients with somatoform disorder and anxiety and depression can be attributed to the overlap between these two disorders [52]. The major part of impairment in the dimensions of mental and general health and social functioning can be attributed to the combination of somatoform disorder and anxiety/depression.

The unique contribution to impairment of somatoform disorder is seen principally in the dimensions of bodily pain, general health and physical functioning.

In a detailed US-based study, Harris and colleagues found in multivariate analyses that a high number of somatic symptoms was independently associated with impairment of function (social function and impairment of daily activities), but that depressive disorder and several physical illnesses (notably heart failure and peripheral vascular disease) were also independently associated with impairment [165]. In other words, the more of these disorders that a person has, the greater their disability. In a further multivariate analysis to determine the correlates of work limitations for health reasons, a high number of somatic symptoms and medical comorbidity were the only independent correlates after adjustment for demographic variables. This is rather similar to the findings in severe functional somatic syndromes (see below).

Impairment in functional somatic syndromes

It is well recognised that people who have one or more of the functional somatic syndromes have impairment of health status or health-related quality of life [166;167;168]. For example, a systematic review found that people with fibromyalgia had mental and physical health summary scores one and two standard deviations below the general population, respectively. People with fibromyalgia also had similar or significantly lower scores on all eight SF-36 health status domains compared with people with other specific pain conditions, including rheumatoid arthritis, osteoarthritis, osteoporosis and systemic lupus erythematosus [166]. A similar pattern has been found in irritable bowel syndrome patients, who show greater impairment on all eight scales of the SF-36 questionnaire than healthy comparison groups; the impairment in health status for irritable bowel syndrome is similar to that recorded for diabetes, depression or gastro-oesophageal reflux disease [169;170].

A systematic review reported consistent findings across studies that chronic fatigue syndrome is associated with impairment of physical functioning and unemployment [167]. Patients with chronic fatigue syndrome were less likely to be employed than healthy controls. The situation is complex in chronic fatigue, however, as the definition of chronic fatigue syndrome includes 'substantial reduction in level of occupational, educational, social and all personal activities' [76].

Less severe forms of medically unexplained fatigue have been identified that are much more common than chronic fatigue syndrome – these have been described as 'chronic disabling fatigue', 'chronic fatigue syndrome-like' or 'suspected chronic fatigue syndrome' [85;171;172]. Although they are far more numerous than chronic fatigue syndrome, people classified as having chronic fatigue syndrome-like have been shown to be quite markedly disabled and a high proportion are unemployed [171]. The disability associated with these lesser degrees of unexplained fatigue must be included in any assessment of impairment due to chronic fatigue.

In a population study in UK, it was found that 9% of the population had unexplained chronic fatigue for at least 6 months [91]. This was associated with increased disability but much of this disability could be accounted for by the presence of accompanying psychiatric disorder. Another study identified two groups of patients with chronic fatigue syndrome. One group had more prolonged illness, was more severely disabled and a greater proportion had depressive illness; the group also had numerous somatic symptoms in addition to fatigue [173]. This suggests that the presence of depression and numerous body symptoms are strongly associated with disability and that within the chronic fatigue spectrum there is a range of severity with associated disability.

Impairment is greatest when there is accompanying somatisation

The two studies just mentioned suggest that not everyone with a functional somatic syndrome is severely disabled. There appear to be subgroups of patients that are far more severely impaired than the remainder [91;173]. A large population-based study in Germany (n = 2500) identified two groups of individuals with widespread pain [174]. The two groups were similar in terms of the diagnosis, a female predominance, low socioeconomic status and older age, but only one group was markedly impaired according to the SF-36 physical and mental component summary scores. This group also reported multiple somatic symptoms and depression; these are the key factors associated with marked impairment of health-related quality of life in widespread pain (fibromyalgia).

Clinical studies of fibromyalgia and irritable bowel confirm that subgroups of patients can be defined who have a low susceptibility to pain, high levels of anxiety, depression, history of sexual abuse and tendency to catastrophise in relation to pain; it is these subgroups who have the greatest impairment of health status [175;176]. These features are those associated with the highest somatisation score [113].

In a primary care sample of irritable bowel syndrome patients, numerous somatic symptoms were associated with impairment assessed by physical and mental component summary scores [111]. The proportion on a disability pension (34%) was highest for the group with most somatic symptoms and 10% for the remainder (p<0.001). In secondary care, health status of patients with irritable bowel syndrome is closely associated with number of somatic symptoms and severity of abdominal pain [177;178;179;180]. Number of somatic symptoms was also the most powerful predictor of health status at one-year follow-up [113;181]. The only independent correlate of unemployment through health problems was somatic symptom score [180].

Healthcare use and costs

This section reviews evidence that medically unexplained symptoms, somatoform disorders and functional somatic syndromes are associated with increased costs. Such costs may involve healthcare – frequent doctor visits, numerous investigations and admissions – and may involve societal costs, such as time missed from work and unemployment through illness, and the costs associated with carers.

Costs associated with medically unexplained symptoms and somatoform disorders

Data from the UK Department of Health indicate that the diagnosis of 'Signs, symptom and ill-defined conditions' (ICD diagnosis ICD code 780–789) accounts for the most costly diagnostic category of outpatients in UK and the fourth most expensive category in primary care. It was noted above that in USA this is the fifth most frequent reason for visiting a doctor (p. 3) [22]. In the Netherlands, this diagnosis is the fifth most expensive diagnostic category (Table 1.8) [182]. The costs appear to be higher than those incurred by stroke and cancer. The high healthcare costs do not include time lost from work and the reduced productivity, nor time of carers.

Figure 1.4 shows that the number of doctor visits increased linearly with number of somatic symptoms in a US-based study also described above [54]. Figure 1.5 shows the same pattern observed in a UK secondary care study, which also showed that the relationship

Table 1.8 The 10 most expensive diagnostic groups in Netherlands [182].

Diagnostic groups	Per cent of total healthcare costs
Mental handicap/Down's syndrome	8.1
Musculoskeletal	6.0
Dementia	5.6
Other mental disorders[a]	5.0
Symptoms, signs; ill-defined conditions	**4.8**
Dental diseases	4.2
Stroke	3.2
Cancer	3.2
Pregnancy	2.6
Coronary heart diseases	2.5

[a] Dementia, schizophrenia, depression, alcohol and drugs, mental handicap.

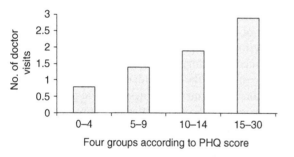

Figure 1.4 Number of doctor visits over previous three months, adjusted for number of physical illness and other confounders, made by four groups of patients based on somatisation score (as Figure 1.2) [54]. PHQ, Patient Health Questionnaire.

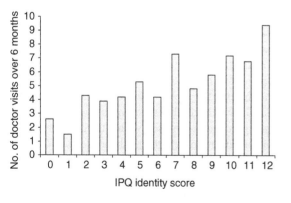

Figure 1.5 Number of doctor visits during the six months after clinic visit according to number of bodily symptoms [31]. IPQ identity score = number of bodily symptoms; IPQ, Illness Perception Questionnaire.

between number of somatic symptoms and doctor visits is similar for medically explained and unexplained symptoms [31]. In both studies, patients in the top 10% of somatic symptom score make approximately four times as many doctor visits as patients with a very low somatic symptom score.

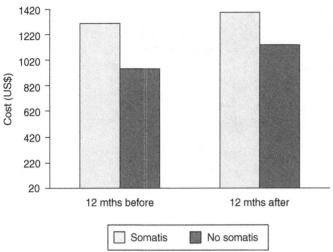

Figure 1.6 Annual adjusted healthcare costs for somatising and non-somatising patients for 12 months before and 12 months after index clinic visit [58].

In the UK primary care setting, the number of somatic symptoms has been shown to be an independent predictor of frequency of consultation over the subsequent year after adjustment for chronic physical illness, psychiatric disorder, illness behaviour, health anxiety and demographic variables [183]. In American primary care, patients in the top 14% of somatic symptom scores incurred higher costs than the remainder[58]. After adjustment for the effect of demographic factors and concurrent medical illnesses, these patients with numerous somatic symptoms made approximately three outpatient visits per year more than the remainder, and total outpatient costs were approximately US$300 greater per year (Figure 1.6).

A similar American primary care study adjusted for the effect of depressive, anxiety and panic disorders in addition to demographic features and concurrent medical illnesses [53]. Compared with the remainder, patients in the top 20% of somatic symptom scores made more primary care and medical specialist visits, more visits to the emergency department and had more hospital admissions; their adjusted, annual total healthcare cost was US$5678 per patient, which was US$2734 higher than that for the remaining patients. This study estimated that if these findings were extrapolated to the whole of USA then US$256 billion a year in medical costs could be attributed to the effect of somatisation alone, i.e. after adjusting for the effect of concurrent medical and psychiatric illnesses. The importance of this study is that it adjusted for both medical and psychiatric illnesses, so that the additional cost quoted above is the unique contribution of somatisation to high healthcare costs.

In the UK, where GPs act as 'gatekeepers' to secondary care, a similar picture has been noted [31]. Medical outpatients who scored in the top 25% of somatic symptom scores made an additional seven visits to primary and secondary care over an 18-month period compared with those with lower somatisation scores (19.7 (standard deviation (SD) 12.1) versus 12.7 (8.9)).

Another way of demonstrating the relationship between medically unexplained symptoms and healthcare use is through the correlates of frequent attendance (top 10%) at primary care. In a large Dutch study, 25% of persistent frequent attenders over a three-year period had medically unexplained symptoms, compared with 13% of frequent attenders over a one-year period only and 6.8% of non-frequent attenders [184]. In secondary care, a quarter of medical outpatients who attended very frequently (median of 18 visits over three years) had consulted for medically unexplained symptoms [185]. The costs of investigations (principally computed tomography (CT) brain scan, exercise electrocardiogram (ECG), endoscopy and abdominal ultrasound) was twice as high in the frequent attenders with medically unexplained symptoms as the other frequent attenders, whose symptoms were explained by organic disease (mean = £244 versus £124, respectively) [185;186].

Shaw and Creed found, among patients referred to a psychiatrist because of medically unexplained symptoms, the range of expenditure on investigations for possible organic disease ranged from £25 to £2300 (median £286) [187]. The determinants of costs included the diagnostic difficulties of the presenting symptom, the attitude of both patient and doctor towards organic disease as an explanation for symptoms and any resistance on either's part to adopting a psychological view of the symptoms. It was independent of the view expressed in the GP's referral letter. In a German trial, the direct costs (–36.7%) and indirect costs (–35.3%) were to be reduced greatly in a controlled study with somatoform patients undergoing an inpatient treatment with cognitive behavioural therapy (CBT) ([188]).

Costs associated with functional somatic symptoms

It has been recognised for some time that patients with functional somatic syndromes incur greater healthcare costs and greater societal costs than many other diagnostic groups. Recently there have been some large surveys.

Fibromyalgia (chronic widespread pain)

A recent Spanish study of 63 000 people under the care of a single healthcare provider identified 1.7% who had consulted a primary care physician with fibromyalgia [189]. The 1081 patients with fibromyalgia incurred a mean annual total healthcare costs €613 greater than those without fibromyalgia. The patients with fibromyalgia made, on average, five more GP office visits per annum than the remainder and incurred mean pharmacological costs of €300 more than the remainder. There was a much greater difference (€4396) in the mean annual non-healthcare costs (€6977 versus €2330) as the fibromyalgia patient group had a mean of 21 days sick leave per annum compared with 8.0 for the remainder, and 29.5% took premature retirement compared with 9.5% of the remainder. Overall, the mean total costs, including health and societal costs, showed a difference of €5010: €8654 (SD €9645) for fibromyalgia patients and €3265 (6421) for patients without fibromyalgia.

These results concur with those of a large US study, which found that annual healthcare costs were US$5945 for people whose health claims included fibromyalgia compared with US$2486 for non-fibromyalgia claimants [173]. The prevalence of disability was twice as high among fibromyalgia claimants than that for the workforce in general and the costs for absenteeism and disability were equal to or greater than the direct healthcare costs. This study revealed that many of the claims in the fibromyalgia group were not for fibromyalgia itself but numerous other illnesses, most commonly unspecified disorders of the back, osteoarthritis/rheumatoid arthritis, chest symptoms, abdominal pain, depression and other mental disorders; all of these occurred at least twice as often in the fibromyalgia claimants group as the remainder of the sample. The healthcare and disability costs for these disorders far outweighed the costs incurred for fibromyalgia. In other words, it is the numerous comorbidities associated with fibromyalgia that lead to the high costs and many of these comorbid disorders are themselves functional somatic symptoms.

A similar study divided the fibromyalgia sample into two groups according to the presence of depression [190]. Nine per cent of the fibromyalgia patients had also been treated for depression during the study period. This subgroup had a greater number of comorbidities. Chronic fatigue syndrome was recorded for 27% of patients with fibromyalgia and depression, 14% of those who had fibromyalgia without depression and 2.5% of those without fibromyalgia. The respective proportions for abdominal pain were 50%, 32% and 6% (irritable bowel syndrome was diagnosed in 12%, 5% and 0.6%). It is clear that the presence of depression in fibromyalgia is an important marker of the subgroup of fibromyalgia patients who have multiple concurrent functional somatic symptoms and syndromes.

Another way to quantify the costs associated with a diagnosis of fibromyalgia is to compare them with the costs incurred by people with rheumatoid arthritis. One large study found that the mean annual expenditures for fibromyalgia and rheumatoid arthritis patients were similar (US$10911 (SD US$16075) versus US$10716 (US$16860)) [191]. Time off work and disability costs were also similar for the two conditions. Once again this study found that patients with fibromyalgia had a greater burden of comorbid conditions than patients with rheumatoid arthritis, notably diseases of the respiratory, digestive, musculoskeletal and connective tissue systems, back and neck pain, symptoms, signs, and ill-defined conditions and many painful neuropathies.

Irritable bowel syndrome

A systematic review found high costs associated with irritable bowel syndrome in both the USA and the UK [192]. In the UK, it has been estimated that irritable bowel syndrome costs the National Health Service (NHS) £224.11 million (US$358 million) per year [193]. In the USA, irritable bowel syndrome is among the 10 most costly gastrointestinal diseases, with a total estimated cost of $US1353 million for direct and $US205 million for indirect costs [194]. A detailed American study indicated that the age- and gender-adjusted mean total annual direct costs in irritable bowel syndrome patients (US$4376) were similar to those in patients with gastro-oesophageal reflux (US$5144) but lower than costs for patients with inflammatory bowel disease (US$ 7237) [195].

The variation in healthcare costs for irritable bowel syndrome is also considerable. In the largest UK primary care study, healthcare costs for these patients were £123 greater than in comparison patients, but there was considerable variation between individuals [193]. In the detailed American study mentioned in the previous paragraph, mean total annual healthcare costs were just over US$4000 (compared with US$2719 for comparison group), but the standard deviation was US$7739 [195]. In this study only 33% of the costs were attributable to symptoms of the lower gastrointestinal tract; the remaining costs concerned comorbid conditions.

Similar findings emerged in an intensive Norwegian study of 200 primary-care patients with irritable bowel syndrome [196]. During a six-month follow-up period costs directly related to irritable bowel syndrome amounted to 1049 (SD 6574) Norwegian kroner, while the costs incurred for comorbid conditions were 14856 (30570) kroner. The mean number of sick leave days related to irritable bowel syndrome was 1.7 (SD 16) days compared with 16.3 (43) days for comorbid conditions [196]. Thus, with regards to societal costs, irritable bowel syndrome is not in itself associated with much time missed from work, but impaired productivity occurs mostly in the people with irritable bowel syndrome who also have extraintestinal comorbidities, such as chronic fatigue syndrome, fibromyalgia and interstitial cystitis [82].

When the Norwegian primary care irritable bowel syndrome sample was subdivided into three groups according to number of somatic symptoms, the patients with the highest somatic symptom score made the most visits to the GP and they also included the highest proportion who were receiving a disability pension [111]. In multivariate analysis the three independent predictors of healthcare costs were age, number of organic illnesses and number of bodily symptoms scored on a checklist [196]. Thus the situation is similar to that already observed in fibromyalgia: a large proportion of costs associated with a functional somatic syndrome is attributable to comorbid disorders, and number of somatic symptoms is an independent predictor of costs.

For patients attending a gastroenterology clinic with irritable bowel syndrome, it has been shown that retrospective healthcare costs vary linearly with number of somatic symptoms recorded on a questionnaire (Symptom Checklist-90-R (SCL-90R) somatisation subscale) [197]. Patients with a somatic symptom score two or more standard deviations above the mean incurred healthcare costs of US$2481 more than average, whereas those with very few bodily symptoms (i.e. irritable bowel syndrome but no additional bodily symptoms) incurred US$1699 less than the average costs.

Another clinic-based study of patients with severe irritable bowel syndrome showed that all patients incurred high costs but the top 25% scorers on the SCL-90R somatisation subscale (eight or more somatic symptoms outside of the gastrointestinal tract) had greatly increased costs [113]. This top quarter incurred total costs for the year prior to entering a trial of £2010 (standard error (SE) 214) compared with £1080 (SE=124) for the remainder after adjusting for demographic features and concurrent medical illnesses [113]. The patients in this study were in a treatment trial and the very high costs were reduced for those who received active treatment (Figure 1.7).

Chronic fatigue syndrome

It can be seen from Table 1.9 that the few studies that have examined costs in chronic fatigue syndrome indicated very high costs associated with this condition. Although there is considerable variation, two of the American studies suggest that US$7–9 billion are spent on this condition each year. Reynolds and colleagues [172] calculated that approximately a quarter of people with chronic fatigue syndrome stopped working and, for those who continued working, their income was reduced by a third. These authors estimated that the annual total value of lost productivity in the USA was US$9.1 billion, which is comparable with the annual total value lost on account of digestive diseases.

McCrone and colleagues [198] calculated in detail the costs of chronic fatigue syndrome over three months in a primary-care sample. They estimated this to be £3515 (SD 4360) for those with chronic fatigue syndrome and £1176 (2369) for those with disabling chronic fatigue. The latter group was twice as numerous as those with chronic fatigue syndrome but in the Reynolds study they were much more numerous. It is clear that chronic fatigue syndrome, although relatively rare, is extremely expensive to society, mostly because of time lost from work and support from carers. Disabling chronic fatigue, however, is much more common and is less expensive than chronic fatigue syndrome, but must account for very considerable total costs.

Not surprisingly, the costs of chronic fatigue syndrome are associated with functional impairment. Contact with doctors can be reassuring and supportive or may actually

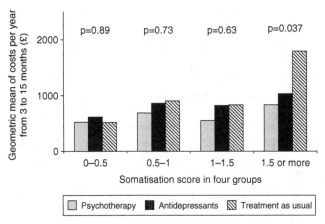

Figure 1.7 Total costs over 15 months after entry into a trial [113]. The sample has been divided into four quartiles according to somatisation score at baseline (0–0.5 represents the low scores, 1.5 or more represents the patients with highest somatisation scores). The costs are shown by treatment group for each quartile. In the highest somatisation group (right-hand side of figure) costs remain very high (at pre-trial levels) in the usual treatment group, whereas they are reduced in the psychotherapy and antidepressant groups to levels comparable with the lower somatisation groups.

Table 1.9 Chronic fatigue syndrome (CFS): estimates of mean annual costs

Study	Sample	Direct healthcare costs	Total costs including societal costs	Extrapolation to population
McCrone et al., 2003 [198]	Primary care	£808[a]	£14 060[a] per patient	
Lloyd and Pender, 1994 [199]		AU$2000	AU$9436 per patient	AU$25 million (government) AU$50 million to society
Bombardier and Buchwald, 1996 [200]	Referral clinic	US$1013		
Reynolds et al., 2008 [172]	Population-based		US$20 000 per affected individual	US$9.1 billion
Jason et al., 2008 [201]	CFS from population-based study	US$2342 versus US$1333 for controls		US$2.0 million
Jason et al., 2008 [201]	Tertiary care	US$8675 (SD 8854)		US$7 billion

[a] Extrapolated from three months' costs.

Table 1.10 The cause of long-term sickness absence (≥8 weeks) according to GP sick notes (n = 2076, Denmark) [205]

Categories of illness as reason for disability pension	Per cent of total
Functional disorders	14
Mental disorders (depression and anxiety)	22
Stress, including 'burn-out'	7
Subjective organic, i.e. conditions for which no certain clinical findings are expected, e.g. migraine, frozen shoulder, tennis elbow	4
Probable organic, i.e. diagnostically less certain = slipped disc, angina, unclarified organic (the disorder is under examination)	6
Definite organic disease	41
Data unavailable	6

exacerbate the patient's difficulties. This may occur when the doctor appears to deny the validity of the patients' symptoms or orders investigations for possible organic disease which carry the risk of heightening the patient's health anxiety, especially when the result is normal. Doctors who accept patients' model of their symptoms and are perceived as supportive appear to be most helpful [202;203].

Costs of sickness benefits due to MUS/somatoform or functional disorders

In Sweden, fatigue is the most common reason for sickness absence [204]. In a Danish study based on one county (Aarhus), all individuals with eight weeks of sickness absence during one year (n = 2076, 54% females) were studied (Table 1.10) [205]. According to GP sick note diagnoses, 14% of the absences were definitely due to a functional disorder. However, this is an minimum figure as many of the stress-related and 'subjective organic' categories may include medically unexplained conditions. Definite organic disorders included only about half of all illness episodes.

Disability benefit/early retirement pension

In a study of 191 consecutive patients aged 18–50 years attending their family GP, it was found that 37.5% of the patients with an ICD-10 somatoform disorder received social security, pension or disability benefit against only 10.8% (p>0.003) among other patients [206]. In a study of 1785 consecutive patients aged 18–50 years consulting their GP, 4.9% received early retirement pension/disability benefit [204]. In patients whose problems were regarded by the GP as 'medically unexplained', the figure was 7.8% [207; P. Fink, personal communication, 2010]. A Danish register study of data on disability benefit/early retirement pensions in the period 1 July 1998 to 31 December 2000 reported that among all individuals who were granted pension in that period in Denmark, 8.3% had a functional somatic syndrome diagnosis; 11 % of the women and 5 % of the men [205]. Table 1.11 shows data from the same patient register, but for the period 2000–2005 and the figures are broken down on selected functional somatic syndromes and somatoform disorders. It appears that these diagnoses account for about 5.8–9.8% of all early retirement pensions/disability benefits in Denmark per year [12].

Table 1.11 Syndrome cases: early retirement pension/disability benefit grants at county level according to diagnosis and year [205]

	2000	2001	2002	2003	2004	2005
Somatoform disorder	56	31	79	65	68	74
Chronic fatigue syndrome	40	36	33	32	9	13
Fibromyalgia	305	262	336	262	227	203
Symphysis pubis dysfunction	12	12	13	10	8	3
Chronic pain	27	15	29	36	34	39
Whiplash	293	276	337	229	251	227
Total of above	**733**	**632**	**827**	**634**	**597**	**559**
Total pensions/benefits	14110	14971	17404	15173	15835	14706
Percentage of all pensions for functional disorders	**5.2**	**4.2**	**4.7**	**4.2**	**3.8**	**3.8**

Somatoform disorders and disability

It is likely that there is very considerable variation across European countries regarding the causes for receipt of incapacity benefits. For example, in the UK, the most common reason for sickness absence used to be musculoskeletal disorders (23% of sickness certification) [208]. Over recent years, however, there has been a shift away from musculoskeletal disorders to mental health disorders and in Glasgow, where there is a very high rate of claiming sickness benefits, 33.6% were claiming because of mental and behavioural disorders, with a corresponding reduction in claims for musculoskeletal disorders [209].

Depressive, anxiety and other neurotic disorders account for approximately 70% of the mental and behavioural disorders given as reasons for claiming sickness benefits; somatoform disorders is a diagnostic label that is never used [209]. The importance of this lies in the lack of specific treatment. A Cochrane systematic review of interventions to prevent workplace disability identified only interventions to prevent musculoskeletal disorders and one for adjustment disorders [210]. It is likely that the opportunity to intervene, probably with cognitive behavioural therapy tailored to somatoform disorders, should be included in the repertoire of interventions to reduce disability. If this diagnosis is never used, however, this is unlikely to occur.

Conclusion

In this chapter we have seen that medically unexplained symptoms are very common in the general population, and in primary care they may lead to high healthcare costs because they are responsible for so many consultations. Most medically unexplained symptoms are transient, however, and only a small proportion become persistent and are potentially disabling and expensive to healthcare and society. It is these persistent symptoms that are diagnosed as somatoform disorder. The one study that has attempted to estimate the prevalence of somatoform disorder in Europe found that 18.9 million residents aged

18–65 years in the EU population were affected by these disorders within the previous 12 months [69].

The functional disorders are similarly common and the Declaration of the European Parliament (2009) states that fibromyalgia affects 14 million persons in the EU. Similar high costs have been estimated for irritable bowel syndrome and chronic fatigue syndrome. More detailed studies have shown that the uncomplicated functional somatic syndromes (or single-organ type of bodily distress syndrome) are not, in themselves, seriously disabling or particularly expensive. It is the functional somatic syndrome that is accompanied by numerous somatic symptoms ('complicated' functional somatic syndrome or multiorgan type of bodily distress syndrome) that is associated with much time off work, frequent healthcare seeking and consequent high healthcare and societal costs.

There is little doubt that somatoform disorders, or bodily distress syndromes, are an important and challenging group of conditions that are expensive in terms of healthcare use and time missed from work. The rest of this book aims to demonstrate what is currently known about these disorders and the measures required to improve the care of patients who suffer from them. As indicated in later chapters, there is little current recognition of this problem across the EU.

References

1. Nimnuan C, Hotopf M, Wessely S. Medically unexplained symptoms: how often and why are they missed? *QJM – Monthly Journal of the Association of Physicians* 2000; **93**(1): 21–8.

2. Van Hemert AM, Hengeveld MW, Bolk JH, Rooijmans HG, Vandenbroucke JP. Psychiatric disorders in relation to medical illness among patients of a general medical out-patient clinic. *Psychological Medicine* 1993; **23**(1): 167–73.

3. Hamilton J, Campos R, Creed F. Anxiety, depression and management of medically unexplained symptoms in medical clinics. *Journal of the Royal College of Physicians of London* 1996; **30**(1): 18–20.

4. Nimnuan C, Hotopf M, Wessely S. Medically unexplained symptoms: an epidemiological study in seven specialities. *Journal of Psychosomatic Research* 2001; **51**(1): 361–7.

5. Fiddler M, Jackson J, Kapur N, Wells A, Creed F, Fiddler M et al. Childhood adversity and frequent medical consultations. *General Hospital Psychiatry* 2004; **26**(5): 367–77.

6. Kooiman CG, Bolk JH, Rooijmans HG, Trijsburg RW. Alexithymia does not predict the persistence of medically unexplained physical symptoms. *Psychosomatic Medicine* 2004; **66**(2): 224–32.

7. Targosz SA, Kapur N, Creed F. Medically unexplained symptoms, illness perception and childhood experience in neurology outpatients. *Irish Journal of Psychological Medicine* 2001; **18**(1): 16–20.

8. Carson AJ, Ringbauer B, MacKenzie L, Warlow C, Sharpe M. Neurological disease, emotional disorder, and disability: they are related: a study of 300 consecutive new referrals to a neurology outpatient department. *Journal of Neurology Neurosurgery and Psychiatry* 2000; **68**(2): 202–6.

9. Stone J, Carson A, Duncan R, Coleman R, Roberts R, Warlow C et al. Symptoms 'unexplained by organic disease' in 1144 new neurology out-patients: how often does the diagnosis change at follow-up? *Brain* 2009; **132**: 2878–88.

10. Mangwana S, Burlinson S, Creed F. Medically unexplained symptoms presenting at secondary care – a comparison of white Europeans and people

of south Asian ethnicity. *International Journal of Psychiatry in Medicine* 2009; **39**(1): 33–44.

11. Kroenke K, Mangelsdorff AD. Common symptoms in ambulatory care – incidence, evaluation, therapy, and outcome. *American Journal of Medicine* 1989; **86**(3): 262–6.

12. Fink P, Toft T, Morten SH, Ørnbøl E, Olesen F. Symptoms and syndromes of bodily distress: An exploratory study of 978 internal medical, neurological, and primary care patients. *Psychosomatic Medicine* 2007; **69**: 30–9.

13. Sharpe M, Stone J, Hibberd C, Warlow C, Duncan R, Coleman R *et al*. Neurology outpatients with symptoms unexplained by disease: illness beliefs and financial benefits predict 1-year outcome. *Psychological Medicine* 2010; **40**:689–98.

14. Mumford DB, Devereux TA, Maddy PJ, Johnston JV. Factors leading to the reporting of functional somatic symptoms by general-practice attenders. *British Journal of General Practice* 1991; **41**(352): 454–8.

15. Peveler R, Kilkenny L, Kinmouth AL. Medically unexplained physical symptoms in primary care: a comparison of self-report screening questionnaires and clinical opinion. *Journal of Psychosomatic Research* 1997; **42**: 245–52.

16. Kirmayer LJ, Robbins JM. Three forms of somatization in primary care: prevalence, co-occurrence, and sociodemographic characteristics. *Journal of Nervous and Mental Disease* 1991; **179**: 647–55.

17. Palsson N. Functional somatic symptoms and hypochondriasis among general-practice patients – a pilot-study. *Acta Psychiatrica Scandinavica* 1988; **78**(2): 191–7.

18. Kisely S, Goldberg D, Simon G. A Comparison between somatic symptoms with and without clear organic cause: results of an international study. *Psychological Medicine* 1997; **27**(5): 1011–19.

19. Duddu V, Husain N, Dickens C. Medically unexplained presentations and quality of life: a study of a predominantly South Asian primary care population in England. *Journal of Psychosomatic Research* 2008; **65**(4): 311–17.

20. Burton C. Beyond somatisation: a review of the understanding and treatment of medically unexplained physical symptoms (MUPS). *British Journal of General Practice* 2003; **53**(488): 231–9.

21. Rosendal M, Bro F, Fink P, Christensen KS, Olesen F, Rosendal M *et al*. Diagnosis of somatisation: effect of an educational intervention in a cluster randomised controlled trial. *British Journal of General Practice* 2003; **53**(497): 917–22.

22. Cherry DK, Woodwell DA, Rechsteiner EA. *National Ambulatory Medical Care Survey: 2005*. Hyattsville, MD: US Dept of Health and Human Services, Centres for Disease Control and Prevention, National Centre for Health Statistics.

23. Kroenke K, Price RK. Symptoms in the community – prevalence, classification, and psychiatric comorbidity. *Archives of Internal Medicine* 1993; **153**(21): 2474–80.

24. Hiller W, Rief W, Brahler E, Hiller W, Rief W, Brahler E. Somatization in the population: from mild bodily misperceptions to disabling symptoms. *Social Psychiatry and Psychiatric Epidemiology* 2006; **41**(9): 704–12.

25. Simon G, Gureje O. Stability of somatisation disorder and somatisation symptoms among primary care patients. *Archives of General Psychiatry* 1999; **56**: 90–5.

26. Gureje O, Simon GE. The natural history of somatization in primary care. *Psychological Medicine* 1999; **29**(3): 669–76.

27. olde Hartman TC, Borghuis MS, Lucassen PL, van de Laar FA, Speckens A, van Weel C. Medically unexplained symptoms, somatisation disorder and hypochondriasis: Course and prognosis. A systematic review. *Journal of Psychosomatic Research* 2009; **66**: 363–77.

28. Leiknes KA, Finset A, Moum T, Sandanger I. Course and predictors of medically unexplained pain symptoms in the general population. *Journal of Psychosomatic Research* 2007; **62**(2): 119–28.

29. Escobar JI, Cook B, Chen CN, Gara MA, Alegría M, Interian A *et al*. Whether

medically unexplained or not, three or more concurrent somatic symptoms predict psychopathology and service use in community populations. *Journal of Psychosomatic Research* 2010; **69**(1): 1–8.

30. Verhaak PF, Meijer SA, Visser AP, Wolters G. Persistent presentation of medically unexplained symptoms in general practice. *Family Practice* 2006; **23**(4): 414–20.

31. Jackson J, Fiddler M, Kapur N, Wells A, Tomenson B, Creed F *et al.* Number of bodily symptoms predicts outcome more accurately than health anxiety in patients attending neurology, cardiology, and gastroenterology clinics. *Journal of Psychosomatic Research* 2006; **60**(4): 357–63.

32. American Psychiatric Association. *Diagnostic and Statistical Manual of Mental Disorders – DSM-IV*, 4th edn. Washington, DC: American Psychiatric Association; 1994.

33. World Health Organization. *The ICD-10 Classification of Mental and Behavioural Disorders Clinical Descriptions and Diagnostic Guidelines*. Geneva: World Health Organization; 1992: XII+362P.

34. Rief W, Heuser J, Mayrhuber E, Stelzer I, Hiller W, Fichter MM. The classification of multiple somatoform symptoms. *Journal of Nervous and Mental Disease* 1996; **184**(11): 680–7.

35. Escobar JI, Gara M, Silver RC, Waitzkin H, Holman A, Compton W. Somatisation disorder in primary care. *British Journal of Psychiatry* 1998; **173**: 262–6.

36. Kroenke K, Spitzer RL, deGruy FV III, Hahn SR, Linzer M, Williams JB *et al.* Multisomatoform disorder. An alternative to undifferentiated somatoform disorder for the somatizing patient in primary care. *Archives of General Psychiatry* 1997; **54**(4): 352–8.

37. Creed FH, Barsky A. A systematic review of somatisation and hypochondriasis. *Journal of Psychosomatic Research* 2004; **56**: 391–408.

38. Gureje O, Ustun TB, Simon GE. The syndrome of hypochondriasis: a cross-national study in primary care.

Psychological Medicine 1997; **27**(5): 1001–10.

39. Looper KJ, Kirmayer LJ, Looper KJ, Kirmayer LJ. Hypochondriacal concerns in a community population. *Psychological Medicine* 2001; **31**(4): 577–84.

40. Frohlich C, Jacobi F, Wittchen HU, Frohlich C, Jacobi F, Wittchen HU. DSM-IV pain disorder in the general population. An exploration of the structure and threshold of medically unexplained pain symptoms. *European Archives of Psychiatry and Clinical Neuroscience* 2006; **256**(3): 187–96.

41. Schaefert R, Laux G, Kaufmann C, Schellberg D, Bolter R, Szecsenyi J *et al.* Diagnosing somatisation disorder (P75) in routine general practice using the International classification of primary care. *Journal of Psychosomatic Research* 2010; **69**(3): 267–77.

42. Ruddy R, House A. Psychosocial interventions for conversion disorder. *Cochrane Database of Systematic Reviews* 2005; **4**: CD005331.

43. Veale D. Cosmetic procedures. In: Lloyd GG, Guthrie E, eds. *Handbook of Liaison Psychiatry*. Cambridge: Cambridge University Press; 2007: 617–31.

44. Phillips KA, Wilhelm S, Koran LM, Didie ER, Fallon BA, Feusner J *et al.* Body dysmorphic disorder: some key issues for DSM-V. *Depression and Anxiety* 2010; **27**(6): 573–91.

45. Phillips KA, Didie ER, Feusner J, Wilhelm S. Body dysmorphic disorder: treating an underrecognized disorder. *American Journal of Psychiatry* 2008; **165**(9): 1111–18.

46. Fink P, Sorensen L, Engberg M, Holm M, Munk-Jorgensen P. Somatization in primary care. Prevalence, health care utilization, and general practitioner recognition. *Psychosomatics* 1999; **40**: 330–8.

47. de Waal MW, Arnold IA, Eekhof JA, van Hemert AM. Somatoform disorders in general practice: prevalence, functional impairment and comorbidity with anxiety and depressive disorders. *British Journal of Psychiatry* 2004; **184**: 470–6.

48. Toft T, Fink P, Oernboel E, Christensen K, Frostholm L, Olesen F. Mental disorders in primary care: prevalence and co-morbidity among disorders. Results from the functional illness in primary care (FIP) study. *Psychological Medicine* 2005; **35**(8): 1175–84.

49. Hanel G, Henningsen P, Herzog W, Sauer N, Schaefert R, Szecenyi J *et al.* Depression, anxiety, and somatoform disorders: vague or distinct categories in primary care? Results from a large cross-sectional study. *Journal of Psychosomatic Research* 2009; **67**: 189–97.

50. Jackson JL, Kroenke K. Prevalence, impact, and prognosis of multisomatoform disorder in primary care: a 5-year follow-up study. *Psychosomatic Medicine* 2008; **70**(4): 430–4.

51. Ustun TB, Sartorius N. *Mental Illness in General Health Care. An International Study.* Chichester: Wiley; 1995.

52. Lowe B, Spitzer RL, Williams JB, Mussell M, Schellberg D, Kroenke K *et al.* Depression, anxiety and somatization in primary care: syndrome overlap and functional impairment. *General Hospital Psychiatry* 2008; **30**(3): 191–9.

53. Barsky AJ, Orav EJ, Bates DW. Somatization increases medical utilization and costs independent of psychiatric and medical comorbidity. *Archives of General Psychiatry* 2005; **62**(8): 903–10.

54. Kroenke K, Spitzer RL, Williams JB. The PHQ-15: validity of a new measure for evaluating the severity of somatic symptoms. *Psychosomatic Medicine* 2002; **64**(2): 258–66.

55. World Health Organisation, Division of Mental Health. *Schedules for Clinical Assessment in Neuropsychiatry.* Geneva: World Health Organization; 1994.

56. Spitzer RL, Williams JB, Kroenke K, Linzer M, deGruy FV III, Hahn SR *et al.* Utility of a new procedure for diagnosing mental disorders in primary care. The PRIME-MD 1000 study. *Journal of the American Medical Association* 1994; **272**(22): 1749–56.

57. Wittchen HU. Reliability and validity studies of the WHO – Composite International Diagnostic Interview (CIDI): a critical review. *Journal of Psychiatric Research* 1994; **28**(1): 57–84.

58. Barsky AJ, Ettner SL, Horsky J, Bates DW. Resource utilization of patients with hypochondriacal health anxiety and somatization. *Medical Care* 2001; **39**(7): 705–15.

59. Kolk AM, Schagen S, Hanewald GJ. Multiple medically unexplained physical symptoms and health care utilization: outcome of psychological intervention and patient-related predictors of change. *Journal of Psychosomatic Research* 2004; **57**(4): 379–89.

60. Fink P, Hansen MS, Oxhoj ML. The prevalence of somatoform disorders among internal medical inpatients. *Journal of Psychosomatic Research* 2004; **56**(4): 413–18.

61. Harter M, Baumeister H, Reuter K, Jacobi F, Hofler M, Bengel J *et al.* Increased 12-month prevalence rates of mental disorders in patients with chronic somatic diseases. *Psychotherapy and Psychosomatics* 2007; **76**: 354–60.

62. Essau CA. Course and outcome of somatoform disorders in non-referred adolescents. *Psychosomatics* 2007; **48**(6): 502–9.

63. Essau CA, Conradt J, Petermann F. Course and outcome of anxiety disorders in adolescents. *Journal of Anxiety Disorder* 2002; **16**: 67–81.

64. Lieb R, Zimmermann P, Friis RH, Hofler M, Tholen S, Wittchen HU. The natural course of DSM-IV somatoform disorders and syndromes among adolescents and young adults: a prospective-longitudinal community study. *European Psychiatry: Journal of the Association of European Psychiatrists* 2002; **17**(6): 321–31.

65. Lieb R, Isensee B, von Sydow K, Wittchen HU. The early developmental stages of psychopathology study (EDSP), a methodological update. *European Addiction Research* 2000; **6**: 170–82.

66. Leiknes KA, Finset A, Moum T, Sandanger I. Current somatoform disorders in

Norway: prevalence, risk factors and comorbidity with anxiety, depression and musculoskeletal disorders. *Social Psychiatry and Psychiatric Epidemiology* 2007; 42(9): 698–710.

67. Jacobi F, Wittchen HU, Holting C, Hofler M, Pfister H, Muller N *et al.* Prevalence, co-morbidity and correlates of mental disorders in the general population: results from the German Health Interview and Examination Survey (GHS). *Psychological Medicine* 2004; 34(4): 597–611.

68. Wittchen HU, Jacobi F. Size and burden of mental disorders in Europe – a critical review and appraisal of 27 studies. *European Neuropsychopharmacology* 2005; 15(4): 357–76.

69. Wittchen HU, Nelson CB, Lachner G. Prevalence of mental disorders and psychosocial impairments in adolescents and young adults. *Psychological Medicine* 1998; 28: 109– 26.

70. Kringlen E, Torgersen S, Cramer V. Mental illness in a rural area – a Norwegian psychiatric epidemiological study. *Social Psychiatry and Psychiatric Epidemiology* 2006; 41(9): 713–19.

71. Kringlen E, Torgersen S, Cramer V. A Norwegian psychiatric epidemiological study. *American Journal of Psychiatry* 2001; 158(7): 1091–8.

72. Sandanger I, Nygard JF, Ingebrigtsen G, Sorensen T, Dalgard OS. Prevalence, incidence and age at onset of psychiatric disorders in Norway. *Social Psychiatry and Psychiatric Epidemiology* 1999; 34(11): 570–9.

73. Rief W, Hessel A, Braehler E. Somatization symptoms and hypochondriacal features in the general population. *Psychosomatic Medicine* 2001; 63(4): 595–602.

74. Rief W, Rojas G, Rief W, Rojas G. Stability of somatoform symptoms – implications for classification. *Psychosomatic Medicine* 2007; 69(9): 864–9.

75. Drossman DA, ed. *Rome III: The Functional Gastrointestinal Disorders*, 3rd edn. McLean, VA: Degnon Associates; 2006.

76. Fukuda K, Straus SE, Hickie I, Sharpe MC, Dobbins JG, Komaroff A *et al.* The chronic

fatigue syndrome – a comprehensive approach to its definition and study. *Annals of Internal Medicine* 1994; 121(12): 953–9.

77. Wolfe F, Smythe HA, Yunus MB, Bennett RM, Bombardier C, Goldenberg DL *et al.* The American College of Rheumatology 1990 criteria for the classification of fibromyalgia. Report of the Multicenter Criteria Committee. *Arthritis and Rheumatism* 1990; 33(2): 160–72.

78. Wessely S, Nimnuan C, Sharpe M. Functional somatic syndromes: one or many? *The Lancet* 1999; 354(9182): 936–9.

79. Aaron LA, Buchwald D. A review of the evidence for overlap among unexplained clinical conditions. *Annals of Internal Medicine* 2001; 134: 868–81.

80. Aggarwal V, McBeth J, Zakrzewska JM, Lunt M, Macfarlane GJ. The epidemiology of chronic syndromes that are frequently unexplained: do they have common associated factors? *International Journal of Epidemiology* 2006; 35: 468–76.

81. Thompson WG, Heaton KW, Smyth GT, Smyth C. Irritable bowel syndrome in general practice: Prevalence, characteristics, and referral. *Gut* 2000; 46: 78–82.

82. American College of Gastroenterology Task Force on Irritable Bowel Syndrome; Brandt LJ, Chey WD, Foxx-Orenstein AE, Schiller LR, Schoenfeld PS *et al.* An evidence-based position statement on the management of irritable bowel syndrome. *American Journal of Gastroenterology* 2009; 104(Suppl 1): S1–S35.

83. Cathebras PJ, Robbins JM, Kirmayer LJ, Hayton BC. Fatigue in primary care – prevalence, psychiatric comorbidity, illness behavior, and outcome. *Journal of General Internal Medicine* 1992; 7(3): 276–86.

84. Fuhrer R, Wessely S. The epidemiology of fatigue and depression – a French primary-care study. *Psychological Medicine* 1995; 25(5): 895–905.

85. Darbishire L, Ridsdale L, Seed PT. Distinguishing patients with chronic fatigue from those with chronic fatigue syndrome: a diagnostic study in UK

primary care. *British Journal of General Practice* 2003; **53**(491): 441–5.

86. Rohrbeck J, Jordan K, Croft P. The frequency and characteristics of chronic widespread pain in general practice: a case-control study. *British Journal of General Practice* 2007; **57**(535): 109–15.

87. Nimnuan C, Rabe-Hesketh S, Wessely S, Hotopf M, Nimnuan C, Rabe-Hesketh S *et al.* How many functional somatic syndromes? *Journal of Psychosomatic Research* 2001; **51**(4): 549–57.

88. Buskila D, Neumann L, Odes LR, Schleifer E, Depsames R, Abu-Shakra M. The prevalence of musculoskeletal pain and fibromyalgia in patients hospitalized on internal medicine wards. *Seminars in Arthritis and Rheumatism* 2001; **30**(6): 411–17.

89. Reeves WC, Jones JF, Maloney E, Heim C, Hoaglin DC, Boneva RS *et al.* Prevalence of chronic fatigue syndrome in metropolitan, urban, and rural Georgia. *Population Health Metrics* 2007; **5**: 5.

90. Wessely S, Chalder T, Hirsch S, Wallace P, Wright D. The prevalence and morbidity of chronic fatigue and chronic fatigue syndrome: A prospective primary care study. *American Journal of Public Health* 1997; **87**(9): 1449–55.

91. Skapinakis P, Lewis G, Meltzer H. Clarifying the relationship between unexplained chronic fatigue and psychiatric morbidity: results from a community survey in Great Britain. *American Journal of Psychiatry* 2000; **157**(9): 1492–8.

92. Lawrence RC, Felson DT, Helmick CG, Arnold LM, Choi H, Deyo RA *et al.* Estimates of the prevalence of arthritis and other rheumatic conditions in the United States. *Arthritis and Rheumatism* 2008; **58**(1): 26–35.

93. Wolfe F, Ross K, Anderson J, Russell IJ, Hebert L. The prevalence and characteristics of fibromyalgia in the general population. *Arthritis and Rheumatism* 1995; **38**(1): 19–28.

94. White KP, Speechley M, Harth M, Ostbye T. The London fibromyalgia epidemiology study: The prevalence of fibromyalgia

syndrome in London, Ontario. *Journal of Rheumatology* 1999; **26**(7): 1570–6.

95. Coster L, Kendall S, Gerdle B, Henriksson C, Henriksson KG, Bengtsson A. Chronic widespread musculoskeletal pain – a comparison of those who meet criteria for fibromyalgia and those who do not. *European Journal of Pain* 2008; **12**(5): 600–10.

96. Branco JC, Bannwarth B, Failde I, Carbonell JA, Blotman F, Spaeth M *et al.* Prevalence of fibromyalgia: a survey in five European countries. *Seminars in Arthritis and Rheumatism* 2010; **39**(6): 448–53.

97. Croft P. The epidemiology of chronic widespread pain. *Journal of Musculoskeletal Pain* 2002; **10**: 191–9.

98. Andersson HI, Ejlertsson G, Leden I, Rosenberg C. Characteristics of subjects with chronic pain, in relation to local and widespread pain report – a prospective study of symptoms, clinical findings and blood tests in subgroups of a geographically defined population. *Scandinavian Journal of Rheumatology* 1996; **25**(3): 146–54.

99. Ledingham J, Doherty S, Doherty M. Primary fibromyalgia syndrome – an outcome study. *British Journal of Rheumatology* 1993; **32**(2): 139–42.

100. Kroenke K, Wood DR, Mangelsdorff AD, Meier NJ, Powell JB. Chronic fatigue in primary care – prevalence, patient characteristics, and outcome. *Journal of the American Medical Association* 1988; **260**(7): 929–34.

101. Thompson WG. A world view of IBS. In: Camilleri M, Spiller RC, eds. *Irritable Bowel Syndrome. Diagnosis and Treatment.* Edinburgh: WB Saunders; 2002: 17–26.

102. Joyce J, Hotopf M, Wessely S. The prognosis of chronic fatigue and chronic fatigue syndrome: a systematic review. *QJM – Monthly Journal of the Association of Physicians* 1997; **90**(3): 223–33.

103. McBeth J, Symmons DP, Silman AJ, Allison T, Webb R, Brammah T *et al.* Musculoskeletal pain is associated with a long-term increased risk of cancer and cardiovascular-related mortality. *Rheumatology* 2009; **48**(4): 459.

104. McBeth J, Symmons DP, Silman AJ, Webb R, Macfarlane GJ. Comment on: Musculoskeletal pain is associated with a long-term increased risk of cancer and cardiovascular-related mortality: reply. *Rheumatology* 2009; **48**(5): 595.

105. Macfarlane GJ, McBeth J, Silman AJ. Widespread body pain and mortality: prospective population-based study. *BMJ* 2001; **323**(7314): 662–4B.

106. Dreyer L, Kendall S, Danneskiold-Samsøe B, Bartels EM, Bliddal H. Mortality in a cohort of Danish patient with fibromyalgia – increased suicide, liver disease and cerebrovascular disease. *Arthritis and Rheumatism* 2010; **62**(10): 3101–8.

107. Nisenbaum R, Jones JF, Unger ER, Reyes M, Reeves WC. A population-based study of the clinical course of chronic fatigue syndrome. *Health and Quality of Life Outcomes* 2003; **1**: 49.

108. McBeth J, Macfarlane GJ, Hunt IM, Silman AJ. Risk factors for persistent chronic widespread pain: a community-based study. *Rheumatology* 2001; **40**(1): 95–101.

109. Koloski NA, Boyce PM, Talley NJ. Somatization an independent psychosocial risk factor for irritable bowel syndrome but not dyspepsia: a population-based study. *European Journal of Gastroenterology and Hepatology* 2006; **18**(10): 1101–9.

110. Locke GR, Weaver AL, Melton LJ, Talley NJ. Psychosocial factors are linked to functional gastrointestinal disorders: a population-based nested case-control study. *American Journal of Gastroenterology* 2004; **99**(2): 350–7.

111. Vandvik PO, Wilhelmsen I, Ihlebaek C, Farup PG. Comorbidity of irritable bowel syndrome in general practice: a striking feature with clinical implications. *Alimentary Pharmacology and Therapeutics* 2004; **20**(10): 1195–203.

112. North CS, Downs D, Clouse RE, Alrakawi A, Dokucu ME, Cox J et al. The presentation of irritable bowel syndrome in the context of somatization disorder. *Clinical Gastroenterology and Hepatology* 2004; **2**(9): 787–95.

113. Creed F, Tomenson B, Guthrie E, Ratcliffe J, Fernandes L, Read N et al. The relationship between somatisation and outcome in patients with severe irritable bowel syndrome. *Journal of Psychosomatic Research* 2008; **64**: 613–20.

114. Whitehead WE, Palsson O, Jones KR. Systematic review of the comorbidity of irritable bowel syndrome with other disorders: what are the causes and implications? *Gastroenterology* 2002; **122**(4): 1140–56.

115. Riedl A, Schmidtmann M, Stengel A, Goebel M, Wisser AS, Klapp BF et al. Somatic comorbidities of irritable bowel syndrome: a systematic analysis. *Journal of Psychosomatic Research* 2008; **64**(6): 573–82.

116. Baad-Hansen L, Leijon G, Svensson P, List T, Baad-Hansen L, Leijon G et al. Comparison of clinical findings and psychosocial factors in patients with atypical odontalgia and temporomandibular disorders. *Journal of Orofacial Pain* 2008; **22**(1): 7–14.

117. Plesh O, Sinisi SE, Crawford PB, Gansky SA. Diagnoses based on the Research Diagnostic Criteria for Temporomandibular Disorders in a biracial population of young women. *Journal of Orofacial Pain* 2005; **19**(1): 65–75.

118. Yunus MB, Yunus MB. Central sensitivity syndromes: a new paradigm and group nosology for fibromyalgia and overlapping conditions, and the related issue of disease versus illness. *Seminars in Arthritis and Rheumatism* 2008; **37**(6): 339–52.

119. Palmer KT, Calnan M, Wainwright D, Poole J, O'Neill C, Winterbottom A et al. Disabling musculoskeletal pain and its relation to somatization: a community-based postal survey. *Occupational Medicine (Oxford)* 2005; **55**(8): 612–17.

120. Zaman MS, Chavez NF, Krueger R, Talley NJ, Lembo T. Extra-intestinal symptoms in patients with irritable bowel syndrome (IBS). *Gastroenterology* 2001; **120**(Suppl 1):A636.

121. Lembo AJ, Zaman M, Krueger RF, Tomenson B, Creed FH. Psychiatric

disorder,irritable bowel syndrome, and extra-intestinal symptoms in a population-based sample of twins. *American Journal of Gastroenterology* 2009; **104**(3): 686–94.

122. Henningsen P, Herzog W, Henningsen P, Herzog W. Irritable bowel syndrome and somatoform disorders. *Journal of Psychosomatic Research* 2008; **64**(6): 625–9.

123. Alpers DH, Alpers DH. Multi-dimensionality of symptom complexes in irritable bowel syndrome and other functional gastrointestinal disorders. *Journal of Psychosomatic Research* 2008; **64**(6): 567–72.

124. Henningsen P, Zipfel S, Herzog W. Management of functional somatic syndromes. *The Lancet* 2007; **369**(9565): 946–55.

125. Creed FH. Somatisation and pain syndromes. In: Mayer EA, Bushnell MC, eds. *Functional Pain Syndromes: Presentation and Pathophysiology*. Seattle, WA: IASP; 2009: 227–44.

126. Fink P, Schroeder A. One single diagnosis, Bodily distress syndrome, succeeded to capture ten diagnostic categories of functional somatic syndromes and somatoform disorders. *Journal of Psychosomatic Research* 2010; **68**: 415–26.

127. Deary V, Chalder T, Sharpe M, Deary V, Chalder T, Sharpe M. The cognitive behavioural model of medically unexplained symptoms: a theoretical and empirical review. *Clinical Psychology Review* 2007; **27**(7): 781–97.

128. Mayou R, Bass C, Sharpe M. Overview of epidemiology, classification and aetiology. In: Mayou R, Bass C, Sharpe M, eds. *Treatment of Functional Somatic Symptoms*. Oxford: Oxford University Press; 1995: 42–65.

129. Katon W, Sullivan M, Walker E. Medical symptoms without identified pathology: relationship to psychiatric disorders, childhood and adult trauma, and personality traits. *Annals of Internal Medicine* 2001; **134**: 917–25.

130. Barsky AJ, Peekna HM, Borus JF. Somatic symptom reporting in women and men. *Journal of General Internal Medicine* 2001; **16**(4): 266–75.

131. Gillespie NA, Zhu G, Heath AC, Hickie IB, Martin NG. The genetic aetiology of somatic distress. *Psychological Medicine* 2000; **30**(5): 1051–61.

132. Kato K, Sullivan P, Evengard B, Pedersen N. A population-based twin study of functional somatic syndromes. *Psychological Medicine* 2009; **39**: 487–505.

133. Hotopf M, Mayou R, Wadsworth M, Wessely S, Hotopf M, Mayou R et al. Childhood risk factors for adults with medically unexplained symptoms: results from a national birth cohort study. *American Journal of Psychiatry* 1999; **156**(11): 1796–800.

134. Hotopf M, Wilson-Jones C, Mayou R, Wadsworth M, Wessely S. Childhood predictors of adult medically unexplained hospitalisations. Results from a national birth cohort study. *British Journal of Psychiatry* 2000; **176**: 273–80.

135. De Gucht V. Neuroticism, alexithymia, negative affect and positive affect as predictors of medically unexplained symptoms in primary care. *Acta Neuropsychiatrica* 2002; **14**(4): 181–5.

136. Watson D, Pennebaker JW, Watson D, Pennebaker JW. Health complaints, stress, and distress: exploring the central role of negative affectivity. *Psychological Review* 1989; **96**(2): 234–54.

137. Rosmalen JG, Neeleman J, Gans RO, de Jonge P, Rosmalen JGM, Neeleman J et al. The association between neuroticism and self-reported common somatic symptoms in a population cohort. *Journal of Psychosomatic Research* 2007; **62**(3): 305–11.

138. LeResche L, Mancl LA, Drangsholt MT, Huang G, Von Korff M, LeResche L et al. Predictors of onset of facial pain and temporomandibular disorders in early adolescence. *Pain* 2007; **129**(3): 269–78.

139. VonKorff M, LeResche L, Dworkin SF. First onset of common pain symptoms

– a prospective-study of depression as a risk factor. *Pain* 1993; **55**(2): 251–8.

140. Eek F, Karlson B, Osterberg K, Ostergren PO. Factors associated with prospective development of environmental annoyance. *Journal of Psychosomatic Research* 2010; **69**(1): 9–15.

141. Leiknes KA, Finset A, Moum T, Sandanger I. Overlap, comorbidity, and stability of somatoform disorders and the use of current versus lifetime criteria. *Psychosomatics* 2008; **49**(2): 152–62.

142. Rief W, Nanke A, Emmerich J, Bender A, Zech T. Causal illness attributions in somatoform disorders: associations with comorbidity and illness behavior. *Journal of Psychosomatic Research* 2004; **57**(4): 367–71.

143. Rief W, Broadbent E, Rief W, Broadbent E. Explaining medically unexplained symptoms-models and mechanisms. *Clinical Psychology Review* 2007; **27**(7): 821–41.

144. Jackson JL, Passamonti M. The outcomes among patients presenting in primary care with a physical symptom at 5 years. *Journal of General Internal Medicine* 2005; **20**(11): 1032–7.

145. Barsky AJ, Borus JF. Functional somatic syndromes. *Annals of Internal Medicine* 1999; **130**(11): 910–21.

146. Henningsen P, Zimmermann P. Medically unexplained physical symptoms, anxiety, and depression: a meta-analytic review. *Psychosomatic Medicine* 2003; **65**(4): 528–33.

147. Watanabe N, Stewart R, Jenkins R, Bhugra DK, Furukawa TA, Watanabe N et al. The epidemiology of chronic fatigue, physical illness, and symptoms of common mental disorders: a cross-sectional survey from the second British National Survey of Psychiatric Morbidity. *Journal of Psychosomatic Research* 2008; **64**(4): 357–62.

148. Lerdal A, Wahl AK, Rustoen T, Hanestad BR, Moum T. Fatigue in the general population: a translation and test of the psychometric properties of the Norwegian version of the fatigue severity scale.

Scandinavian Journal of Public Health 2005; **33**(2): 123–30.

149. Ahlberg K, Ekman T, Gaston-Johansson F, Mock V. Assessment and management of cancer-related fatigue in adults. *The Lancet* 2003; **362**(9384): 640–50.

150. Dunlop SP, Jenkins D, Spiller RC. Distinctive clinical, psychological, and histological features of postinfective irritable bowel syndrome. *American Journal of Gastroenterology* 2003; **98**(7): 1578–83.

151. Gwee KA, Leong YL, Graham C, McKendrick MW, Collins SM, Walters SJ et al. The role of psychological and biological factors in postinfective gut dysfunction. *Gut* 1999; **44**(3): 400–6.

152. Spence MJ, Moss-Morris R, Spence MJ, Moss-Morris R. The cognitive behavioural model of irritable bowel syndrome: a prospective investigation of patients with gastroenteritis. *Gut* 2007; **56**(8): 1066–71.

153. Spence M, Moss-Morris R. To 'lump' or to 'split' the functional somatic syndromes: can infectious and emotional risk factors differentiate between the onset of chronic fatigue syndrome and irritable bowel syndrome? *Psychosomatic Medicine* 2006; **68**(3): 463–9.

154. Hamilton WT, Gallagher AM, Thomas JM, White PD. Risk markers for both chronic fatigue and irritable bowel syndromes: a prospective case-control study in primary care. *Psychological Medicine* 2009; **39**:1913–21.

155. Petersen I, Thomas JM, Hamilton WT, White PD. Risk and predictors of fatigue after infectious mononucleosis in a large primary-care cohort. *QJM – Monthly Journal of the Association of Physicians* 2006; **99**(1): 49–55.

156. Prins JB, van der Meer JWM, Bleijenberg G. Chronic fatigue syndrome. *The Lancet* 2006; **367**(9507): 346–55.

157. Harvey SB, Wessely S, Kuh D, Hotopf M. The relationship between fatigue and psychiatric disorders: Evidence for the concept of neurasthenia. *Journal of Psychosomatic Research* 2009; **66**(5): 445–54.

158. Nijrolder I, van der Horst H, van der Windt D. Prognosis of fatigue. A systematic review. *Journal of Psychosomatic Research* 2008; **64**: 335–49.

159. van Dulmen AM, Fennis JF, Mokkink HG, Van der Velden HG, Bleijenberg G. Doctor-dependent changes in complaint-related cognitions and anxiety during medical consultations in functional abdominal complaints. *Psychological Medicine* 1995; **25**(5): 1011–18.

160. Ware JE Jr., Sherbourne CD. The MOS 36-item short-form health survey (SF-36). I. Conceptual framework and item selection. *Medical Care* 1992; **30**(6): 473–83.

161. Katon W, Lin EH, Von Korff M, Russo J, Lipscomb P, Bush T. Somatization: a spectrum of severity. *American Journal of Psychiatry* 1991; **148**: 34–40.

162. Hansen MS, Fink P, Frydenberg M, Oxhoj ML. Use of health services, mental illness, and self-rated disability and health in medical inpatients. *Psychosomatic Medicine* 2002; **64**(4): 668–75.

163. Smith RC, Gardiner JC, Lyles JS, Sirbu C, Dwamena FC, Hodges A *et al.* Exploration of DSM-IV criteria in primary care patients with medically unexplained symptoms. *Psychosomatic Medicine* 2005; **67**(1): 123–9.

164. Koch H, van Bokhoven MA, ter Riet G, van der WT, Dinant GJ, Bindels PJ. Demographic characteristics and quality of life of patients with unexplained complaints: a descriptive study in general practice. *Quality of Life Research* 2007; **16**(9): 1483–9.

165. Harris AM, Orav EJ, Bates DW, Barsky AJ. Somatization increases disability independent of comorbidity. *Journal of General Internal Medicine* 2009; **24**(2): 155–61.

166. Hoffman DL, Dukes EM. The health status burden of people with fibromyalgia: a review of studies that assessed health status with the SF-36 or the SF-12. *International Journal of Clinical Practice* 2008; **62**:115–26.

167. Ross SD, Estok RP, Frame D, Stone LR, Ludensky V, Levine CB. Disability and chronic fatigue syndrome – a focus on function. *Archives of Internal Medicine* 2004; **164**(10): 1098–107.

168. El Serag HB, Olden K, Bjorkman D. Health-related quality of life among persons with irritable bowel syndrome: a systematic review. *Alimentary Pharmacology and Therapeutics* 2002; **16**(6): 1171–85.

169. El Serag HB. Impact of irritable bowel syndrome: prevalence and effect on health-related quality of life. *Reviews in Gastroenterological Disorders* 2003; **3**(Suppl 2): S3–11.

170. Gralnek IM, Hays RD, Kilbourne A, Naliboff B, Mayer E. The impact of irritable bowel syndrome on health-related quality of life. *Gastroenterology* 2000; **119**(3): 655–60.

171. Solomon L, Nisenbaum R, Reyes M, Papanicolaou DA, Reeves WC. Functional status of persons with chronic fatigue syndrome in the Wichita, Kansas population. *Health and Quality of Life Outcomes* 2003; **1**: 48.

172. Reynolds KJ, Vernon SD, Bouchery E, Reeves WC. The economic impact of chronic fatigue syndrome. *Cost Effectiveness and Resource Allocation* 2008; **2**(1): 4.

173. Robinson RL, Birnbaum HG, Morley MA, Sisitsky T, Greenberg PE, Claxton AJ. Economic cost and epidemiological characteristics of patients with fibromyalgia claims. *Journal of Rheumatology* 2003; **30**(6): 1318–25.

174. Hauser W, Schmutzer G, Brahler E, Glaesmer H. A cluster within the continuum of biopsychosocial distress can be labeled 'fibromyalgia syndrome' – evidence from a representative German population survey. *Journal of Rheumatology* 2009; **36**(12): 2806–12.

175. Guthrie E, Creed F, Fernandes L, Ratcliffe J, Van Der JJ, Martin J *et al.* Cluster analysis of symptoms and health-seeking behaviour differentiates subgroups

of patients with severe irritable bowel syndrome. *Gut* 2003; **52**(11): 1616–22.

176. Giesecke T, Williams DA, Harris RE, Cupps TR, Tian X, Tian TX *et al.* Subgrouping of fibromyalgia patients on the basis of pressure-pain thresholds and psychological factors. *Arthritis and Rheumatism* 2003; **48**(10): 2916–22.

177. Naliboff BD, Balice G, Mayer EA. Psychosocial moderators of quality of life in irritable bowel syndrome. *European Journal of Surgery Supplements* 1998; **583**: 57–9.

178. Spiegel BM, Gralnek IM, Bolus R, Chang L, Dulai GS, Mayer EA *et al.* Clinical determinants of health-related quality of life in patients with irritable bowel syndrome. *Archives of Internal Medicine* 2004; **164**(16): 1773–80.

179. Creed F, Ratcliffe J, Fernandes L, Palmer S, Rigby C, Tomenson B *et al.* Outcome in severe irritable bowel syndrome with and without accompanying depressive, panic and neurasthenic disorders. *British Journal of Psychiatry* 2005; **186**:507–15.

180. Creed F, Ratcliffe J, Fernandez L, Tomenson B, Palmer S, Rigby C *et al.* Health-related quality of life and health care costs in severe, refractory irritable bowel syndrome. *Annals of Internal Medicine* 2001; **134**: 860–8.

181. Creed F, Guthrie E, Ratcliffe J, Fernandes L, Rigby C, Tomenson B *et al.* Does psychological treatment help only those patients with severe irritable bowel syndrome who also have a concurrent psychiatric disorder? *Australian and New Zealand Journal of Psychiatry* 2005; **39**(9): 807–15.

182. Meerding WJ, Bonneux L, Polder JJ, Koopmanschap MA, van der Maas PJ, Meerding WJ *et al.* Demographic and epidemiological determinants of health-care costs in Netherlands: cost of illness study. *British Medical Journal* 1998; **317**(7151): 111–15.

183. Kapur N, Hunt I. Psychosocial and illness related predictors of consultation rates in primary care – a cohort study. *Psychological Medicine* 2004; **34**(4): 719–28.

184. Smits FT, Brouwer HJ, van Weert. Epidemiology of frequent attenders: a 3-year historic cohort study comparing attendance, morbidity and prescriptions of one-year and persistent frequent attenders. *BMC Public Health* 2009; **9**: 36.

185. Reid S, Whooley D, Crayford T, Hotopf M. Medically unexplained symptoms – GPs' attitudes towards their cause and management. *Family Practice* 2001; **18**(5): 519–23.

186. Reid S, Wessely S, Crayford T, Hotopf M. Frequent attenders with medically unexplained symptoms: service use and costs in secondary care. *British Journal of Psychiatry* 2002; **180**: 248–53.

187. Shaw J, Creed F. The cost of somatization. *Journal of Psychosomatic Research* 1991; **35**(2–3): 307–12.

188. Hiller W, Kroymann R, Leibbrand R, Cebulla M, Korn HJ, Rief W *et al.* Effects and cost-effectiveness analysis of inpatient treatment for somatoform disorders. *Fortschritte der Neurologie-Psychiatrie* 2004; **72**(3): 136–46.

189. Sicras-Mainar A, Rejas J, Blanca M, Morcillo A, Larios R, Velasco S *et al.* Treating patients with fibromyalgia in primary care settings under routine medical practice: a claim database cost and burden of illness study. *Arthritis Research and Therapy* 2009; **11**(2): R54.

190. Robinson RL, Birnbaum HG, Morley MA, Sisitsky T, Greenberg PE, Wolfe F. Depression and fibromyalgia: treatment and cost when diagnosed separately or concurrently. *Journal of Rheumatology* 2004; **31**(8): 1621–9.

191. Silverman S, Dukes EM, Johnston SS, Brandenburg NA, Sadosky A, Huse DM. The economic burden of fibromyalgia: comparative analysis with rheumatoid arthritis. *Current Medical Research and Opinion* 2009; **25**(4): 829–40.

192. Maxion-Bergemann S, Thielecke F, Abel F, Bergemann R, Maxion-Bergemann S, Thielecke F *et al.* Costs of irritable bowel syndrome in the UK and US. *Pharmacoeconomics* 2006; **24**(1): 21–37.

193. Akehurst RL, Brazier JE, Mathers N, O'Keefe C, Kaltenthaler E, Morgan A

et al. Health-related quality of life and cost impact of irritable bowel syndrome in a UK primary care setting. *Pharmacoeconomics* 2002; **20**(7): 455–62.

194. Sandler RS, Everhart JE, Donowitz M, Adams E, Cronin K, Goodman C *et al.* The burden of selected digestive diseases in the United States. *Gastroenterology* 2002; **122**(5): 1500–11.

195. Levy RL, Von Korff M, Whitehead WE, Stang P, Saunders K, Jhingran P *et al.* Costs of care for irritable bowel syndrome patients in a health maintenance organization. *American Journal of Gastroenterology* 2001; **96**(11): 3122–9.

196. Johansson PA, Farup PG, Bracco A, Vandvik PO. How does comorbidity affect cost of health care in patients with irritable bowel syndrome? A cohort study in general practice. *BMC Gastroenterology* 2010; **10**: 31.

197. Spiegel BM, Kanwal F, Naliboff B, Mayer E. The impact of somatization on the use of gastrointestinal health-care resources in patients with irritable bowel syndrome. *American Journal of Gastroenterology* 2005; **100**(10): 2262–73.

198. McCrone P, Darbishire L, Ridsdale L, Seed P. The economic cost of chronic fatigue and chronic fatigue syndrome in UK primary care. *Psychological Medicine* 2003; **33**(2): 253–61.

199. Lloyd A, Pender H. Chronic fatigue syndrome: does it need more healthcare resources? *Pharmacoeconomics* 1994; **5**(6): 460–4.

200. Bombardier CH, Buchwald D. Chronic fatigue, chronic fatigue syndrome, and fibromyalgia. Disability and health-care use. *Medical Care* 1996; **34**(9): 924–30.

201. Jason LA, Benton MC, Valentine L, Johnson A, Torres-Harding S. The economic impact of ME/CFS: individual and societal costs. *Dynamic Medicine* 2008; **7**: 6.

202. Salmon P, Peters S, Stanley I. Patients' perceptions of medical explanations for somatisation disorders: qualitative analysis. *British Medical Journal* 1999; **318**(7180): 372–6.

203. Salmon P. Why do primary care physicians propose medical care to patients with medically unexplained symptoms? A new method of sequence analysis to test theories of patient pressure. *Psychosomatic Medicine* 2006; **68**(2): 269–76.

204. Fink P, Sorensen L, Engberg M, Holm M, Munk-Jorgensen P. Somatization in primary care. Prevalence, health care utilization, and general practitioner recognition. *Psychosomatics* 1999; **40**(4): 330–8.

205. Stenager EN, Svendsen MA, Stenager E. Disability retirement pension for patients with syndrome diagnoses: a register study on the basis of data from the Social Appeal Board. (Article in Danish). *Ugeskr Laeger* 2003; **165**(5): 469–74.

206. Fink p, Ørnbøl E, Tomas T, Sparle KC, Frostholm L, Olesen F. A new empirically established hypochondriasis diagnosis. *American Journal of Psychiatry* 2004; **161**: 1680–91.

207. Frostholm L, Ørnbøl E, Christensen KS, Toft T, Olesen F, Weinman J *et al.* Do illness perceptions predict health outcomes in primary care patients? A 2-year follow-up study. *Journal of Psychosomatic Research* 2007; **62**(2): 129–38.

208. Waddell G. Preventing incapacity in people with musculoskeletal disorders. *British Medical Bulletin* 2006; **77–78**: 55–69.

209. Brown J, Hanlon P, Turok I, Webster D, Arnott J, Macdonald EB. Mental health as a reason for claiming incapacity benefit – a comparison of national and local trends. *Journal of Public Health* 2009; **31**(1): 74–80.

210. van Oostrom SH, Driessen MT, de Vet HC, Franche RL, Schonstein E, Loisel P *et al.* Workplace interventions for preventing work disability. *Cochrane Database of Systematic Reviews* 2009; **2**: CD006955.

Terminology, classification and concepts

Peter Henningsen, Per Fink, Constanze
Hausteiner-Wiehle and Winfried Rief

Introduction

Patients who suffer from persistent bodily complaints such as pain, dizziness or fatigue, without obvious explanation of this suffering through structural pathology of bodily organs or body systems, are challenging not least because of the difficulties they pose for classification and terminology. Patients with identical clinical presentations are described in different terms and receive different diagnostic labels depending on the specialty or interest of the doctor they consult [1;2;3]. As a consequence, the problems related to unclear and inconsistent terminology and classification can be seen as major barriers to improved care for these patients (see Chapter 5). The topic is complicated, and this chapter deals with several inter-related aspects of the general question 'What exactly are we talking about?'.

In the first part of the chapter, we discuss the terminology, stressing the difficulties of the words and concept 'medically unexplained symptoms' (MUS), and discussing the pros and cons of alternative terms. We will then, in the second part, deal with classification in five respects: (i) we briefly present the problems of the current negative classification and its history; (ii) we introduce and evaluate current alternative terms; (iii) we discuss the importance of positive psychobehavioural criteria for disorders in this field; (iv) we briefly give recommendations regarding the preliminary classification as long as the clinical significance of the symptoms is unknown; and lastly (v) we discuss two current proposals for a new classification for clinically significant bodily symptoms, i.e. 'complex somatic symptom disorder' under DSM-V, and 'bodily distress syndrome'. In the last part of the chapter, we discuss some conceptual aspects of classification and nosology in general. We also discuss what it means to have bodily sensations that are not primarily indicators of underlying organic disease and what the relation of central and peripheral factors is in the aetiology and maintenance of these symptoms.

All in all, we hope to make clear that, on the one hand, there is no easy solution to the problems around terminology, classification and concepts, but, on the other hand, there is much room for improvement, starting with good knowledge of the complexities involved.

Terminology
Medically unexplained symptoms

The term 'medically unexplained symptoms' (sometimes also called 'medically unexplained physical symptoms' (MUPS), has gained some popularity during recent years among general

Medically Unexplained Symptoms, Somatisation and Bodily Distress, ed. Francis Creed, Peter Henningsen and Per Fink. Published by Cambridge University Press. © Cambridge University Press 2011.

practitioners and others to describe the bodily complaints of their patients when the aetiology is unclear. The term implies that the complaints cannot be fully explained by structural bodily pathology. Used in this way, the term 'medically unexplained symptoms' is like a pre-diagnostic statement: it implies that currently there is no 'organic cause' for the problem but it leaves open the potential aetiology of the problem [4].

As the term is so widely known, 'medically unexplained symptoms' appears in the title of this book. However, unfortunately, any advantage of using this term in a purely descriptive, diagnostically non-committal way is outweighed by a number of disadvantages that should discredit its further use. From a clinical point of view the phrase 'medically unexplained' is a negative statement, withholding from the patient that which he or she usually seeks most – a positive explanation for their symptom(s) and support [5;6]. Conceptually, referring to a symptom as 'medically unexplained' is ambiguous in at least two senses [4]:

- It is not sufficiently clear what counts as a medical explanation of a symptom. This might refer to a good correlation between the nature of the symptom and proven organic pathology, described in functional anatomical and pathophysiological terms. Alternatively, it might refer to a description of central nervous system (CNS) dysfunctions associated with a subjective symptom, such as pain, even though this may not implicate the CNS in direct causation.
- It is not clear whether describing a symptom as 'medically' unexplained implies that medicine has nothing to offer the patient who has such a symptom. By labelling the symptom in this way it may appear that the doctor is dismissing the patient because he or she is unable to help. Even if this is not what the doctor intends, it may be understood by patients in this way [7].

A more fundamental problem with the concept underlying 'medically unexplained symptoms' is the dualism it fosters. A patient's symptom is seen *either* as an organic one ('medically explained') *or* 'medically unexplained', which may be taken to imply a psychological cause. This dualism is still enshrined in our classifications of diseases (The International Classification of Diseases (ICD) has a separate chapter for 'mental' disorders and the *Diagnostic and Statistical Manual of Mental Disorders* (DSM) is only concerned with mental disorders), despite the fact that we know now that human illness is determined by a mixture of biological, psychological and social factors.

Ten criteria to evaluate terminology

There is a long list of other terms that are currently used, or discussed as future concepts, to describe the group of symptoms frequently referred to as 'medically unexplained'. The most important ones are: somatoform disorder, functional disorder or functional somatic syndrome, bodily distress syndrome/disorder or bodily stress syndrome/disorder, (complex) somatic symptom disorder, psychophysical/psychophysiological disorder, psychosomatic disorder and symptom-defined illness/ syndrome. Apart from these categorical terms, the tendency to experience and communicate somatic distress in response to psychosocial stress and to seek medical help for it is referred to as 'somatisation' in a dimensional way, i.e. as a feature that can be present in different degrees.

In order to judge the value of these terms, 10 criteria seem to be useful [4]. Obviously, this list of criteria does not claim to be exhaustive, but it captures the most important aspects. The criteria are that the term:

1. is acceptable to patients
2. is acceptable and usable by doctors and other healthcare professionals, making it likely that they will use it in daily practice
3. does not reinforce unhelpful dualistic thinking
4. can be used readily in patients who also have pathologically established disease
5. can be adequate as a standalone diagnosis
6. has a clear core theoretical concept
7. will facilitate the possibility of multidisciplinary (medical and psychological) treatment
8. has similar meaning in different cultures
9. is neutral with regard to aetiology and pathology
10. has a satisfactory acronym.

In view of these criteria, the term currently used in the classification systems ICD-10 and DSM-IV, 'somatoform disorders', is problematic. It implies psychogenic origin, therefore is little acceptable to patients, and it enforces dualistic thinking. However, it has to be noted that the acceptability of this term is better in some countries, e.g. Germany, than in others, e.g. the UK or the USA. The term 'symptom-defined illness/ syndrome' is unlikely to be widely accepted among patients and doctors alike; it lacks a clear core concept and does not easily fit with a concurrent pathologically established disease.

'(Complex) somatic symptom disorder' rightly addresses the complexity of the issue by acknowledging that the condition is defined by somatic symptoms, but that there are also other aspects (such as disproportionate suffering, or psychobehavioural characteristics) [8]. It has, however, an uncertain core concept, dubious wide acceptability across cultures and does not promote multidisciplinary treatment. In addition, it seems odd to call something a symptom and a disorder at the same time, and the notion 'complex' is unclear without reference to a 'simple' category. Nevertheless, the DSM-V workgroup currently proposes to rename 'somatoform disorders' as 'somatic symptom disorders' (in combination with 'psychological factors affecting medical condition' and 'factitious disorders'), and subsume former somatoform disorder subtypes under a 'complex somatic symptom disorder' (see below) [8]. Apparently, the terms that fit most closely the criteria set out above are: bodily distress (or stress) syndrome/disorder, psychosomatic or psychophysical disorder and functional (somatic) syndrome/disorder.

The term 'bodily distress disorder' fulfils most criteria from the list above with the exception of criterion 10 (the acronym BDD is in use already to indicate body dysmorphic disorder) [1]. In a discussion among international specialists in the field it became clear that there is a semantic uncertainty as to the notion of distress: in Danish and German, this term does not necessarily imply a psychological component (there can be distress solely in the form of bodily complaints such as pain and dizziness), whereas in Britain the notion of distress seems to be inextricably linked to a psychological state (pain and other bodily complaints 'causing' distress, not being a form of distress) [4].

The term 'psychosomatic disorder' also fulfils most criteria. Although it is accurate in describing the problem in terms of both psychological and somatic components, it generally has negative connotations outside of some, especially German-speaking, countries [9;10]. This difference may be because in Anglophone countries the term is exclusively linked to the more or less Freudian tradition of psychogenic explanations of disease. In these countries, the term 'psychosomatic medicine' does seem to be more generally acceptable and those psychiatrists who offer 'psychosomatic medicine' or 'psychological medical' clinics find that patients are not put off by these labels. Thus there seems to be a difference according to whether we use the term 'psychosomatic' to describe symptoms/disorder or a type of health-care. The term 'psychophysical/psychophysiological disorder' is similar in its immediate meaning to 'psychosomatic disorder'. It has the advantage that it is not bound to the tradition of assuming a psychogenic origin. However, 'physical' is not a widely used description for bodily complaints.

The term 'functional somatic disorder/syndrome' fulfils most criteria; it is reasonably widely accepted because it is neutral as to mental or organic backgrounds [10]. There is some confusion regarding its core concept as it may refer to a functional disturbance of the organs implied in the bodily complaints (the traditional understanding) or a functional disturbance of the brain systems underlying symptom experience (the currently favoured view).

Classification
Current classification in DSM-IV and ICD-10

The current classification of patients with persistent bodily complaints without clear organic pathology to explain them is to be found in the fourth edition of the *Diagnostic and Statistical Manual* of the American Psychiatric Association (DSM-IV) and in the tenth edition of the International Classification of Diseases of the World Health Organization (ICD-10).

Somatoform disorders

The 'locus classicus' for the classification of these patients as having a mental disorder is within the category of 'somatoform disorders' in the DSM-IV and in block F (mental disorders) of the ICD-10. Over the past years, this category has encountered not only fundamental criticism, including the suggestion to abolish it altogether, but also suggestions for reform [11;12]. Meanwhile, the process of transforming it in forthcoming editions of DSM and ICD (expected around 2013) is well under way. Therefore we will not discuss the current classification in more detail and will only briefly hint at four of these problems (see also the discussion concerning the term 'somatoform', above):

- *Lack of a medium severe category*: 'Somatisation disorder' as the rare end point in a spectrum of severity has dominated epidemiological research in most large studies, leading to vast underestimations of the effects on functioning, disability and healthcare use of patients with persistent bodily distress. The 'Somatisation Disorder' diagnosis has been shown to be too rigid for clinical use as only the most severe cases with a specific predefined symptom profile fulfil the diagnostic criteria, and the majority of patients with multiple symptoms fall into one of the residual categories of 'undifferentiated' or 'not otherwise specified' somatoform disorders [12;13]. Since the appearance of ICD-10 and DSM-IV, several suggestions have been made (see below).

- *Lack of positive psychobehavioural features in the definition of somatoform disorders*: The definition of somatoform disorders is primarily based on one central negative criterion, the exclusion of organic pathology that can explain the extent of the bodily complaints. This in itself is problematic, as discussed above for the term 'medically unexplained symptoms'. What is more or less completely lacking in the classification, though, are psychobehavioural features that positively define the patients with these complaints (see below) [12].

- *Internal inconsistencies*: There are many inconsistencies within and between the DSM-IV and ICD-10 categories of somatoform disorders. 'Conversion disorder' is part of this category in DSM-IV, but not in ICD-10, where it is part of the dissociative disorders. 'Neurasthenia' is a diagnosis in ICD-10 that is related to somatoform disorders, but it is not part of this category. 'Somatoform autonomic dysfunction' is a subcategory in ICD-10, but not in DSM-IV. 'Pain disorder' in DSM-IV is different from 'persistent somatoform pain disorder' in ICD-10, etc.
- *Unclear relation to depression and anxiety*: Innumerable studies have shown that patients with somatoform disorders or functional somatic syndromes have higher rates of depression and anxiety than not only healthy persons but also patients with organically explained bodily problems [14]. Epidemiologically, overlap of these categories is not the exception, but the rule – this renders the concept of 'comorbidity' somewhat ill-fitting. On the other hand, concepts such as 'masked depression' as a description of patients with persistent bodily distress also fail because a significant subgroup of these patients does not display raised depressivity and/or anxiety.

Functional somatic syndromes

The term 'functional somatic syndrome' (FSS) is not a fixed one, and authors disagree on which syndromes to subsume under this heading. Three syndromes are always mentioned as prototypic examples of FSS: 'irritable bowel syndrome' (IBS) (ICD-10 K58), 'fibromyalgia' (FM) (ICD-10 M79.7) and 'chronic fatigue syndrome' (CFS) (ICD-10 provides only a category for 'postviral fatigue syndrome', G93.3) – probably because they attract most research and there are elaborate research diagnostic criteria outside the official diagnostic system ICD-10 for them (e.g. the Rome criteria for IBS, American College of Rheumatology (ACR) criteria for FM, Centers for Disease Control and Prevention criteria for CFS). Others are also frequently mentioned, although for most of them research diagnostic criteria do not exist: 'multiple chemical sensitivity' (MCS), 'tension headache', 'temporomandibular joint disorder', 'non-specific chest pain', 'non-ulcer dyspepsia' and many more. Some syndromes such as 'interstitial cystitis' or 'tinnitus' are only rarely subsumed here. Entities also fall out of fashion, while others are newly proposed (Table 2.1) [15]. FSS are to be found outside the mental disorders section, in texts which refer to different organs and organ systems, e.g. in the sections on gastroenterological or musculoskeletal diseases. There is widespread agreement that there is no clear logic behind the parallel classification of certain conditions as either 'somatoform disorder' or 'functional somatic syndrome', and it is clearly, as mentioned above, mostly a question of who makes the diagnosis and not of what the condition is like, whether a patient, e.g. with chronic widespread pain, is diagnosed as having 'persistent somatoform pain disorder' or 'fibromyalgia' [15].

In addition, there is also widespread agreement that the separation of single FSS is problematic: first of all, there is considerable overlap in symptoms between different FSS (e.g. muscle pain in CFS and FM); secondly, although there are cases where patients only have symptoms belonging to one FSS (e.g. 'uncomplicated' IBS), many others fulfil criteria for more than one FSS. Thirdly, different FSS respond to the same types of treatments, i.e. psychotherapy, antidepressants and multimodal treatments. As a result, most researchers are convinced that single FSS are primarily artefacts of the specialised diagnostic and treatment services in our healthcare systems [2;15;16;17;18].

Table 2.1 Functional somatic syndromes grouped according to medical specialty (selection) [15]

Medical specialty	Functional somatic syndrome
Gastroenterology	Irritable bowel syndrome, non-ulcer dyspepsia
Gynaecology	Pelvic arthropathy, premenstrual syndrome, chronic pelvic pain
Rheumatology	Fibromyalgia, chronic lower back pain
Cardiology	Atypical or non-cardiac chest pain
Respiratory medicine	Hyperventilation syndrome
Infectious diseases	Chronic fatigue syndrome (CFS/ME)
Neurology	Tension headache, pseudo-epileptic seizure
Dentistry	Temporomandibular joint dysfunction, atypical facial pain
Ear, nose and throat	Globus syndrome
Allergy	Multiple chemical sensitivity
Orthopaedics	Whiplash-associated disorder
Anaesthesiology	Chronic benign pain syndrome
Psychiatry	Somatoform disorders, neurasthenia, conversion

ME, myalgic encephalopathy.

History of current classification

The 'somatisation disorder' diagnosis has its origin in the concept of hysteria. It was introduced in DSM-III in 1980 as a diagnosis in the new somatoform disorder group; it arose
from an exploratory study by Perley and Guze in the early 1960s [19]. On the basis of symptoms reported by 39 female patients admitted to a psychiatric ward and diagnosed with
'Hysteria', they set up diagnostic criteria for hysteria later named 'Briquet's syndrome' [19].
From a factor analysis of all symptoms, they listed 59 physical and psychological symptoms
distributed in 10 groups: 25 of the symptoms from nine groups were required to qualify for
the diagnosis of Briquet's syndrome. This was a pioneer study as it was one of the first to
use factor analyses to identify symptom clustering. However, as the criteria were developed
in highly unrepresentative samples, the study severely violates representativeness, and the
symptom structure may more reflect the setting, the gender of the patients and what was
believed to be hysteria at that time, rather than a characteristic of the illness. 'Briquet's syndrome' was modified when introduced in the DSM-III to the 'somatisation disorder' diagnosis in the way that all psychological symptoms were eliminated to avoid overlapping with
other psychiatric diagnoses.

The diagnostic criteria underwent a major revision in the DSM-IV, and according
to these criteria, symptoms from three of four symptom groups (pain, gastrointestinal,
sexual and pseudo-neurological) are required. It is unclear on what basis this diagnosis
was founded. The somatoform diagnosis category was included in ICD-10 in 1992, but
(confusingly) the ICD-10 criteria list different symptoms and require a different number
of symptoms compared with the corresponding DSM criteria, and the diagnoses are different. Although the diagnostic criteria have been modified in later permutations of the DSM
classifications, its heritage is unmistakable. The basis of the other somatoform diagnoses in
the DSM and the ICD is obscure.

To increase the sensitivity of the 'somatisation disorder' diagnosis, Escobar *et al.* [20] introduced an abridged somatisation index. This required four symptoms for males and six symptoms for females out of the 37 somatic symptoms listed in the DSM-III, compared with 12 and 14 symptoms, respectively, for the full DSM-III somatisation disorder diagnosis. Kroenke *et al.* [21] have suggested a diagnosis of 'multisomatoform disorder', defined as three or more MUPS from a 15-symptom checklist along with at least a two-year history of somatisation.

However, these abridged versions share the same basic problem as the original ones, namely that the chosen number of symptoms to qualify for the individual diagnoses is arbitrary and not empirically based. Furthermore, many studies have relied on predefined symptom lists derived from the DSM-III symptom lists, and widely used diagnostic instruments such as the Composite International Diagnostic Interview (CIDI) and the layperson version of the CIDI, the Diagnostic Interview Schedule (DIS), only explore symptoms included in the DSM-III symptom checklist. This means that criteria that go beyond the original ones are not explored. Few studies have used instruments such as the Present State Examination (PSE)/Schedule of Clinical Assessment in Neuropsychiatry (SCAN) or tailored instruments that are not diagnosis bound.

Positive description of cognitions and behaviour

Because of the manifold problems inherent to the current terminology and classification of MUS, future classifications must take a fundamentally different approach. As an important step, it has been suggested to include positive psychobehavioural criteria [12;22;23]. A recent population-based study identified 10 (binary coded) psychobehavioural variables that identified those people with somatic symptoms who needed medical help and/or were seriously disabled (for example, 'avoidance of physical activities', 'bias for somatic illness attributions', 'self-concept of being physically weak' and 'desperation because of somatic symptoms') [23]. There is also some evidence indicating that psychological symptoms can predict disease course and treatment outcome [22]. A focus on psychobehavioural features during the diagnostic phase may also facilitate their therapeutic modification later on. On the other hand, many patients with MUS present to primary care or specialised 'somatic' settings, where an assessment of psychobehavioural characteristics may demand too much time and expertise. In the following sections, we will discuss the empirical foundation of positive psychobehavioural descriptors, and refer to their suitability as diagnostic criteria in more detail.

Self-focused attention, bodily self-observation

Barsky and others have described the process of 'somatosensory amplification' [24]. They postulate that people with these syndromes focus their attention on somatic perceptions. This process of focused attention increases the perceptual intensity. More intense somatic perceptions in turn increase the risk of more negative and catastrophising interpretations. Barsky's theory was initially based on the results of self-rating scales assessing somatosensory amplification [25]. In most (but not all) subsequent studies, it could be confirmed that 'body scanning' is more pronounced in patients with somatisation and hypochondriasis [26;27]. The process of mental body scanning describes a tendency to check different body parts and body functions mentally to decide whether they are functioning correctly (e.g. checking body parts to search for cancer signs; observing the intensity of existing pain symptoms). Moreover, many patients reduce their social activities and other sources of external stimulation, which further increases the intensity of internal stimuli (e.g. somatic symptoms) and supports the process of persistence of these complaints [23]. Recent studies and reviews on the role of somatosensory amplification for development and maintenance of 'medically unexplained', 'somatoform' or 'functional' symptoms relativise its importance, though [22;23;28].

Meanwhile, neuroimaging studies support the assumption that focusing attention facilitates the perception of somatic symptoms, while distraction reduces the perceptual intensity [29]. The authors were able to show that the brain activation of the pain matrix is lower if people try to distract their attention in contrast to focusing the attention to pain stimuli. However, the continuous focusing of attention on somatic symptoms can lead to neural sensitisation processes that amplify processes of chronicity [30].

Overinterpretation of bodily symptoms

The overinterpretation (catastrophising) of bodily symptoms is another psychobehavioural feature that is partially included in Barsky's somatosensory amplification model. It postulates that patients with somatisation symptoms have a tendency to overinterpret everyday bodily sensations. Although this could be confirmed using self-rating scales [26], the experimental investigation of somatoform-specific interpretation styles when using standardised somatic stimuli is equivocal [31]. However, in research on chronic pain conditions it is a reliable result that patients with a high tendency towards 'catastrophising somatic symptoms' show an increased risk of chronicity [32]. Therefore 'catastrophising' is considered a yellow flag for persisting symptoms and also for healthcare use in the prior 12 months [23]. Even if it should also be mentioned that catastrophising does not seem to be a necessary condition for somatic complaints, recent reviews have come to the conclusion that it constitutes an important descriptor of MUS and 'somatoform disorder diagnoses', and that modification of catastrophising beliefs is associated with positive outcomes [22;31].

Are somatic illness beliefs a necessary condition for somatisation?

It has been frequently suggested that patients with 'medically unexplained', 'somatoform' or 'functional' symptoms are characterised by rigid somatic illness beliefs. Many therapists in psychiatry, psychosomatic medicine and clinical psychology struggled with patients who overemphasised their somatic illness beliefs. However, the empirical data point to a somewhat different conclusion. Patients with rigid somatic illness beliefs are certainly challenging and constitute a difficult group, but many patients with MUS do not only have a single, monocausal illness explanation. In fact, several studies have shown that they report several different illness explanations including psychological ones [33;34]. Moreover, the more psychological illness explanations patients report, the more disabled they are. Therefore it is not the overemphasis of single somatic explanations for their symptoms, but perhaps a kind of inflexibility of using different explanations for somatic complaints. All current reviews conclude that patients with 'medically unexplained', 'somatoform' or 'functional' symptoms usually have no monocausal simplistic explanations, even if they have more organic attributions than depressed patients [22;28;31]. However, this aspect needs to be investigated further.

Self-concept of bodily weakness

It has been shown that patients with chronic 'unexplained' symptoms report a negative self-concept of being weak, not tolerating stress and not tolerating any physical challenges [26;27]. This concept should not be confused with a 'catastrophising style of interpreting somatic perceptions'. While the latter focuses on episodes of interpreting current symptoms, a negative self-concept is a variable trait which persists over time, even in the absence of somatic perception. Therefore it can be considered to be a chronic and continuous risk factor. A re-analysis of previous data indicated that a negative self-concept is one of the strongest predictors of poor outcome in psychological intervention trials, yet this result has to be further replicated using longitudinal investigations. In a population-based study, a self-concept of bodily weakness independently identified those people with somatic symptoms who needed medical help and/or were seriously disabled [23].

Expectation and memory

The expectation of symptoms provokes a state of facilitated perception of bodily complaints – both lead to an activation of highly similar brain structures [35;36]. Brown's model of rogue perception of symptoms [37;38] postulates that existing memory traces for symptom perception can be triggered by other external and internal stimuli. This provocation of rogue perceptions is more pronounced in patients with 'medically unexplained' symptoms. Although the participation of memory processes in the development and persistence of somatic symptoms needs further investigation, it is an extremely exciting and highly relevant approach [31].

Health anxiety and health concerns

Health anxiety (also referred to as illness worries) is the central feature of hypochondriasis. However, even in 'medically unexplained', 'somatoform' or 'functional' symptoms *without* hypochondriasis, many patients describe increased scores for health anxiety [22;27;31]. Based on their population data about identifiers of clinically significant MUS, Rief *et al.* suggested that new classifications should include ruminations about physical complaints, worrying about health and illness issues [23]. But again, health anxiety itself is not a necessary, yet a frequent condition in these patients. Some patients are well reassured by their doctors, believe that their symptoms are not based on a life-threatening disease, but still have the somatic complaints.

Abnormal illness behaviour

Pilowsky [39] introduced the concept of abnormal illness behaviour, and postulated that it is a characteristic feature of patients with somatisation and hypochondriasis. However, it is difficult to use his broad and multifaceted construct of illness behaviour as positive criteria for the classification of patients with 'medically unexplained', 'somatoform' or 'functional' symptoms. Illness behaviour is highly depending on the healthcare system, interaction patterns of the doctors, time and personal skills of healthcare professionals, etc. Nevertheless, several studies have shown that healthcare utilisation is closely related to the number of somatic symptoms described by the patient [40]. Increased healthcare use by patients with somatoform symptoms is not explained by comorbid depression [41;42]. Moreover, illness behaviour can be highly heterogeneous. While some patients report an increased need for medical reassurance (e.g. repeated verification of diagnosis), others describe the need for medical intervention (e.g. medication), while a third group communicates the symptoms to their social network and reports increased disability [43]. Increased healthcare use is not specific for 'medically unexplained', 'somatoform' or 'functional' symptoms, since it also occurs in hypochondriasis, depression and anxiety disorders as well as physical diseases [31]. In summary, there appears to be a relationship between MUS and abnormal or dysfunctional illness behaviour, but it is complex and not sufficiently understood [28]. The originally introduced concept of abnormal illness behaviour has to be modified and has to consider this diversity of individual needs.

Avoidance of physical activity and of other stimuli seen as symptom-provoking

Avoidance of physical activities was the most powerful discriminator between patients with somatic complaints needing medical help and feeling disabled, and those with somatic complaints but without healthcare needs or disability [23]. This result of somatisation is well confirmed by studies in pain research. The reduction of physical activity when suffering from complaints is one of the best predictors of a continuous pain experience [44]. However, avoidance of physical activities is not only limited to a general avoidance, but can also focus on some specific body parts (disuse syndromes of body parts etc.). The 'pain avoidance model' outlines how avoidance of physical activities transforms to aspects of physical deconditioning and facilitates the perception of somatic complaints [45]. While some patients with hypochondriasis obsessively collect information on health issues, others completely avoid any news about health and illness. Moreover, many patients with somatisation and/or hypochondriasis report some kind of 'safety behaviour'. They avoid not only activities, but locations, information or social contacts that are supposed to elicit symptoms.

Interpersonal problems

There is also an important interpersonal dimension to 'medically unexplained', 'somatoform' or 'functional' symptoms that particularly shows up in satisfaction with healthcare; many patient–doctor relationships are described as problematic, in fact by both the doctors and the patients. Somatising patients tend to be less satisfied with their medical care than subjects with severe organic illness or affective disorders, even when length, type and intensity of care are taken into account [27;46;47]. This dissatisfaction also leads to dysfunctional healthcare utilisation, i.e. frequent change of care providers, discontinuation of treatment, concealment of previous findings. Our healthcare system is definitely not well prepared to care for patients with somatoform disorders – and patients may be rightly dissatisfied (see Chapter 5). It has been shown, however, that there is probably more to this raised level of dissatisfaction than just a reaction to inadequate treatments. Somatising patients genuinely tend to have a more insecure attachment style that contributes to a tendency to experience attempts by others to help them as unsatisfactory. These observations argue for more profound disturbances of personality development and not just reactive interpersonal problems [48].

Summing up, there appear to be a set of defining psychobehavioural features that help to characterise this patient group. This can be of enormous help with regard to earlier identification and also to planning personalised treatment that focuses on the modification of these (often dysfunctional) cognitions and behaviours. Nevertheless, it is unclear whether the empirical data on psychobehavioural characteristics allow their use as diagnostic criteria. Further, psychobehavioural characteristics should not be confused with causality factors. Their aetiological role in the process of symptom development and persistence is far from clear: many of the psychobehavioural features mentioned can not only be conditions preceding symptom onset, but also be consequences of the symptoms or predictors of poor outcome.

It is agreed that the DSM-V (like the DSM-IV) will be based on phenomenological rather than aetiological statements. If positive psychobehavioural characteristics are included as mandatory for classificatory case definitions, they must be taken as pure descriptors. Currently, the classification proposal for DSM-V ('complex somatic symptom disorder',

CSSD (see below)) includes positive psychobehavioural characteristics [8]. In view of the limited evidence concerning the sensitivity and specificity of psychobehavioural criteria, and their somewhat more complicated assessment especially in somatic and primary care settings, a *different* classification approach could refrain completely from listing psycho-behavioural characteristics. A current proposal for such an approach that relies on bodily symptoms only, but without demanding their 'medical inexplicability', is 'bodily distress syndrome' (BDS), introduced by Fink *et al.* [1] (see below).

Before we discuss these two classification approaches in more detail, we will address another important issue: the clinical significance of MUS can rarely be determined at their onset, or their first presentation. Therefore, suggestions for the *preliminary* classification of 'medically unexplained', 'somatoform' or 'functional' symptoms are needed.

The preliminary classification of 'medically unexplained symptoms' before a diagnosis can be established

Most people suffer from some sort of bodily discomfort on many occasions. Usually, these symptoms are self-limited and do not cause significant impairment and/or suffering. Therefore, it takes a certain (subjective) severity, and usually a duration of several months, to classify these symptoms as a 'disorder'.

The *preliminary* classification of 'medically unexplained', 'somatoform' or 'functional' symptoms is mainly a problem in primary care (where such 'banal', potentially transient sensations or symptoms are quite prevalent) and early in the diagnostic process. Basically, we recommend simply using the neutral name 'symptom' or even 'idiopathic symptom' for these phenomena, according to the ICD-10 block R00-R99. The International Classification of Primary Care (ICPC)-2 addresses this problem by the 'symptom component' of diagnoses. Symptom diagnoses thus include symptoms that are yet unclarified, symptoms that do not require further examination or treatment and persistent symptoms that do not match a specific ICD-10 diagnosis. Patients presenting with bodily sensations and mild cases are included as symptom diagnoses. This seems to be a pragmatic solution, as long as the patients do not misunderstand the 'diagnosis' as being evidence of disease. However, it could lead to problems if primary care physicians are reluctant to use the more 'severe' psychiatric diagnoses, such as 'somatisation disorder', and instead prefer to use this less stigmatising symptom diagnosis [49].

Since there is wide diagnostic variation in the labelling of symptoms as 'physical disorders' or MUS [49], it has been suggested that a category called 'multiple symptoms' should be introduced in the ICPC as a diagnosis of early or mild conditions. Because the 'multiple symptom' diagnosis is not in the psychiatric section, it may be more acceptable to both physicians and patients. This is a way to use a multi-dimensional approach in the borderland between normal and clearly pathological. It is suggested that the 'multiple symptom' diagnosis is used when a patient displays a repeated pattern of primary care consultation for three or more symptoms during a six-month period. In this way, the diagnosis is also intended as a yellow flag for the more severe, clinically significant diagnoses.

Two new proposals for the classification of clinically significant MUS

Complex somatic symptom disorder

In early 2010, the DSM-V Somatic Symptom Disorders Work Group proposed significant changes to the categories currently subsumed under the heading of 'somatoform disorders' [8].

At the time of writing, it is not clear to what extent they will change, therefore we will discuss them only briefly. The new proposal for CSSD consists of four major changes (Table 2.2):

- *One new name for all disorders formerly subsumed under the heading of somatoform disorders:* (somatisation disorder, undifferentiated somatoform disorder, hypochondriasis, pain disorder associated with both psychological factors and a general medical condition, and pain disorder associated with psychological factors).

  (This suggestion is an improvement insofar as the new term CSSD is probably as acceptable to patients as to doctors, that it does not imply unsubstantiated causal assumptions, and that it emphasises that this condition presents with bodily symptoms.)

- *Definition of positive psychobehavioural criteria in addition to bodily symptoms:* For the first time, it is required that a patient displays distinct psychobehavioural characteristics. Verbatim, the current proposal demands 'one or more somatic symptoms that are distressing and/or result in significant disruption in daily life' and 'at least two out of three psychobehavioural features (health-related anxiety, disproportionate and persistent concerns, excessive time and energy devoted to the symptoms or health concerns)' (Table 2.2) [8].

  (This part of the new definition is an important step forward, even if the choice of positive psychobehavioural criteria appears to be somewhat arbitrary and therefore is still under discussion.)

- *Omission of the central criterion of the symptoms being medically unexplained:* This is the most important of all changes in the new proposal. In the description of the category it is said that 'the symptoms may or may not be associated with a known medical condition' [8]. This means that also patients with, for instance, multiple sclerosis, who experience distressing fatigue and have fear of progression (high health anxiety) and a persistent organic attribution of their fatigue, qualify for the diagnosis of CSSD, if other conditions (chronicity etc.) are met. It is unclear yet whether this removal of any reference to the symptoms not having a typical organic explanation leads to a loss of discriminatory value of the category. An alternative, potentially less radical formulation could have been: 'the extent of suffering and complaints is not related to the extent of organic pathology demonstrable in these patients'.

- In addition, the CSSD proposal also suggests three optional specifiers, and it is recommended to assess the disorder's severity with established dimensional measures (Table 2.2).

In summary, this proposal demands a 'combination of distressing (often multiple) symptoms and an excessive or maladaptive response to these symptoms or associated health concerns'. The patient's suffering is seen as authentic, whether or not it is 'medically explained' [8]. Its major advantages lie in the abandonment of dualistic symptom allocation and the acknowledgement of a psychobehavioural dimension. The most important disadvantage is the still insufficient evidence base for the selected psychobehavioural criteria. A recent review stated that of all diagnostic proposals, CSSD has the best construct and descriptive validity as it reflects all dimensions of current biopsychosocial models of somatisation and goes beyond somatic symptom counts by including psychological and behavioural symptoms [22].

Bodily distress syndrome

Recently, 'bodily distress syndrome' was introduced as an alternative, empirically based diagnosis that may help solve the problem of diagnostic confusion [1]. The hallmark of BDS is that the patients suffer from various physical symptoms of bodily distress.

Table 2.2 DSM-V proposal: diagnostic criteria for 'complex somatic symptom disorder' (reproduced with permission from the American Psychiatric Association) [8]

To meet criteria for CSSD, criteria A, B, and C are necessary	
A. Somatic symptoms	One or more somatic symptoms that are distressing and/or result in significant disruption in daily life
B. Excessive thoughts, feelings, and behaviours related to these somatic symptoms or associated health concerns	At least two of the following are required to meet this criterion: *(1) High level of health-related anxiety* *(2) Disproportionate and persistent concerns about the medical seriousness of one's symptoms* *(3) Excessive time and energy devoted to these symptoms or health concerns* *
C. Chronicity	Although any one symptom may not be continuously present, the state of being symptomatic is chronic (at least 6 months)
For patients who fulfill the CSSD criteria, the following **optional specifiers** may be applied to a diagnosis of CSSD where one of the following dominates the clinical presentation:	XXX.1 Predominant somatic complaints (previously, Somatisation Disorder) XXX.2 Predominant health anxiety (previously, hypochondriasis). If patients present solely with health-related anxiety with minimal somatic symptoms, they may be more appropriately diagnosed as having an anxiety disorder. XXX.3 Predominant Pain (previously Pain Disorder). This classification is reserved for individuals presenting predominantly with pain complaints who also have many of the features described under criterion B. Patients with other presentations of pain may better fit other psychiatric diagnoses such as adjustment disorder or psychological factors affecting a medical condition.

*According to the Somatic Symptom Disorders Work Group, criterion B is still under active discussion. For assessing **severity** of CSSD, metrics are available for rating the presence and severity of somatic symptoms (such as the PHQ [50]). Scales are also available for assessing severity of the patient's misattributions, excessive concerns and preoccupations (such as Whiteley inventory [51]).

A large diagnostic study in various different medical settings provided the empirical foundation for the diagnostic criteria of BDS [1]. It showed that no single symptoms stood out as distinctive for patients with multiple symptoms. However, principal component factor analysis identified three symptom clusters: cardiopulmonary, including autonomic symptoms, musculoskeletal and gastrointestinal (Table 2.3). Although the symptoms could be grouped into three clusters, a latent class analysis showed that these clusters did not divide the patients into distinct groups, as some patients had unspecific general symptoms, i.e. common symptoms such as fatigue, headache, dizziness and concentration difficulties, which were related to all of the three identified symptom clusters. However, a latent class analysis including the three symptom groups plus a group of five additional general, unspecific symptoms allowed construction of clinical diagnostic criteria for a BDS, dividing patients into three classes: a group not suffering from bodily distress, a severe, multiorgan

Table 2.3 Symptoms of and diagnostic criteria for 'bodily distress syndrome' [1]

Yes	No	Symptom groups
		≥3 cardiopulmonary/autonomic arousal
		Palpitations/heart pounding, precordial discomfort, breathlessness without exertion, hyperventilation, hot or cold sweats, trembling or shaking, dry mouth, churning in stomach/'butterflies', flushing or blushing
		≥3 gastrointestinal arousal
		Abdominal pains, frequent loose bowel movements, feeling bloated/full of gas/distended, regurgitations, constipation, diarrhoea, nausea, vomiting, burning sensation in chest or epigastrium
		≥3 musculoskeletal tension
		Pains in arms or legs, muscular aches or pains, pains in the joints, feelings of paresis or localised weakness, back ache, pain moving from one place to another, unpleasant numbness or tingling sensations
		≥3 general symptoms
		Concentration difficulties, impairment of memory, excessive fatigue, headache, dizziness
		≥4 symptoms from one of the above groups

Diagnostic criteria:
1–3:'yes': Moderate or single-organ system 'bodily distress syndrome'
4–5:'yes': Severe or multiorgan system 'bodily distress syndrome'.

type of bodily distress (prevalence 3.3%) and a modest, single-organ type, with symptoms primarily from one organ system (prevalence 25.3%) (Table 2.3). The single-organ type was further divided into four subtypes: cardiopulmonary, gastrointestinal, musculoskeletal and general symptoms. It is worth noting that these symptom profiles are in line with various other studies using quite different approaches, and the structure has also been confirmed in a population-based confirmatory study (Table 2.4) [3;52;53;54;55; Rosmalen, personal communication, 2009]. On this basis, the finding of BDS subtypes seems to be quite robust.

In a later analysis of the same dataset, it was tested if patients diagnosed with one of six functional somatic syndromes (i.e. CFS, FM, IBS, non-cardiac chest pain, hyperventilation syndrome, pain syndrome) or DSM-IV somatoform disorders characterised by physical symptoms were captured by the new diagnosis [56]. It was shown that BDS included all patients with FM, CFS and hyperventilation syndrome, 98% of those with IBS and at least 90% of patients with non-cardiac chest pain, pain syndrome or any somatoform disorder (Figure 2.1). The overall agreement of BDS with any of these diagnostic categories was 95% (95% CI 93.1–96.0; kappa 0.86). BDS therefore seems to cover most of the relevant 'somatoform' or 'functional' syndromes presenting with physical symptoms not explained by well-recognised medical illness. This may resolve the much-discussed problem of comorbidity between various functional somatic syndromes [2].

It is remarkable that the BDS diagnosis (i.e. that based on an exploratory statistical approach) includes most patients with somatoform disorders, despite psychological symptoms or behavioural characteristics not being part of the diagnostic criteria. It appears from Table 2.5, that emotional/behavioural symptoms are just as, or even more, frequent among

Table 2.4 Symptom clusters or factors in patients presenting with 'medically unexplained symptoms' (exploratory and interview-based studies only)

DSM-IV/ICD-10	Gara et al. [53] N = 1456	Simon et al. [52] N = NA	Fink et al. [1] N = 978	Rosmalen et al. (personal communication, 2009)*
Assessment instrument	CIDI, DIS	CIDI	SCAN	CIDI
Setting: Symptom cluster:	Primary care	Primary care	Primary care neurological, internal medicine	General population
Gastrointestinal + +	+	+	+	+
Musculoskeletal + (+)	+	+	+	+
Cardiopulmonary +	+	+	+	+
Urogenital +	+	–		
Neurological +	–	+	–	
Sexual +	–	–	–	
Headache	+	–	–	
Higher hierarchy cluster, i.e. multisymptomatic	+	NA	+	–

* Confirmatory analyses of symptom cluster model suggested by Fink et al. (personal communication, 2010). CIDI, Composite International Diagnostic Interview; SCAN, Schedule of Clinical Assessment in Neuropsychiatry; DIS, Diagnostic Interview Schedule.

patients diagnosed with various functional syndromes as among patients with a somatoform disorder [56;57]. This criterion does not seem to discriminate between the syndromes, i.e. nothing indicates that there is a group of 'psychiatric' and 'non-psychiatric' syndromes. The patient groups may be different in sociodemographic characteristics, and there are no differences in outcome [55]. This does not mean that psychobehavioural characteristics are unimportant, but it does raise questions about their necessity for the classification. A pragmatic solution to this problem may be to specify for the BDS concept if it is associated with emotional or behavioural symptoms, for example, it could be specified whether the disorder is associated with somatic symptoms or not in depressive disorder.

The BDS concept provides a common, non-specialty-specific basis on which to understand the phenomenon of persistent and disabling physical symptoms not attributable to well-defined medical disease, which will make it easier to communicate and collaborate across specialties. It may have the potential to facilitate patient care, given that very similar treatments have been shown to be effective in various functional somatic syndromes and somatoform disorders [15;58;59;60;61;62]. It may be easier to deliver these treatments if patients currently receiving various diagnostic labels are given the same diagnosis.

The BDS concept is based on symptom counts from symptom clusters. Previous research has shown that symptom lists are quite useful to identify clinically relevant MUS. In particular, the number of somatic symptoms has been found to be a strong predictor of disability

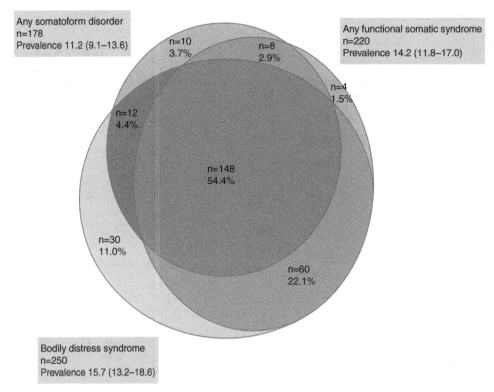

Figure 2.1 Diagnostic overlap of 'bodily distress syndrome' with functional somatic syndromes and selected somatoform disorder categories [1:56]

[22]. On the other hand, the use of symptom patterns (as in current somatisation disorder) has been shown to reduce clinical utility [22].

Psychobehavioural characteristics are not included in the BDS criteria, which according to some authors may be seen as a weakness of the diagnosis [63]. However, this may actually be one of the major advantages of the BDS concept: the vast majority of (non-psychiatric) physicians, who are often unfamiliar with exploring complicated or 'hidden' psychobehavioural phenomena, could benefit from the new diagnosis, and it may also be acceptable to physicians and patients who are reluctant to give or accept a psychiatric diagnosis for physical symptoms.

Taking all of this together, the empirically based BDS concept provides an economic alternative for the CSSD concept and may be more practical in somatic or primary care settings. It identifies patients in need of intensified care, but does not directly address the dimensions of impairment and dysfunctional cognitions and behaviours. Even if *phenomenologically* it focuses on bodily instead of psychosocial distress, it is based on the majority (57%) of somatic symptoms that can be described as 'functional', i.e. representing bodily distress rather than well-recognised medical illness. In contrast to CSSD, however, it does *not* include psychobehavioural features as positive indicators for the diagnosis; instead the positive diagnosis of BDS depends on the presence of certain symptom *patterns* and the exclusion of mental and organic *differential* diagnoses (not organic explanations for the symptoms in question).

Table 2.5 Depression and anxiety comorbidity in various syndromes [56]

	Fibromyalgia	Chronic fatigue syndrome	Irritable bowel syndrome	Chest pain	Hyperventilation syndrome	Pain syndrome
	(n = 58)	(n = 54)	(n = 43)	(n = 129)	(n = 49)	(n = 130)
	pr[a] = 3.7 (2.6–5.3)	pr = 2.9 (2.2–3.8)	pr = 2.8 (1.9–4.3)	pr = 7.7 (6.2–9.5)	pr = 2.6 (1.9–3.5)	pr = 8.6 (6.7–10.9)
	n/%	n/%	n/%	n/%	n/%	n/%
Depression (n = 181)	21	23	19	51	25	43
(total 18.5%)	36.2	42.6	44.2	39.5	51.0	33.1
Anxiety (n = 181)	16	21	21	46	33	44
(total 18.5%)	27.6	38.9	48.8	35.7	67.3	33.8

[a] Prevalences (95% CI) in the original sample of consecutive patients from primary care, internal medicine and neurology (n = 2277).

In summary, the two proposals for the classification of 'medically unexplained symptoms', CSSD and BDS, are clear improvements over the vague, heterogeneous and dualistic approaches of former terminologies and classifications. Yet the two constructs are fundamentally different: CSSD requires the exploration of additional findings (significant impairment through the symptoms, and psychobehavioural characteristics), whereas BDS is deliberately based on the neutral/non-judgemental retrieval of bodily symptoms only.

Conceptual issues

Thus far, we have discussed terminology and classification of patients with persistent and disabling bodily complaints without further reference to the underlying *conceptual* issues. These are at least twofold:

- It is important to be aware of what it means to classify patients and, more generally, what the status of nosology is in this field.
- Although current classifications claim to be atheoretical, some idea of the pathopsychophysiological processes involved in the experience of these bodily complaints is useful.

We briefly discuss both of these points below.

Nosology and the value of a classification

Let us start with what it means to establish a classification in our field. A classification ought to be based on something more valid than 'what the professor says', expert panels or consensus [64]. Robins and Guze [65], and later Kendell [66], have listed a range of strategies to scientifically establish the validity of clinical syndromes (Table 2.6): the first is to identify and describe the syndrome by 'clinical intuition' or cluster analysis; the second is to demonstrate boundaries or 'point of rarity' between related syndromes by statistical methods; the third to perform follow-up studies to establish a distinct course or outcome; the fourth to conduct therapeutic trials to establish a distinct treatment response; the fifth to conduct family studies establishing that the syndrome 'breeds true'; and, finally, to demonstrate the association with some more fundamental abnormalities, i.e. anatomical, biochemical or molecular. Three more rules should however be added to the list: first, the patients have to be sampled from appropriate populations; second, it is necessary to confirm the results in cross-validation studies; and, third, the patients must be assessed by an appropriate method [64].

Some authors have stressed that the most important aspect of diagnoses is their utility [67]. Undoubtedly, utility is of key importance, but it may not necessarily warrant a diagnosis' validity. In the functional somatic syndromes such as IBS, MCS, CFS and FM, they are supported by strong patient organisations, pharmaceutical companies, a huge network of complementary therapists, clinics specialised in a specific 'diagnosis' and insurance companies. The diagnoses have a high utility for some of these groups as they make money on it, others earn academic merits and for the patients the diagnoses represent acceptance that their illness is 'real' and not a mental disorder [68]. However, in the management of patients with these disorders, the diagnoses seem to have very low utility as they may hinder appropriate treatment.

We have to bear in mind that even for the most traditional and seemingly clear cut diagnoses in psychiatry, establishing their validity and utility has proven very difficult; for

Table 2.6 Validators of clinical syndromes [64;65;66]

Validator	Scientific method
Identification and description of the syndrome	By 'clinical intuition' or by cluster analysis
Identification of boundaries or 'points of rarity' between related syndromes	By discriminant function analysis, latent class analysis, etc.
Follow-up studies	In follow-up studies establishing a distinctive course or outcome
Therapeutic trials	By establishing a distinctive treatment response
Family studies	By establishing that the syndrome 'breeds true'
Biological correlates	By showing an association with some more fundamental abnormality (histological, psychological, biochemical or molecular)
Specific exposure	
Patients have to be sampled in representative or appropriate populations	
Results must be confirmed in cross-validation studies	
Patients must be assessed by an appropriate method (not questionnaire)	

instance, there seems to be no clear boundary or 'point of rarity' even between schizophrenia and bipolar disorder [67]. There is also considerable criticism of the 'diagnostic literalism' and 'scientific progressivism' induced by the DSM system: slightly changed, seemingly 'better' criteria create new syndromes, other constellations suddenly fall out of the range of diagnosable disorders – a change that will certainly also happen when the new concept of CSSD is introduced, replacing 'somatoform disorders'. At the same time 'richer' phenomenological accounts of disorders are discouraged by this diagnostic system.

In their paper with the telling title 'The incredible insecurity of psychiatric nosology', Kendler and Zachar discuss, as a possible way out of this dilemma, having broader, higher order diagnostic classes [69]. These higher order constructs are less vulnerable to either changes in the diagnostic system or to changes in the context-dependent appearance of disorders. In the field we are discussing here, one possibility for a higher order construct is based on the fact that overlap of somatic, depressive and anxiety symptoms is the rule rather than an exception. With this fact in mind, several authors have argued for dimensional models within the spectrum of what is frequently called 'internalising disorders'. Whereas the first models concentrated on anxiety and depression only, newer models also include somatic symptoms or somatisation as one dimension. They suggest one rather large common general factor (mostly called 'negative affectivity') and specific factors differentiating between depression and somatisation, for instance [70].

Another possibility for a broader higher order diagnostic class could be 'general medicine–psychiatry interface disorders'. In principle, this construct of 'interface disorders' remains problematic because it is linked to a dualistic perspective of either psychological or organic disorders. Pragmatically, however, it could serve as a useful overarching category under which all 'functional somatic syndromes', 'somatoform disorders' or, in future, 'complex somatic symptom disorders' or 'bodily distress syndromes' could be subsumed – justified by the fact that they are neither clearly mental nor organic disorders and have their own common characteristics in terms especially of treatment (concentrating on bodily symptoms *and*, at the same time, on subjective experience and behaviour).

Classification and pathopsychophysiology

An important conceptual issue concerns the influence on classification of the psychophysiological models we have for the experience of disabling bodily symptoms. Although 'officially' the DSM and ICD classification systems claim to be 'atheoretical' and descriptive, it is clear that this claim is an idealisation and that pathophysiological models have influenced the classification in significant ways. A particularly good example of this is the category of 'somatoform autonomic disorder' which by its name implies a dysfunction of the autonomic nervous system as a basis for complaints related to heart, respiration, digestion, etc., although to date there is no sound evidence that such a dysfunction is relevant. Another example is the category of 'conversion disorder', which by its name and also by the criterion that psychological factors have to be seen as causally relevant at the onset, clearly implies a definite, i.e. psychogenic, aetiology.

Addressing the issue of psychophysiological models involves two questions: what type of phenomenon or experience is it to suffer from disabling bodily complaints, and what is the most likely physiological basis for it? Typically, the first question does not get sufficient attention, and trying to explain the aetiology of a phenomenon of something we cannot define in the first place, may be misleading. So what can be said, in brief, about the phenomenon of bodily complaints?

Bodily *signals* or *sensations* are a part of everyday life and a necessity for the survival of human beings. The body tells us that we need a rest when running, that something we touch is warm so we can avoid burns, that we have to move on the chair to avoid muscle strains, etc. Human beings may also react to life stressors with bodily sensations or symptoms such as musculoskeletal pain or headache, in the same way as they can react when upset, depressed or nervous. A parallel can be drawn between emotional and bodily reactions to stress, and bodily symptoms should be viewed as a direct reaction to a stressor and not something secondary to emotions – they may sometimes, e.g. when somebody reacts to a threatening stressor with trembling without experiencing anxiety, be seen as bodily correlate of an emotion, but even then they are not 'somatised' emotional reactions. It is an age-old understanding that bodily symptoms are a less mature reaction in people who cannot express their feelings, and usually the symptoms do not represent a masked emotional reaction.)

Bodily sensations and reactions such as these are not, and ought not be, included in the classification. They become symptoms (and hence potentially objects for classification) when sensations attract medical attention or become disturbing, or are interpreted by the patient or the doctor as illness. It is a problem that in everyday language and also in medical practice, we often do not make this distinction between symptoms and sensations: using the word '*symptoms*' for both phenomena lowers the threshold for viewing sensations as symptoms of an illness – and using a word like sensations, or similar words for both, adds to the neglect of the severity of symptoms of bodily *distress* in many severely ill patients.

Once sensations attract medical attention, they also become a differential diagnostic issue. Doctors and patients alike may be inclined to think primarily in a biomedical frame of reference, meaning that symptoms are seen as indicators of organic disease. Patients often prefer this view because they see a biomedical description or even an explanation of their complaints as proof of the legitimacy of their complaints. If the doctors do not consider the possibility that the symptoms are stress reactions or otherwise based on altered perceptions, they may inflict iatrogenic harm to the patients by unnecessary examinations, tests and treatment attempts that will be fruitless, but not always harmless. It is still not well enough known that for enduring and disabling bodily symptoms a purely biomedical explanation of the extent of the symptoms is hardly ever appropriate. This does not mean that an interpretation as stress reaction is usually fully adequate either, for two reasons: First, enduring and disabling bodily symptoms very often occur independent of any obvious context that could allow for an explanation of them as bodily correlates of an emotion (i.e. a context with positive or negative valence for the person, inducing a combination of motivation, e.g. to approach or to avoid, and sensation). Only in some of these cases, further course and in particular psychotherapeutic treatment later reveals relevant context information which with hindsight make it likely that the bodily symptoms are correlates of emotional reactions to threatening or other conflictual contexts that initially were not consciously experienced as such. Second, for maintenance of these symptoms many stress-independent mechanisms may come into play, on a psychosocial level (e.g. operant conditioning) as well as on a neuro-biological level (e.g. neural plasticity).

So, in a very general sense, the phenomenon of enduring bodily complaints may be described as an expression of disturbed homoeostasis of the organism, be it a purely bodily type of emotional reaction in the sense of Craig's description of pain as a homoeostatic emotion, or a disturbance of homoeostasis induced by other mechanisms best described on a psychological or a neurobiological level [71;72].

From this general description, several important things follow which are relevant for the search for a physiological basis for classification as well as a psychological one. First of all, pathological peripheral stimuli are not the primary physiological cause of enduring bodily complaints conceptualised as disturbed homoeostasis. Such a view of 'normal' central processing of 'pathological' peripheral processes would 'fit' typical organic disease, but not 'medically unexplained', 'somatoform' or 'functional' symptoms. Instead, undoubtedly nowadays the most obvious physiological dysfunctions of patients with such *bodily distress* can be found in the CNS, with a lot of evidence from functional and structural neuroimaging supporting this view. But, and this is often overlooked, assigning a central pathopsychophysiological role to the CNS conceptually fits with two rather different and not easily compatible models: the presently more popular one sees the CNS dysfunction as an altered, augmented processing of normal peripheral stimuli, variously called, for example, sensitisation or amplification. This augmented processing is conceptually close to psychological descriptions of altered attention, focusing, thinking about bodily processes, etc., thereby maintaining the old psycho–physical dichotomy. The other model sees the CNS dysfunction not as falsely indicating a peripheral problem, but as a consequence and expression of an altered homoeostasis, with peripheral stimuli playing a subordinate and more arbitrary role, like a provider of material for the more autonomous central processes [73]. In this second model, the experience of bodily distress is more a unitary psychophysical or organismic process, not easily separated into bodily and cognitive–emotional components.

Assigning a central role to dysfunctional CNS processes makes it clear why bodily distress co-occurs so often with depression and anxiety, as they are syndromes of abnormal stress reactions with emotional content where dysfunctional CNS processes are also seen as centrally relevant. In terms of classification, our main topic, this proximity should also be reflected, for instance by avoiding the term 'comorbidity' for a co-occurrence which epidemiologically is the rule rather than the exception. As an alternative, dimensional models including anxiety, depression and bodily distress as three correlated, but non-identical, dimensions offer a better classification basis [70]. Nevertheless, for classification purposes, there are still differences between the two 'CNS-type models' briefly sketched above. The first implicitly fits with keeping clinically relevant 'medically unexplained', 'somatoform' or 'functional' symptoms (i.e. bodily distress syndromes) under the heading of 'mental disorders' because the assumed pathopsychophysiology is a psychological one (cognitive–emotional processes underlying 'sensitisation and amplification'). The second model fits with the suggestion of creating a supraordinate interface category for bodily distress syndromes between 'normal' somatic medicine and 'normal' psychological medicine, because these 'organismic dysfunctions' fit neither and are equally distant to both [15;74].

Returning to the task of improving the terminology and classification of clinically relevant 'medically unexplained', 'somatoform' or 'functional' symptoms, these reflections allow several conclusions: Both new concepts, CSSD as well as BDS, are acceptable proposals. With regard to the term itself, CSSD is somewhat more cautious insofar as it stays close to the *phenomenon* 'somatic symptoms', and also acknowledges ('complex') how little is really known about their aetiology. BDS is also a rather descriptive term, but also dares an *aetiological* statement for the symptoms being an expression of distress. In accordance with our hitherto limited knowledge about the role of the CNS in the development and maintenance of MUS, neither term implies 'mental' processes warranting classification as 'mental disorders'.

As far as the classification proposals behind these two terms are concerned, CSSD acknowledges the patients' suffering and thus (correctly) brings in a subjective component. Further, by requiring bodily as well as psychobehavioural 'symptoms', it still separates the bodily from the psychological dimension, but nevertheless strongly promotes a biopsychosocial illness model. The diagnosis CSSD is meant as a categorical one (either present or not); dimensional assessments are encouraged only half-heartedly.

Initially BDS does not seem much of an advance on former symptom lists assessing 'somatisation disorder' or 'somatisation'. However, its plain requirement of bodily symptoms without judging their 'explicability' is radically anti-dualistic, making no statement at all about the symptoms' aetiology. The acknowledgement of the multi-dimensional nature of 'BDS' is inherent to its (simple) approach of a symptom count, at least in its defining a 'moderate' versus a 'severe' type.

Conclusion

At the end of this '*tour d'horizon*' across practical and theoretical aspects of the classification of patients with persistent and disabling bodily complaints, we conclude that:

– Classification needs to be valid and useful; it should be accessible for patients, and for as many different specialties and levels of care in medicine as possible. In view of these requirements, the current classification of somatoform disorders and functional somatic syndromes is not adequate. It can only be understood through its history, not through any kind of systematic approach.

– Before the clinical relevance of MUS with respect to their duration and severity can be confirmed, they should be classified as 'plain (idiopathic) symptoms' as in the ICD-10 block R or the symptom component of the ICPC-2.

- For the terminology and classification of clinically relevant MUS, both new proposals, CSSD and BDS, are improvements in many respects. Given the combination of its being a feasible term, our limited knowledge about 'watertight' psychobehavioural criteria, and its practicability in various settings, BDS might currently have a few more advantages. By implementing the pathopsychophysiological model of 'bodily distress' explicitly in its name, it promotes a plausible, forward-looking and integrative terminology.
- Consequently, even if we do not adopt the specific concept of BDS in this book, we will use the term *bodily distress syndromes* as an umbrella term for the large, yet ill-defined group of formerly called 'medically unexplained', 'somatoform' or 'functional' symptoms and syndromes.

References

1. Fink P, Toft T, Hansen MS, Ørnbøl E, Olesen F. Symptoms and syndromes of bodily distress: an exploratory study of 978 internal medical, neurological, and primary care patients. *Psychosomatic Medicine* 2007; **69**: 30–9.

2. Wessely S, Nimnuan C, Sharpe M. Functional somatic syndromes: one or many? *Lancet* 1999; **354**(9182): 936–9.

3. Fink P, Rosendal M, Olesen F. Classification of somatisation and functional somatic symptoms in primary care. *Australian and New Zealand Journal of Psychiatry* 2005; **39**: 772–81.

4. Creed F, Guthrie E, Fink P, Henningsen P, Rief W, Sharpe M *et al.* Is there a better term than 'medically unexplained symptoms'? *Journal of Psychosomatic Research* 2010; **68**: 5–8.

5. Ring A, Dowrick CF, Humphris GM, Salmon P. The somatising effect of clinical consultation: what patients and doctors say and do not say when patients present medically unexplained physical symptoms. *Social Science and Medicine* 2005; **61**: 1505–15.

6. Salmon P, Humphris GM, Ring A, Davies JC, Dowrick CF. What do general practice patients want when they present medically unexplained symptoms, and why do their doctors feel pressurized? *Journal of Psychosomatic Research* 2005; **59**: 255–60.

7. Salmon P, Peters S, Stanley I. Patients' perceptions of medical explanations for somatisation disorders: qualitative analysis. *British Medical Journal* 1999; **318**: 372–6.

8. DSM-V Somatic Disorders Work Group. *Current Proposal for Somatoform Disorders.* Available at: www.dsm5. org/ProposedRevisions/Pages/ SomatoformDisorders.aspx (Accessed November 25, 2010).

9. Stone J, Colyer M, Feltbower S, Carson A, Sharpe M. 'Psychosomatic': a systematic review of its meaning in newspaper articles. *Psychosomatics* 2004; **45**: 287–90.

10. Stone J, Wojcik W, Durrance D, Carson A, Lewis S, MacKenzie L *et al.* What should we say to patients with symptoms unexplained by disease? The number needed to offend. *BMJ* 2002; **325**: 1449–50.

11. Mayou R, Kirmayer LJ, Simon G, Kroenke K, Sharpe M. Somatoform disorders: time for a new approach in DSM-V. *American Journal of Psychiatry* 2005; **162**: 847–55.

12. Kroenke K, Sharpe M, Sykes R. Revising the classification of somatoform disorders: key questions and preliminary recommendations. *Psychosomatics* 2007; **48**: 277–85.

13. Murphy MR. Classification of the somatoform disorders. In: Bass C, ed. *Somatisation: Physical Symptoms & Psychological Illness.* Oxford: Blackwell; 1990: 10–39.

14. Henningsen P, Zimmermann T, Sattel H. Medically unexplained physical symptoms, anxiety, and depression: a meta-analytic review. *Psychosomatic Medicine* 2003; **65**: 528–33.

15. Henningsen P, Zipfel S, Herzog W. Management of functional somatic syndromes. *The Lancet* 2007; **369**(9565): 946–95.

16. Barsky AJ, Borus JF. Functional somatic syndromes. *Annals of Internal Medicine* 1999; **130**: 910–21.

17. Aaron LA, Buchwald D. A review of the evidence for overlap among unexplained clinical conditions. *Annals of Internal Medicine* 2001; **134**: 868–81.

18. Nimnuan C, Rabe-Hesketh S, Wessely S, Hotopf M. How many functional somatic syndromes? *Journal of Psychosomatic Research* 2001; **51**: 549–57.

19. Perley MJ, Guze SB. Hysteria – The stability and usefulness of clinical criteria. A quantitative study based on a follow-up period of six to eight years in 39 patients. *New England Journal of Medicine* 1962; **266**: 421–6.

20. Escobar JI, Manu P, Matthews D, Lane T, Swartz M, Canino G. Medically unexplained physical symptoms, somatisation disorder and abridged somatization: studies with the Diagnostic Interview Schedule. *Psychiatric Development* 1989; 7: 235–45.

21. Kroenke K, Spitzer RL, deGruy FV, Hahn SR, Linzer M, Williams JB et al. Multisomatoform disorder. An alternative to undifferentiated somatoform disorder for the somatizing patient in primary care. *Archives of General Psychiatry* 1997; **54**: 352–8.

22. Voigt K, Nagel A, Meyer B, Langs G, Braukhaus C, Löwe B. Towards positive diagnostic criteria: a systematic review of somatoform disorder diagnoses and suggestions for future classification. *Journal of Psychosomatic Research* 2010; **68**: 403–14.

23. Rief W, Mewes R, Martin A, Glaesmer H, Braehler E. Are psychological features useful in classifying patients with somatic symptoms? *Psychosomatic Medicine* 2010; **72**: 648–55.

24. Barsky AJ, Wyshak GL. Hypochondriasis and somatosensory amplification. *British Journal of Psychiatry* 1990; **157**: 404–9.

25. Barsky AJ. Amplification, somatisation, and the somatoform disorders. *Psychosomatics* 1992; **33**: 28–34.

26. Rief W, Hiller W, Margraf J. Cognitive aspects of hypochondriasis and the somatisation syndrome. *Journal of Abnormal Psychology* 1998; **107**: 587–95.

27. Hausteiner C, Bornschein S, Bubel E, Groben S, Lahmann C, Grosber M et al. Psychobehavioral predictors of somatoform disorders in patients with suspected allergies. *Psychosomatic Medicine* 2009; **71**: 1004–11.

28. Duddu V, Isaac MK, Chaturvedi SK. Somatization, somatosensory amplification, attribution styles and illness behaviour: a review. *International Review of Psychiatry* 2006; **18**: 25–33.

29. Bantick SJ, Wise RG, Ploghaus A, Clare S, Smith SM, Tracey I. Imaging how attention modulates pain in humans using functional MRI. *Brain* 2002; **125**: 310–19.

30. Smith BW, Tooley EM, Montague EQ, Robinson AE, Cosper CJ, Mullins PG. Habituation and sensitization to heat and cold pain in women with fibromyalgia and healthy controls. *Pain* 2008; **140**: 420–8.

31. Rief W, Broadbent E. Explaining medically unexplained symptoms-models and mechanisms. *Clinical Psychology Review* 2007; **27**: 821–41.

32. Bishop SR, Warr D. Coping, catastrophizing and chronic pain in breast cancer. *Journal of Behavioral Medicine* 2003; **26**(3): 265–81.

33. Rief W, Nanke A, Emmerich J, Bender A, Zech T. Causal illness attributions in somatoform disorders – associations with comorbidity and illness behavior. *Journal of Psychosomatic Research* 2004; **57**: 367–71.

34. Groben S, Hausteiner C. Somatoform disorder patients in an allergy department: Do somatic causal attributions matter? *Journal of Psychosomatic Research* 2011; **70**: 229–38.

35. Witthöft M, Hiller W. Psychological approaches to origins and treatments of somatoform disorders. *Annual Review of Clinical Psychology* 2010; **6**: 257–83.

36. Keltner JR, Furst A, Fan C, Redfern R, Inglis B, Fields HL. Isolating the modulatory of expectation on pain transmission: a functional magnetic resonance imaging study. *Journal of Neuroscience* 2006; **26**: 4437–43.

37. Koyama T, McHaffie JG, Laurienti PJ, Coghill RC. The subjective experience of pain: where expectations become reality. *Proceedings of the National Academy of Sciences of the U S A* 2005; **102**: 12950–5.

38. Brown RJ. Psychological mechanisms of medically unexplained symptoms: an integrative conceptual model. *Psychological Bulletin* 2004; **130**: 793–812.

39. Pilowsky I. Aspects of abnormal illness behaviour. *Psychotherapy and Psychosomatics* 1993; **60**: 62–74.

40. Al-Windi A. The influence of complaint symptoms on health care utilisation, medicine use, and sickness absence. A comparison between retrospective and prospective utilisation. *Journal of Psychosomatic Research* 2005; **59**: 139–46.

41. Barsky AJ, Orav J, Bates DW. Somatization increases medical utilization and costs independent of psychiatric and medical morbidity. *Archives of General Psychiatry* 2005; **62**: 903–10.

42. Rief W, Martin A, Klaiberg A, Brähler E. Specific effects of depression, panic, and somatic symptoms on illness behavior. *Psychosomatic Medicine* 2005; **67**: 596–601.

43. Rief W, Ihle D, Pilger F. A new approach to assess illness behaviour. *Journal of Psychosomatic Research* 2003; **54**: 405–14.

44. Heneweer H, Vanhees L, Picavet HSJ. Physical activity and low back pain: a U-shaped relation? *Pain* 2009; **143**: 21–5.

45. Vlaeyen JWS, Linton SJ. Fear-avoidance and its consequences in chronic musculoskeletal pain: a state of the art. *Pain* 2000; **85**: 317–32.

46. Noyes R Jr, Langbehn DR, Happel RL, Sieren LR, Muller BA. Health attitude survey. A scale for assessing somatizing patients. *Psychosomatics* 1999; **40**: 470–8.

47. Hahn SR. Physical symptoms and physician-experienced difficulty in the physician–patient relationship. *Annals of Internal Medicine* 2001; **134**: 897–904.

48. Waller E, Scheidt CE. Somatoform disorders as disorders of affect regulation: a development perspective. *International Review of Psychiatry* 2006; **18**: 13–24.

49. Rosendal M, Bro F, Fink P, Christensen KS, Olesen F. General practitioners' diagnosis of somatisation: effect of an educational intervention in a cluster randomised controlled trial. *British Journal of General Practice* 2003; **53**(497): 917–22.

50. Kroenke K, Spitzer RL, Williams JB. The PHQ-15: validity of a new measure for evaluating the severity of somatic symptoms. *Psychosomatic Medicine* 2002; **64**: 258–66.

51. Pilowsky I. Dimensions of hypochondriasis. *British Journal of Psychiatry* 1967; 113(494): 89–93.

52. Simon G, Gater R, Kisely S, Piccinelli M. Somatic symptoms of distress: an international primary care study. *Psychosomatic Medicine* 1996; **58**: 481–8.

53. Gara MA, Silver RC, Escobar JI, Holman A, Waitzkin H. A hierarchical classes analysis (HICLAS) of primary care patients with medically unexplained somatic symptoms. *Psychiatry Research* 1998; **81**: 77–86.

54. Kato K, Sullivan PF, Evengard B, Pedersen NL. A population-based twin study of functional somatic syndromes. *Psychological Medicine* 2009; **39**: 497–505.

55. Schröder A, Fink P. The proposed diagnosis of somatic symptom disorders in DSM-V: two steps forward and one step backward? *Journal of Psychosomatic Research* 2010; **68**: 95–6.

56. Fink P, Schröder A. One single diagnosis, Bodily Distress Syndrome, succeeded to capture 10 diagnostic categories of functional somatic syndromes and somatoform disorders. *Journal of Psychosomatic Research* 2010; **68**: 415–26.

57. Price J, Leaver L. ABC of psychological medicine: beginning treatment. *BMJ* 2002; **325**(7354): 33–5.

58. Price JR, Mitchell E, Tidy E, Hunot V. Cognitive behaviour therapy for chronic fatigue syndrome in adults. *Cochrane Database of Systematic Reviews* 2008; **3**: CD001027.

59. Ford AC, Talley NJ, Schoenfeld PS, Quigley E, Moayyedi P. Efficacy of anti-depressants and psychological therapies in irritable bowel syndrome: systematic review and meta-analysis. *Gut* 2009; **58**: 367–78.

60. Zijdenbos IL, de Wit NJ, van der Heijden GJ, Rubin G, Quartero AO. Psychological treatments for the management of irritable bowel syndrome. *Cochrane Database of Systematic Reviews* 2009; **1**: CD006442.

61. Kroenke K. Efficacy of treatment for somatoform disorders: a review of randomized controlled trials. *Psychosomatic Medicine* 2007; **69**: 881–8.

62. Allen LA, Woolfolk RL, Escobar JI, Gara MA, Hamer RM. Cognitive-behavioral therapy for Somatisation Disorder: a randomized controlled trial. *Archives of Internal Medicine* 2006; **166**: 1512–18.

63. Fink P. Somatisation – beyond symptom count. *Journal of Psychosomatic Research* 1996; **40**: 7–10.

64. Fink P, Rosendal M. Recent developments in the understanding and management of functional somatic symptoms in primary care. *Current Opinion in Psychiatry* 2008; **21**: 182–8.

65. Robins E, Guze SB. Establishment of diagnostic validity in psychiatric illness: its application to schizophrenia. *American Journal of Psychiatry* 1970; **126**: 983–7.

66. Kendell RE. Clinical validity. *Psychological Medicine* 1989; **19**: 45–55.

67. Kendell R, Jablensky A. Distinguishing between the validity and utility of psychiatric diagnoses. *American Journal of Psychiatry* 2003; **160**: 4–12.

68. Wolfe F. Fibromyalgia wars. *Journal of Rheumatology* 2009; **36**: 671–8.

69. Kendler KS, Zachar P. The incredible insecurity of psychiatric nosology. In: Kendler KS, Parnas J, eds. *Philosophical Issues in Psychiatry: Explanation, Phenomenology and Nosology*. Baltimore, MD; Johns Hopkins University Press; 2008: 370–85.

70. Goldberg DP, Krueger RF, Andrews G, Hobbs MJ. Emotional disorders: cluster 4 of the proposed meta-structure for DSM-V and ICD-11. *Psychological Medicine* 2009; **39**: 2043–59.

71. Craig AD. How do you feel? Interoception: The sense of the physiological condition of the body. *Nature Reviews Neuroscience* 2002; **3**: 655–66.

72. Mayer EA, Naliboff BD, Craig AD. Neuroimaging of the brain-gut axis: from basic understanding to treatment of functional GI disorders. *Gastroenterology* 2006; **131**: 1925–42.

73. Starobinski J. A short history of bodily sensation. *Psychological Medicine* 1990; **20**: 23–33.

74. Strassnig M, Stowell KR, First MB, Pincus HA. General medical and psychiatric perspectives on somatoform disorders: separated by an uncommon language. *Current Opinion in Psychiatry* 2006; **19**: 194–200.

Chapter

3

Evidence-based treatment

Francis Creed, Kurt Kroenke, Peter Henningsen,
Alka Gudi and Peter White

Introduction

This chapter aims to provide an overview of the current state of evidence regarding treatment of medically unexplained symptoms, somatisation and the functional somatic syndromes. We first describe the heterogeneity of the settings and types of treatment that have been used in a wide variety of disorders. The existing evidence is then examined against this background. The data are arranged using the groups of patients described in Chapter 1 and we concentrate on recent systematic reviews where possible. The section on functional somatic symptoms focuses on psychological treatments and antidepressants only; it does not include the numerous symptomatic treatments that are available for these syndromes; they have been reviewed elsewhere [1]. The chapter concludes with a section concerning the commonalities of treatment across all of these disorders, with a view to identifying common, effective ingredients of treatments to indicate how services for these patients may be improved. The chapter does not include a review of the evidence for efficacy of treatment for conversion disorder as the evidence base is so inadequate [2;3].

The different settings of primary and secondary care

There have been several different approaches to improving the care of patients with these disorders. These vary in intensity and are applicable to different parts of the healthcare system. The evidence for each will be considered below.

The first set of approaches involves the training of GPs (primary care physicians) to improve their confidence and skills in managing these patients. Primary care represents the main contact with healthcare systems for many patients with new or persistent symptoms and primary care practitioners are accustomed to dealing with symptoms relating to any body system and ranging in severity from minor to potentially life-threatening. They also have to work in a situation where they may have limited access to diagnostic investigations and only generalist, rather than specialist, knowledge. On the other hand, primary care is also characterised by longitudinal patient–doctor relationships in which considerable effort and trust may be invested by both parties and which have real therapeutic potential. Most studies of efficacy of this approach have involved training GPs in the reattribution model, in which doctors initiate a dialogue to interrogate the possibility that stress or emotional distress may have a role to play in the patient's symptoms [4;5].

Medically Unexplained Symptoms, Somatisation and Bodily Distress, ed. Francis Creed, Peter Henningsen and Per Fink. Published by Cambridge University Press. © Cambridge University Press 2011.

Another approach based in primary care is one where a mental health professional, usually a psychiatrist, interviews the patient on a single occasion with a view to making an assessment and conveying in a conversation and /or letter to the GP a diagnosis and treatment plan. This is known as the 'psychiatric consultation' or 'consultation-liaison' model and has been used for both depression and somatoform disorders [6]. The assessment interview may involve the GP as well as the patient and the psychiatrist. As well as offering treatment suggestions, the recommendations to the GP usually suggest that investigations are kept to a minimum in an attempt to minimise the excessive costs associated with somatisation or bodily distress.

The context of secondary care is quite different from that of primary care. It is usual that patients will undergo investigations for possible organic disease and the results of such investigations are either discussed directly with the patient by the physician or they are conveyed to the GP. By definition, the results of these investigations indicate no evidence of organic disease so the symptoms that are, therefore, described as 'medically unexplained'. The way this is explained to the patient by the physician or the GP is an important issue and brings into question the effectiveness of reassurance (see below). Most doctor–patient contacts in secondary care tend to be brief and many patients with medically unexplained symptoms state that they were informed the investigation 'does not indicate organic disease' but without a positive explanation of the likely cause of symptoms. Sometimes referral to another medical specialist may be suggested, in which case the search for an organic cause continues. Alternatively, the patient may be referred back to the GP, who has primary responsibility for ongoing care, and this includes the decision regarding further investigations. In some healthcare systems the patient has direct access to the specialist physician so it is the patient who decides whether further investigations are sought.

Both primary and secondary care studies have been performed to assess the efficacy of psychological interventions, most commonly cognitive behaviour therapy administered by a mental health professional, or antidepressants, prescribed by the patient's usual doctor. One systematic review compared primary and secondary care and found that patients with functional somatic syndromes (see below) did better in interventions conducted in secondary care than primary care [7]. This may be because patients in primary care have mild disorders with a high spontaneous response rate. Alternatively, more intensive treatment might have been used in secondary care compared to those used in primary care [7]. Also, patients accepting referral to secondary care may be a selected group more willing to accept and adhere to psychological treatments. In the next section the trials to test efficacy of these interventions will be examined by disorder.

Overview of the evidence for effective treatments

Kroenke's comprehensive review of the evidence up to 2006 included 34 randomised controlled trials [3]. Ten trials included patients with medically unexplained symptoms, four with somatisation disorder and nine with 'abridged' somatisation (see Chapter 1, p. 5). There were five studies of hypochondriasis, and three each of body dysmorphic disorder and conversion disorder. Thirteen trials evaluated cognitive behaviour therapy, five evaluated antidepressants, four the effect of a consultation letter to the general practitioner (GP) and three the training of GPs. It is difficult to draw general conclusions from such a heterogeneous group of studies.

The review used a liberal measure of positive outcome – benefit in any one of three patient-centred outcomes (improved symptoms or functioning, or reduction in psychological distress) was regarded as a positive result. The mean effect sizes were 0.92 for antidepressants (five studies), 1.43 for behavioural therapy (four studies) and 1.78 for cognitive behavioural therapy (CBT) (five studies). Since effect sizes of 0.8 or greater are considered large therapeutic effects, these are clinically significant results [3]. An additional important outcome measure was reduction of healthcare costs, which was achieved in about a quarter of studies.

Kroenke's review suggested that positive results were more often obtained in trials including the more severe conditions than medically unexplained symptoms, which so often resolve spontaneously. The review included 10 randomised controlled trials for *medically unexplained symptoms*; only those which involved CBT showed some improvement in symptoms, function and/or healthcare utilisation. Thirteen studies included patients with some form of *somatisation disorder* (including the abridged or multisomatoform types; see Chapter 1, p. 5). Benefit was observed in three of four trials evaluating the use of a consultation letter to the GP. CBT was effective in five out of seven trials and antidepressant drugs in three out of four trials.

Kroenke drew attention to the limitations of the current evidence, including heterogeneity of conditions treated, definition of disorders, type of intervention, its intensity, variable duration of follow-up and variable outcome measures. In many trials the comparison group was a usual care or waiting list control, with no attempt to control for attention by the therapist. Thus the conclusion that CBT is consistently effective across a range of somatoform disorders must be regarded with some caution [3]. The evidence is even more tentative regarding a psychiatric consultation letter or antidepressants, and evidence regarding other forms of treatment was negative or inconclusive. Nearly two-thirds of the trials included fewer than 100 participants so this is an area of research that needs more primary research, including large, high-quality trials. Cost-effectiveness trials are almost non-existent in this field. Some of the studies showed reduction of healthcare costs. For some, this is probably a direct result of the consultation letter that asks GPs or other doctors not to order more investigations unless absolutely necessary. But in two studies this letter was also sent to the doctor in the control group, so it cannot be the only explanation [8;9].

Two further systematic reviews included data concerning treatment in primary care [6;10]. The first was a broad systematic review of psychosocial interventions in primary care, which included two high-quality randomised controlled trials aimed at reducing somatisation [10]. One of these involved modified reattribution (two to three sessions) and the other eight sessions of CBT [11;12]. Both showed benefits over usual care with regards to less illness behaviour, less health anxiety, and less sick leave. A third trial of reattribution showed no benefit over usual care [13]. These authors concluded that there is limited evidence of the effectiveness of a reattribution intervention by a GP in terms of consumption of medical resources, subjective health, sick leave and somatisation.

The second relevant systematic review focused on the effect of a psychiatric consultation in primary care, where the patient was seen by a psychiatrist, who provided the GP with a diagnosis and treatment plan [6]. There were four relevant studies; the meta-analysis indicated that treatment was superior to usual care (overall effect size = 0.6; 95% CI 0.21–1.02).

The Kroenke review reported four studies of antidepressants. One trial used opipramol, which led to borderline significant advantage over placebo in terms of SL-90 somatisation score, but the trial of St John's wort led to considerable improvement by this outcome measure compared with placebo [14;15]. Both trials lasted only six weeks and excluded patients with concurrent psychiatric disorders. Kroenke, on the other hand, only included people with anxiety or depression as well as multisomatoform disorders and found that venlafaxine was not significantly better than placebo in reducing somatic symptoms burden (Patient Health Questionnaire (PHQ)-15 score) [16]. In view of the short duration of these studies, the reluctance of so many patients to take antidepressants and their unproven efficacy, the role of antidepressants is uncertain, with the possible exception of treating pain (see below).

Recent studies of reattribution

Five recent studies in primary care have included larger numbers than most previous studies [17;18;19;20;21]. They reported conflicting results. The first tested a modification to the reattribution model, which involved providing the patient with a plausible physical explanation for their symptoms (described as an hormonal disturbance in response to stress) [20]. This involved 20 hours of training for the general practitioners in the intervention group compared with three hours of reattribution training for the control GPs. Patients (n = 156) attended five half-hour sessions. In the intervention, doctors used empathy and supportive techniques and provided a physical explanation for the patient symptoms, all of which are known to be helpful to patients with medically unexplained symptoms [22;23]. Patients in both groups made improvements in all dimensions of the Medical Outcome Survey Short Form (SF)-36, but these improvements were significantly greater after the intervention than in the control arm. The intervention included many of the ingredients of brief psychodynamic psychotherapy. Patient recruitment and retention in the trial was good but fewer than half of the GPs who were approached joined the trial, which limits the generalisability of the technique.

By contrast, two recent large trials of the reattribution model showed no efficacy, even though both groups of researchers had reported encouraging results in previous smaller trials [17;21;24;25]. In the Danish study, 38 GPs were randomised to the training arm (training in The Extended Reattribution and Management (TERM) model, see Chapter 9) or the control group; 461 patients with medically unexplained symptoms or somatisation cared for by these GPs were studied [21]. Three hundred and fifty patients with somatoform disorder and 111 patients with medically unexplained somatic symptoms were included and analysed separately. The GP training programme consisted of a two-day residential course followed by three evening sessions in which videotaped consultations were discussed. There was a booster meeting after three months and an outreach visit by a supervisor after six months. The GPs in the control group were informed only of the definitions of functional somatic symptoms and somatoform disorder plus the contents of the questionnaires.

There was a significantly greater improvement in physical functioning (SF-36) at three months for patients managed by trained GPs, compared with patients managed by GPs in the control group. This difference was not maintained at follow-up, however. No such difference was apparent in the patients with medically unexplained symptoms. The study concluded that training GPs may increase physical function for patients with somatoform disorder but the effect is small and may not be clinically significant.

The training of GPs in the TERM model was extensive and this might have been one reason why Fink and colleagues recruited less than 10% of GPs who were approached [21]. The training in the recent UK MUST trial was shorter, only six hours, but, even so, the trial managed to recruit fewer than a quarter of all practices approached [17]. The MUST study found that the training of GPs led to a change in patient–doctor communication but there was no improvement of outcome in patients with medically unexplained symptoms. There were 141 patients in this high-quality trial. Interviews with the GPs who had been involved in a previous reattribution study indicated that they felt reattribution was a useful technique that they had incorporated in their routine work, but it had no impact on frequently attending patients with medically unexplained symptoms. The GPs found that symptom diaries were useful for patients and they continued with this practice [11].

The most recent systematic review of reattribution included seven randomised controlled trials [26]. It appears that skills can be taught satisfactorily, which GPs can then use in routine care. The training seems to lead to a more positive attitude among GPs towards patients with medically unexplained symptoms but, overall, the results in terms of patient outcomes have been disappointing.

The review by Gask highlighted one successful Dutch trial, in which reattribution training was combined with collaborative care including a psychiatric consultation [27]. This model is similar to that used in an American trial of patients with somatisation, in which primary care physicians were trained to use antidepressants, cognitive behavioural techniques and a patient-orientated method of communication that maximised the doctor–patient relationship [28]. These two trials differ from the other trials of reattribution in that they recruited patients with more marked somatisation and a high rate of concurrent psychiatric disorders: 86% and 60%, respectively [27;29]. In the American trial, 68% of participants in the intervention group took full-dose antidepressants and the authors showed that the beneficial effect could be attributed to antidepressants [30]. This may have been the case for the Dutch trial also as such a high proportion had a concurrent psychiatric disorder for which antidepressants were recommended [27]. By contrast, in the UK trials of reattribution, 32% and 24% of patients were prescribed antidepressants [17;24].

Recent studies of CBT

One recent trial found that CBT, as used by Allen and colleagues in secondary care for somatisation [8], was effective in primary care patients with medically unexplained symptoms, most commonly pain conditions [18]. The intervention involved 10 CBT sessions. These focused on the reduction of physical distress and somatic preoccupation, activity regulation, facilitation of emotional awareness, cognitive restructuring and interpersonal communication. This intervention was more effective than treatment as usual. It led to reduced somatic symptoms in half of participants and the benefit remained over time. The intervention also led to improved depression, but this was not maintained and the authors concluded that this improvement in depression did not mediate fewer somatic symptoms [18].

By contrast, a recent trial in Sri Lanka found no difference in outcome between CBT and a control group for primary care patients with medically unexplained symptoms [19]. This trial employed structured care for the control group to control for the effect of the doctor's time and attention in the intervention. This involved a detailed assessment by the specialist, the patient keeping a diary of symptoms and cognitions, and regular visits to the physician. The group of patients was rather similar to that included in the trial mentioned in the previous paragraph, with numerous somatic symptoms and considerable distress. The negative result of the Sri Lankan trial is probably explained by the good response to the structured care; both the CBT and control groups recorded over 40% reduction in symptoms in spite of their prior chronicity (more than three years). The structured care was so elaborate that it might itself have been therapeutic.

Conclusions from studies of interventions of medically unexplained symptoms and somatisation

There is an important lesson in the negative trial discussed in the previous section. Most of the positive trials reported above compared the intervention to unmodified usual care or even waiting list control. The Sri Lankan trial improved usual care to the point that it was beneficial to patients, thus demonstrating the benefits of a structured approach to care of patients with medically unexplained symptoms.

It has become clear from qualitative studies of medically unexplained symptoms that the doctor–patient relationship is important and patients benefit when they feel supported and empowered by the doctor to tackle their problems [22]. Medical care of unexplained symptoms is improved if there are improvements in three inter-related elements: diagnosis, specific treatment strategies and communication [31]. Such improvements may well have occurred in the structured care used in the Sri Lankan trial.

GPs often ignore the psychological cues provided by many patients with medically unexplained symptoms [32]. The doctors' initial response is often to discuss potential medical problems with a view to reassuring the patient, with or without ordering an investigation [33]. On the other hand, if both the patient and the GP discuss psychosocial issues in the consultation, the likelihood of somatic intervention decreases [34]. Similarly, if the doctor shows empathy towards patients who present with medically unexplained symptoms, the patients are more likely to report higher ratings of interpersonal care [35]. The findings from the Sri Lankan trial and these systematic observations made from qualitative studies suggest strongly that improving routine clinical care along the lines recommended by Rosendal and colleagues could greatly improve the management of medically unexplained symptoms [31].

An example can be found in an observational study of patients with irritable bowel syndrome (IBS), who received good clinical care in a gastroenterology clinic [36]. Such care led to an improvement of their bowel symptoms, a reduction in their anxiety about a serious disease, an appreciation that the abdominal symptoms may be stress-related and fewer catastrophic thoughts about their symptoms. All of these would be goals of a psychological intervention for IBS. These changes were not associated with the number of investigations performed, but they were associated with seeing the same doctor on each occasion. The key feature of the consultation that was associated with improvement in symptoms was the doctor's correct perception, at the first consultation, of the patient's view of the cause of the symptoms. This was probably a marker of the quality of the patient–doctor interaction, as it is inevitable that the doctor who ascertains that the patient attributes their symptoms to physical rather than stress-related causes will lead on to a plausible alternative explanation. Such work emphasises the importance of doctors understanding patients' views of their medically unexplained symptoms compared with the importance of performing investigations for possible organic disease.

Interventions for health anxiety (hypochondriasis) reassurance

The commonest intervention for health anxiety or worry about a specific illness is the reassurance that is used daily in clinical practice. It is used in primary care where the doctor uses his or her clinical knowledge and skill. Very often in secondary care it is used after an investigation for possible organic disease proves negative. The evidence suggests, however, that many patients are not reassured by normal test results and the doctor's subsequent explanation [37;38;39;40]. Doctors tend to normalise patients' symptoms either without explanation or with a general explanation, which is insufficient to reassure the patient; only an explanation that is both plausible and clearly linked to the patient's specific concerns appeared to be effective [41].

A recent randomised controlled trial tested whether reassurance for patients with non-cardiac chest pain could be made more effective. The trial tested whether more information, given prior to a diagnostic exercise stress test, would make subsequent reassurance more effective [42]. The information was delivered in the form of a pamphlet with or without a brief discussion about the meaning of normal test results. In the discussion arm a research health psychologist briefly reiterated the main points of the pamphlet – many people with chest pain worry that there might be something wrong with their heart, and a normal test result means that the patient's risk for coronary artery disease is as low as for anyone in the general population. It was also emphasised that just because the pain may not be related to the heart does not mean that it is not real pain and that it is important to keep in mind that many other causes of chest pain are less serious.

One month after the investigation, 69%, 40% and 35% of patients in the discussion, pamphlet and control groups, respectively, reported reassurance. The prevalence of chest pain at this time was 17%, 28% and 36%, respectively, for the three groups. The authors concluded that clinicians can more effectively reassure after normal investigation if they explain the meaning of the test result prior to the test.

Both the Kroenke review [3] and a separate Cochrane review [43] found psychological treatment – usually some form of CBT– to be effective for hypochondriasis (health anxiety), although the evidence is limited by the fact that the control condition was most often a waiting list control. The largest study to date found that a six-session, individual CBT intervention led to long-term (12 months) improvement of hypochondriacal attitudes, concerns, health anxiety and social functioning compared with the control group, even though bodily symptoms changed little [44]. This result was adjusted for coexisting anxiety and depression. In terms of acceptability to patients, over a quarter of eligible patients refused the intervention and a quarter of those allocated to the intervention attended three or fewer sessions.

Summary

There have been a number of systematic reviews but rather sparse primary research in this area. A review of the systematic reviews concerning the evidence for the efficacy of treatments for somatoform disorders found one systematic review of antidepressant medication studies and five systematic reviews of CBT trials [44]. All of the latter concluded that CBT appears to be effective in somatoform disorders and functional somatic syndromes, but all pointed to methodological shortcomings. One review concluded that 'although seemingly beneficial, psychosocial treatments have not yet been shown to have a lasting and clinically meaningful influence on medically unexplained symptoms and somatisation' [45].

Interventions for functional somatic syndromes

In contrast to the relative sparse primary research concerning somatoform disorders, there have been a large number of trials of interventions for specific functional somatic syndromes. Most of these have studied syndrome-specific symptomatic ('peripherally acting') treatments which are outside the scope of this book. We review in this section psychological treatments and the use of antidepressants. We will use three systematic reviews to provide an overview of the evidence of efficacy of interventions for functional somatic symptoms.

Systematic reviews

CBT for functional somatic syndromes

An early systematic review found evidence of the usefulness of CBT in patients with persistent somatic symptoms; this review included studies of specific functional somatic syndromes as well as a few including patients with somatisation or hypochondriasis [46]. The authors considered the outcomes of physical symptoms, psychological distress and functional status. Of these, physical symptoms appeared to be the most responsive. Improvement of physical symptoms was greater in patients treated with CBT than in control subjects in 71% of the studies, whereas a definite advantage of CBT for reducing psychological distress was demonstrated in only 38% of studies. In half of the studies, CBT led to an improvement in functional status compared with the control condition.

The authors noted that improvement in physical symptoms often occurred independent of improvement in psychological distress. They pointed out that CBT for somatic symptoms may require additional treatment for depression, e.g. with antidepressants.

In this review, it was noted that the CBT did not conform to a specific pattern as interventions were multifaceted and flexible. Both individual and group formats were found to be effective and the number of sessions varied between studies. Most of the studies were carried out in referred populations and there was considerable variation in the nature of the symptoms, their severity and chronicity.

The authors of this review noted that acceptability of CBT to such patients is a critical issue that had not really been addressed in many of the studies as they did not include data on participation rates. Since most studies were conducted in specialist referral clinics, patients unwilling to attend such clinics would have been screened out. They suggested that future studies should examine what proportion of primary care patients with persistent somatisation and symptom syndromes who were offered CBT actually accepted and completed therapy.

Antidepressants for functional somatic syndromes

One of the first systematic reviews of the use of antidepressants included 94 randomised controlled trials (6595 patients in all), which most frequently included headache, fibromyalgia, functional gastrointestinal disorders and unexplained pain [47]. Overall, two-thirds of the studies found evidence of benefit for antidepressants as patients receiving these drugs were three times more likely than those receiving placebo to show improvement (odds ratio 3.4; 95% CI 2.6–4.5). This result was recorded for patients with fibromyalgia, headache, chronic fatigue, functional gastrointestinal complaints and idiopathic pain.

The overall quality of studies included in this review was described as fair. Studies were generally of short duration, whereas these symptoms are often chronic. Many studies used a crossover design, which is inappropriate for chronic conditions. Withdrawal rates were high (40% of trials had drop-out rates over 20%), suggesting that antidepressants may not be well tolerated in this population. The number of studies for some conditions was very small. There were inadequate data to decide whether the efficacy of antidepressants was mediated by reduction of depression. The use of antidepressants in particular functional somatic syndromes is discussed below.

Updated systematic review of both CBT and antidepressants

The systematic review of the effectiveness of antidepressants and CBT for functional somatic syndromes has been updated [48]. The strength of evidence is summarized in Table 3.1. The reviewers concluded that CBT was consistently demonstrated to be effective in all of the functional somatic syndromes they examined. There is evidence of efficacy of antidepressants for headaches, fibromyalgia and IBS, with weaker evidence for back pain and a lack of evidence for chronic fatigue syndrome. These authors consider that the effect size of

Table 3.1 Efficacy of antidepressants and cognitive behavioural therapy (CBT) for functional somatic syndromes[a]

Syndrome	TCA	SSRI	SNRI	CBT
Irritable bowel syndrome	++	+		+++
Back pain	+	—	+	++
Headache	++	—		++
Fibromyalgia	++		++	++
Neuropathic pain	++	—	++	
Chronic fatigue syndrome	—	—		++
Tinnitus				+
Menopausal syndrome	+	+		
Other pain syndromes	+	—		

Evidence of benefit: +++ = strong; ++ = moderate; + = modest;
± = inconclusive
– = evidence of lack of benefit.
TCA, tricyclic antidepressants; SSRI, serotonin selective reuptake inhibitor;
SNRI, serotonin and norepinephrine reuptake inhibitor.
[a] Adapted from Jackson et al. [47].

treatment with antidepressants is not as great as that resulting from CBT. They also point out the benefits of CBT: it does not interact with other medication and has few if any side effects. There is also some evidence that CBT has increasing effectiveness over time. The recent review states, once again, that some or all of the effect of antidepressants on somatic symptoms is independent of depression. This appears to be true of CBT also [48].

Antidepressants are more effective than placebo in reducing back pain but not in improving functional status in patients with chronic back pain. The effect size in relation to pain, however, is modest and CBT may achieve better results. With regards to headache, there is reasonable evidence for the efficacy of tricyclic antidepressants (TCAs), but a recent meta-analysis suggests that serotonin selective reuptake inhibitors (SSRIs) were no more effective than placebo for patients with migraine headaches and not as effective as TCAs for tension headaches [49]. CBT, relaxation therapy and biofeedback have been shown to yield considerable improvement in migraine and tension headaches, with beneficial effects persisting over seven years [50].

Preliminary evidence for short-term psychodynamic psychotherapy

A systematic review of short-term psychodynamic psychotherapies (STPP) for somatic symptom disorders found 13 RCTs and 10 case series with pre-post outcome assessments [51]. The studies included a total of 1870 subjects, of which 873 received STPP and 535 served as controls. Six studies involved patients with chronic pain. Others included patients with functional disorders such as IBS, while others focused on somatic symptoms related to more traditional medical disorders such as Crohn's disease, coronary artery disease, emphysema and Sjögren's syndrome. Of the included studies,

21/23 (91.3%), 11/12 (91.6%), 16/19 (76.2%) and 7/9 (77.8%) reported significant or possible effects on physical symptoms, psychological symptoms, social-occupational function and healthcare utilisation, respectively. Meta-analysis was possible for 14 studies and revealed significant effects on physical symptoms, psychiatric symptoms and social adjustment, which were maintained in long-term follow-up. While this review suggests potential benefit for STPP, the heterogeneity among the studies and methodological shortcomings makes the evidence basis for STPP more preliminary and not nearly as convincing yet as that for CBT.

Rationale for psychological and exercise-based treatments of functional somatic syndromes

The rationale for CBT in IBS is based on the notion that the abdominal symptoms may be maintained and intensified by cognitive, behavioural and emotional responses to abdominal discomfort or pain. Such symptoms can precipitate thoughts of serious illness or fear of lack of control. These cognitions may lead to the person paying increased attention to abdominal and other bodily sensations and making more frequent visits to the toilet. She or he may start to avoid certain foods and avoid leaving home unless there is a toilet nearby. Attempting to overcome these feared situations usually leads to increased anxiety, abdominal discomfort and fear of impending diarrhoea. Thus a vicious circle can develop which perpetuates and exacerbates pain and diarrhoea. Cognitive behavioural techniques aim to break this vicious cycle by addressing unhelpful thoughts related to the symptoms, normalising diet and bowel habits, using techniques to reduce symptom focusing and reduce stress and anxiety. CBT aims also to help the person develop coping strategies to permit resumption of normal social activities.

Cognitive behavioural therapy has similar aims of changing the cognitions and associated behaviours found in fibromyalgia. Whereas avoidance of physical activity may be helpful in acute pain, it is unhelpful in chronic pain. CBT challenges the beliefs that pain indicates serious damage and avoidance is necessary to stay pain-free; reductions in catastrophising and helplessness are thought to mediate CBT treatment of pain [52;53]. CBT encourages gradual resumption of normal movements with the aim of increasing activity. Autonomic arousal and associated increased muscle tension are also detrimental in chronic pain, so stress management and relaxation components are also often included. Multicomponent CBT refers to a combination of different techniques, including cognitive restructuring, improved pain-coping, goal setting, increasing activity levels, activity pacing and adjustment of pain-related medication.

The rationale for exercise therapy in fibromyalgia is complex [54]. It is thought that muscle, and other peripheral tissues might contribute to chronic pain in fibromyalgia through initiating and/or maintaining central sensitization [55]. Deconditioning is also thought to be important, so aerobic exercise and strength training may reverse some of these changes. Exercise training can lead to improved depression and better sleep, which are also common in fibromyalgia.

Patients with chronic fatigue syndrome are generally inactive [56]. This inactivity is associated with reduced physical strength and cardiovascular deconditioning [57]. Additional physiological changes may include autonomic nervous system changes, hypothalamic–pituitary axis down-regulation and enhanced perception of visceral phenomena (interoception) [58;59]. Sleep and mood may be consequently affected. A vicious circle of exercise avoidance, deconditioning and increased fatigue after effort may occur, which serves to perpetuate fatigue and hence chronic fatigue syndrome [57]. Other patients have an erratic pattern of activity, responding to symptoms, so that they 'boom and bust'; doing too much when feeling well, developing symptoms to which they respond by doing less [60].

Other cognitive and behavioural factors are important in chronic fatigue syndrome as in other functional somatic syndromes [61]. These include attributing symptoms to physical factors, having a lesser sense of control of symptoms and focusing on bodily symptoms; such features are associated with fatigue severity in chronic fatigue syndrome [62]. CBT is a collaborative approach that helps the patient to examine and challenge any thoughts and beliefs (cognitive element) that may be hindering recovery (e.g. challenging the catastrophic interpretation of symptoms following a transient increase in activity), with an additional graded increase in activity (behavioural element). Graded exercise therapy (GET) focuses on stabilizing and then gradually increasing physical activity, particularly exercise (defined as any physical activity that demands exertion). This initially occurs at a low level of intensity, with little aerobic or metabolic load. Once exercising half an hour a day, the intensity is gradually increased. So, GET starts as a behavioural graded exposure therapy and then moves into a physiological training programme.

Comorbid mood disorders will affect prognosis in any functional somatic syndromes, and need to be treated in their own right [58;63;64] but there is very little research published on the effects of such treatment. Psychodynamic psychotherapy has been used successfully in IBS [65;66]. This form of therapy is based on the assumption that the patient's problems arise from, or are exacerbated by, disturbances of significant personal relationships; the person does not make this link between abdominal symptoms and interpersonal stress. A tentative, encouraging, supportive approach on behalf of the therapist aims to develop a deeper understanding of the patient's sources of stress and, through exploration of feelings and metaphors, help the patient to make this link. The therapist uses the therapeutic and transference relationship to explore psychological problems.

Rationale for the use of antidepressants in functional somatic syndromes

The rationale for using antidepressants in IBS and fibromyalgia lies predominantly in their analgesic and hypnotic action [67]. It is thought that serotonin and norepinephrine transmission, which mediate endogenous analgesic mechanisms via the descending inhibitory pain pathways in the central nervous system, may play a key role in the heightened pain sensitivity found in these disorders. There has been particular interest in the efficacy of the serotonin and norepinephrine reuptake inhibitors (SNRI) as they can lead to improved pain and depression. Since these antidepressants are recommended at low doses, however, they have been evaluated at low doses [68;69]. In clinical practice they may be used at full dose for the many patients who also have depression and/or anxiety, but few trials have evaluated them in this way. TCAs may help diarrhoea through their anticholinergic action. It is not clear how SSRIs benefit IBS patients [70].

It is recommended that antidepressants are used as a second line of treatment in IBS if laxatives, loperamide and antispasmodics have not been helpful [67;71]. In fibromyalgia, TCAs are one of the recommended first-line treatments; the others are aerobic exercise, CBT and multicomponent treatment [72]. There is some doubt about the efficacy of antidepressants beyond 12 weeks in fibromyalgia [73].

There is no convincing research evidence to suggest that pharmacological interventions are useful in helping chronic fatigue syndrome [74]. Low-dose tricyclic and related antidepressants may be useful for both pain and insomnia [74]. SSRIs may help comorbid anxiety or depression. Duloxetine and pregabalin are efficacious central pain modulators in patients with associated fibromyalgia [75;76].

People diagnosed with one functional somatic syndrome often have one of the other functional somatic syndromes as well as concurrent depressive and anxiety disorders [77;78]. An individual treatment plan needs to take into account all of the relevant treatments that would normally be provided for those conditions.

Evidence of efficacy of treatments in specific functional somatic syndromes

Chronic fatigue syndrome

There have been a number of systematic reviews of treatment and a few meta-analyses. All conclude that CBT and GET show the best evidence of efficacy [79;80;81;82].

A meta-analysis of CBT compared with usual care showed a clinically important reduction in fatigue severity in 40% of treated patients compared with 26% of those receiving usual care [82]. Active rehabilitative CBT, which included increasing activity and reducing rest, reduced fatigue severity compared with usual care, but CBT with no focus on change rest/activity made no difference to fatigue. The meta-analysis by Malouff and colleagues did not separate these two models of CBT, but still found evidence in favour of CBT, with an effect size of 0.48 compared with control interventions or usual care [81]. CBT delivered in a group setting seems to be less efficacious, albeit with some improvements [83].

A systematic review of five RCTs of GET found a significant advantage for GET versus various control interventions for both fatigue (standard mean difference (SMD) 0.77) and physical function (SMD 0.64) [80]. There were a greater number of dropouts from GET, however, and there are issues of patient acceptability. This was in spite of the fact that there was no evidence to show that exercise therapy may worsen outcomes. The addition of education to GET was helpful. Pacing has been tested recently in the PACE trial (see below).

Knoop and colleagues studied 96 patients who had CBT to find out whether a full recovery was possible after treatment for chronic fatigue syndrome [84]. The definition of recovery was based on the absence of the standardised criteria for CFS, as well as the normal perception of fatigue and their own health; 23% of the patients were judged to be recovered after a course of CBT. Those patients with comorbid medical conditions recovered less often. Deale and colleagues evaluated the long-term (five years) outcome of CBT versus relaxation therapy for patients with chronic fatigue syndrome [85]. Significantly more patients receiving CBT met criteria for complete recovery (24%), were free of relapse or showed a steady improvement in symptoms. Powell and colleagues showed persistence of improvement two years after GET [86].

Cognitive behavioural therapy was more effective than waiting list control in adolescents [86]. At two years follow-up, those who received CBT were significantly less fatigued, less functionally impaired and had higher school attendance [88]. Long-term fatigue levels were associated with fatigue in mothers. The beliefs of parents may also play a role in determining the beliefs and coping of the child. Family-focused CBT returned adolescents to school more quickly than an equal amount of psycho-education, but there were no significant differences in outcome at six and 12 months [89].

Although patient charities have expressed concern about the safety of treatments for chronic fatigue syndrome, particularly regarding GET, randomised controlled trials suggest little concern over safety as long as treatments are delivered by suitably qualified therapists who have been trained to apply these treatments for chronic fatigue syndrome [74;90]. With

GET, additional precautions should be taken for those with comorbid physical health conditions, such as asthma and low back pain. GET should be tailored to individual disability and the approach needs to start at a low level of activity in those who are bed-bound or house-bound [74]. In the recent PACE trial [91] all patients received specialist medical care; three arms also received individually delivered therapies: adaptive pacing therapy (pacing designed to adapt to the illness; APT), CBT and GET. Compared with standard medical care, patients receiving CBT and GET both improved moderately in fatigue and physical functioning, but those receiving APT did not [91].

Cognitive behavioural therapy is based on the cognitive behavioural model of chronic fatigue syndrome [61;92]. Thus being 'psychologically minded' has been found to predict (moderately) a positive outcome and emotional processing mediated improvement both for CBT as well as counselling [93;94]. Considering that CBT involves a graded return to activity, it is intriguing that increased activity does not seem to mediate improvement [95]. Similarly two studies have found that increased fitness did not mediate improvement with GET [96;97]. This is especially surprising as GET is based on a model of deconditioning and avoidance of activity. Reduced symptom focusing appears to mediate the response to GET [97].

Other moderators of a negative outcome with treatment in CFS patients may include pervasive inactivity, comorbid mood problems, being in dispute over benefits, receipt of benefits and membership of a self-help group [58;98]. These results need replication. There are also intriguing physiological changes which have been reported in relation to improvement following CBT in chronic fatigue syndrome patients. A significant increase in grey matter volume, localized in the lateral prefrontal cortex and normalization of the hypothalamic–pituitary adrenal axis have been reported following CBT, but the significance of these changes is unclear [99;100].

There is no convincing evidence that antidepressants are effective treatments in CFS [75].

Irritable bowel syndrome

The treatment for IBS includes dietary advice, antispasmodics, laxative, antimotility and antidepressants drugs and psychological treatments. Only the last two will be discussed here; the reader should consult appropriate guidance for the other treatments [67;71]. The available evidence regarding efficacy of psychological treatments and antidepressants for IBS has been reviewed recently by the British Society of Gastroenterology, the UK's National Institute for Health and Clinical Excellence (NICE) and independent reviewers (Ford and colleagues) [67;68;71].

The review by Ford and colleagues included 14 studies comparing antidepressants with placebo (in a total of 805 patients) and 19 studies comparing psychological treatment with usual care (total of 1278 patients included) [68]. Both treatments were found to be effective and for each type of treatment the number needed to treat to prevent persistent IBS symptoms was 4. The quality of the studies concerning antidepressants was considered to be good but it was poor for those concerning psychological treatments. The results were presented as the proportion of patients who had persistent or unimproved symptoms of IBS.

Forty-two per cent of patients treated with *antidepressants* continued to have persistent or unimproved IBS symptoms compared with 65% of those receiving placebo. Thus the relative risk of symptoms persisting or remaining unimproved after antidepressant treatment versus placebo was 0.66 (95% CI 0.57–0.79). TCAs and SSRIs appeared to be similarly effective in treating IBS symptoms and there was no significant difference in side effects.

Fifty-one per cent of patients receiving *psychological treatment* had persistent or unimproved IBS symptoms compared with 72.5% of those receiving usual care. Thus the relative

Table 3.2 Relative risk of persisting symptoms following different types of psychological treatment [68]

Type of therapy	No. of studies	Relative risk of symptoms persisting
Tricyclic antidepressants	9	0.68 (95% CI 0.56–0.83)
SSRI antidepressants	5	0.62 (95% CI 0.45–0.87)
Cognitive behavioural therapy	7	0.60 (95% CI 0.42–0.87)
Hypnotherapy	2	0.48 (95% CI 0.42–0.87)
Dynamic psychotherapy	2	0.60 (95% CI 0.39–0.93)
Multicomponent	3	0.69 (95% CI 0.56–0.86)
Relaxation	5	0.82 (95% CI 0.63–1.08)

SSRI, serotonin selective reuptake inhibitor.

risk of IBS symptoms persisting for psychological treatment compared to usual care was 0.67 (95% CI 0.57–0.79). Of the different types of psychological treatment (Table 3.2), the evidence was strongest for CBT but three of the studies came from the same centre and had very small numbers. Once these were excluded, the results ceased to be statistically significant.

Five studies investigated relaxation therapy and the results from these did not quite reach statistical significance; the authors warn that these studies involved small numbers and this could be a type II error. There were two studies each of hypnotherapy and dynamic psychotherapy; each showed a statistically significant benefit of the active treatment. Multicomponent psychological treatment was shown to be effective; there was insufficient evidence for stress management and self-administered CBT.

The evidence presented in this review is more secure for antidepressants than for psychological treatment. The latter was compared, in nearly all studies, with usual care; there was no 'attention-placebo' so there was no attempt to control for therapists' time and attention, which does not occur in usual treatment. There was a significant heterogeneity among the psychological treatment studies. Nearly all studies were short (8–12 weeks); only one was performed in primary care.

The authors quoted four studies, all randomised controlled trials of antidepressants, which showed that the improvement in IBS symptoms was not secondary to improvement in depression [101;102;103;104].

NICE review

The NICE review considered the evidence in relation to severity of IBS as most of the clearest evidence concerned patients with refractory irritable bowel syndrome, i.e. those who had not responded to first-line treatments, some of whom also had depression [67]. The review found reasonable evidence of the efficacy of *both* tricyclic and SSRI antidepressants in the treatment of patients with refractory IBS compared with placebo in terms of showing a significant global improvement in symptoms. Pain and bloating appeared to be the most responsive symptoms when tricyclics were used; this was not so for SSRIs.

This review recommended that TCAs should be used as a second-line of treatment for people with IBS when laxatives, loperamide or antispasmodics have not been helpful. These antidepressants are recommended for their beneficial effect on IBS, not for their antidepressant effect as low doses are recommended. SSRI antidepressants are recommended only if tricyclics are ineffective, but many clinicians would use the former in order to avoid side effects in patients who seem very sensitive to medication.

With regard to *psychological* treatments, the NICE review concluded that there is no adequate evidence supporting the efficacy of relaxation or biofeedback. There is fair evidence showing a significant global improvement both in the short and long term for psychodynamic psychotherapy in addition to medical therapy compared with medical therapy alone in patients with refractory or long-term IBS, approximately half of whom have concurrent anxiety or depressive disorders. In this group of patients, there is good evidence that CBT is effective in improving global improvement in symptoms and moderate evidence that hypnotherapy is similarly effective. The NICE review found evidence that psychodynamic psychotherapy is a cost-effective treatment.

The NICE guideline development group considered CBT, hypnotherapy and psychotherapy as a group of therapies for which the evidence is similar in respect to patients with IBS that has not responded to usual treatments. Thus any of these three psychological interventions should be offered according to patient preference and local availability of therapy.

The NICE guidelines include an IBS algorithm which recommends that people with this syndrome are best helped if they are given a positive diagnosis, after being screened for 'red flag' symptoms which might indicate organic disease (rectal bleeding, marked weight loss, family history of bowel or ovarian cancer and age over 60 years). Patients with IBS should be given information that explains the importance of self-help, general lifestyle, physical activity, diet and symptom-targeted medication. The review indicates that a collaborative multidisciplinary approach should be provided by appropriately trained health professionals. The guidelines recognise, however, that there is variability in availability of specialists who can provide the relevant psychological interventions.

British Society of Gastroenterology review

The British Society of Gastroenterology group that reviewed the evidence to produce guidelines for IBS concluded that CBT and psychodynamic psychotherapy improved patients' coping with their symptoms. Hypnotherapy was considered to benefit patients with refractory IBS with lasting effect. This group considered that the evidence indicated that TCAs benefit pain and SSRIs improved global but not specific symptoms.

The British Society of Gastroenterology guidelines state, in relation to psychological therapies [71]:

> All approaches to managing IBS should be informed by psychological understanding, recognising that the most important aspect of management is the relation between the patient and the physician. Empathic listening, respecting patients' views of symptom causation, and giving honest, clear explanations of the interplay between psychological and physical symptoms are essential. Conversely, collusion in seeking a physical cause and undertaking endless investigations must be resisted.

This review group commented on the potential advantages of treating IBS in primary care including early attention to psychological factors. GPs are familiar with prescribing antidepressants and also tend to take a holistic approach to IBS. They are therefore well placed to explore psychological factors associated with IBS and they may have ready access to counsellors who can offer help with psychological problems. There is evidence that a self-help guidebook that can lead to symptom improvement and reduction of healthcare use in primary care [105]. CBT administered in primary care together with mebeverine helps IBS symptoms in the short term and helps work and social adjustment in the long term [106].

Patient preference is important. There have been few direct comparisons but in one study of IBS, which included randomisation to either an SSRI or brief dynamic psychotherapy,

69% of participants completed the course of psychotherapy compared to 50% of those allocated to an SSRI (p = 0.013) [106]. This suggests, perhaps surprisingly, that patients with severe IBS which has not responded to the usual treatment prefer psychotherapy to antidepressants. Many people with functional somatic syndromes dislike the idea of taking drugs long term and express fears of dependence but, in spite of this, over 80% of people with IBS said they would accept either tablets or diet change [108]. It is clear from this study, however, that patient preference is clearly related to the amount of information patients have about relative effectiveness of different treatments.

Fibromyalgia

The three main forms of treatment for fibromyalgia are drugs, cognitive behaviour therapy and exercise. A recent review of the different published guidelines found that the highest level of recommendation has been made for aerobic exercise, CBT, amitriptyline and multicomponent treatment [109]. Three new drugs have received approval by the Food and Drug Administration (FDA) for treatment of fibromyalgia in the past several years: pregabalin, duloxetine and milnacipran; the latter two are SNRIs [110].

Psychological treatment and exercise

Many studies have combined CBT with exercise but a recent systematic review and meta-analysis examined CBT without exercise [111]. The results showed that CBT led to lasting improvement in pain self-efficacy (SMD 0.90; 95% CI 0.14–1.66). Improvement in depressed mood occurred in the short-term only (SMD –0.24; 95% CI –0.40 to –0.08; p = 0.004) but there was no evidence of efficacy in terms of improved pain, fatigue, sleep disturbances or health-related quality of life [111].

Rather similar results emerged from a review of multimethod CBT; the review found some negative trials and some that reported positive results in the short term only [112]. One study reported positive results in the long term, but this study used inpatient treatment, which is most unusual. It also included distressed patients, who did particularly well with this treatment [113].

A Cochrane review concluded that there was moderate quality evidence that aerobic-only exercise training at the recommended intensity levels has positive effects on global well-being (SMD 0.49; 95% CI 0.23–0.75) and physical function (SMD 0.66; 95% CI 0.41–0.92), and possibly on pain (SMD 0.65; 95% CI –0.09–1.39) [54]. The latest systematic review of the efficacy of aerobic exercise in fibromyalgia comes to rather similar conclusions, namely that it leads to improvements in depressed mood, health-related quality of life and physical fitness both immediately after treatment and at follow-up [114]. Aerobic exercise is efficacious for pain and fatigue at the post-treatment assessment only – continuing exercise is necessary to maintain the positive effect on pain at follow-up. There is no evidence that this treatment has a positive effect on sleep [114].

Antidepressants

A recent systematic review makes it clear that antidepressants are effective in fibromyalgia in the short term [69]. The meta-analysis found clear evidence for an association of antidepressant medications with improvements in pain, depression, sleep disturbances, and health-related quality of life in patients with fibromyalgia. The effect sizes were generally small and that for fatigue was negligible. These results relate to assessment at the end of treatment; the median duration of treatment was eight weeks. No trial had a follow-up assessment.

The effect sizes for pain reduction were large for TCAs (SMD −1.64; 95% CI −2.57 to −0.71), medium for monoamine oxidase inhibitors (SMD −0.54; 95% CI −1.02 to −0.07), and small for SSRIs (SMD −0.39; 95% CI −0.77 to −0.01) and SNRIs (SMD −0.36; 95% CI −0.46 to −0.25). With regard to adherence, the median proportion of patients completing the trials was 71%.

Two of the reports concerning duloxetine showed that the beneficial effects were similar in participants with or without concurrent major depressive disorder [115]. In the two relevant trials, 38% and 26% of participants had major depressive disorder at baseline but duloxetine was not significantly more effective than placebo in treating depression in either trial [115;116;117]. It is clear that the beneficial effects of duloxetine in fibromyalgia can be attributed to its direct analgesic effect rather than its antidepressant effect. In one trial the direct effect of duloxetine (120 mg daily) on the reduction of the mean Brief Pain Inventory score accounted for 86.9% of the total treatment effect (p = 0.0007) [115]. The comparable proportion for the indirect treatment effect through improvement in depressive symptoms accounted was 13.1%. In another trial with a six-month treatment period, these proportions were 82.3% for the direct effect and 17.7% for the indirect effect through reduction of depressive symptoms [117]. This emphasises the point that concurrent depression should be treated effectively in any of these conditions to gain optimal outcomes.

No trial seems to have compared antidepressants and exercise therapy or CBT directly but two trials used similar measures and included patients with similar baseline scores. One used exercise therapy and the other used antidepressants. The trial of exercise therapy for fibromyalgia found that the beneficial effects of exercise could be enhanced by combining it with a fibromyalgia self-help course aimed at increasing understanding of the condition and self-management. The participants in this group improved by 25% on the Fibromyalgia Impact Questionnaire (mean improvement 12.7 points; standard deviation (SD) 13.2). This improvement was similar to that observed in a trial of duloxetine, an SNRI antidepressant which has FDA approval in fibromyalgia [75;116;117].

There were some small differences between these treatments. First, the exercise/self-management group recording greater improvements in physical function and mental health whereas duloxetine was associated with greater improvements in pain [75;116;117;118]. Second, the benefits were maintained six months after baseline in the duloxetine trial only if the drug was continued [117]. Long-term benefit in the case of exercise plus self-management instruction did not appear to be dependent on continuing therapy [118]. Adherence to treatment was slightly better for the exercise plus self-management (78%) than for duloxetine (54–70%).

A combination of optimised antidepressant treatment and pain self-management for patients with joint and back pain and depression has shown greater improvement in both of these parameters compared with usual care [119]. Although this group of patients included arthritis patients, the message that antidepressants should be continued in the long term in order to maintain benefit was clear as two-thirds of the intervention group took antidepressants throughout the whole year of the study compared to 3.9% in the usual care group.

Effectiveness and cost-effectiveness trials in functional somatic syndromes

There are very few effectiveness or cost-effectiveness trials in the functional somatic syndromes. In irritable bowel syndrome it has been shown that the provision of a booklet for self-management significantly reduced costs to the health service by £72 per patient because of a reduction in prescribed drugs, and primary and secondary care visits [105]. CBT in primary care for IBS costs an additional £308 per patient [120]. In this trial there were no cost savings as a result of reduced use of other services or reduced time lost from employment during the trial period or nine months' follow-up. This meant that the treatment was not regarded as cost-effective during the follow-up period.

NICE found that both TCAs and SSRIs are cost-effective treatments for IBS [67]. Psychodynamic psychotherapy was found to be a cost-effective treatment for patients with severe IBS in secondary and tertiary care with a high level of National Health Service (NHS) service use at baseline [67;107] The trial showed that direct healthcare costs were lower in the year following treatment for three months of psychotherapy compared with three months of usual care. This benefit offset the high healthcare costs during the intervention period for psychotherapy [107]. This evidence is unlikely to be applicable to primary care patients except those with refractory IBS. NICE also found hypnotherapy to be a cost-effective treatment for refractory IBS.

A cost-effectiveness study of CBT in chronic fatigue syndrome found that this treatment also led to greater reduction of medical and societal costs than guided support group or usual care [121]. CBT was expensive but, in view of the better clinical outcome was cost-effective. Compared with no treatment, the baseline incremental cost-effectiveness of CBT was €20 516 per chronic fatigue syndrome patient showing clinically significant improvement, and €21 375 per quality-adjusted life-year (QALY).

A study in UK found similar results – the cost of providing CBT or graded exercise was £149 greater than that of usual GP care plus a self-help booklet, but the outcome was better [122]. There was no difference between CBT and graded exercise. When NICE analysed these results, it appeared that the cost per QALY was under £20 000, but the sensitivity analysis suggested the real cost might be higher [74]. This study highlighted the very high informal carer costs associated with chronic fatigue syndrome, which have been described in Chapter 1 (p. 27).

A cost-effectiveness study in fibromyalgia found treatment to be more expensive than treatment as usual, as expected but, in this study there was no difference between intervention and control group at follow-up which meant that the intervention was not cost-effective [123].

Numbers of patients needing treatment

The most cost-effective treatments tend to be those that include patients with very high costs, which are reduced with treatment. The UK IBS trial mentioned above recruited 257 patients from 317 eligible patients (82%) in seven gastroenterology clinics in North West England over three years [107]. Since there are approximately 200 such clinics in the country we could estimate that there are approximately 2670 such patients who might be recruited to psychotherapy or antidepressant treatment each year. In fact, the proportion recruited might be higher if there was not a 'usual care' group which made the trial unattractive to some potential participants. A quarter of the patients recruited had a very high somatic symptom score and in this group the treatment led to a cost saving of over £1000 for the year following treatment. Thus for approximately 620 patients there would be a cost saving of £620 000 nationally per annum.

General ingredients of treatment and a stepped-care model

One major review examined treatment for the functional somatic symptoms across all syndromes and identified five types of treatment [1]. These were: *peripheral pharmacotherapy* (such as antispasmodic drugs for IBS), *central pharmacotherapy* (such as antidepressants for analgesia), *active behavioural interventions* (such as exercise), *passive physical interventions* (such as tender point injections) and, finally, *interventions aimed at changing the doctor's behaviour* (such as reattribution training).

The review found that the benefits of peripheral pharmacotherapy are clear in certain disorders, such as IBS or functional dyspepsia, but not helpful in other disorders. On the other hand, central pharmacotherapy, such as antidepressants, are more widely beneficial across different functional somatic syndromes. With regard to non-pharmacological interventions, the review found evidence of efficacy for those treatments that require patient involvement, such as GET or psychotherapy. There is a problem comparing 'benefit' across these types of treatment, however, as non-pharmacological treatments tend to have greatest impact on functioning and overall health status, whereas pharmacological treatments show greatest benefit in particular symptoms, such as pain or bowel dysfunction.

The review drew a distinction between uncomplicated, organ-specific functional disorders, where the typical pharmacological intervention is usually effective and the multiorgan type where a different approach is required. For the latter type, a cognitive interpersonal intervention is suggested from the outset but the review found that evidence for this is lacking.

Increasingly there is a tendency to adopt a stepped-care model. This has recently been tested in chronic fatigue syndrome and the results indicate that stepped care involving a period of guided self-instruction followed by CBT only if necessary, provided similar overall results to 14 sessions of CBT for all participants: 49% and 48% in each arm of the trial achieved clinically significant improvement [124]. The advantage of the guided self-instruction was that fewer people needed CBT and, when it was needed, fewer sessions were required. It has been noted above that self-management for IBS patients attending primary care leads to improvement in symptoms and a reduction in subsequent primary care consultations [105]. Thus the use of a stepped-care approach led to less need for treatment as well as improvement of symptoms. (See Chapter 8 for more details of this approach.)

With regards to multiorgan type of functional somatic syndrome, some data from one study provides evidence of efficacy of treatment. Patients attending secondary or tertiary care gastroenterology clinics with severe IBS which had not responded to usual treatment were divided into those with and without numerous other somatic symptoms[125]. Half of the patients reported four or more somatic symptoms outside the gastrointestinal tract, most commonly headaches, faintness or dizziness, pain in the lower back, soreness of muscles, trouble with breathing, hot or cold spells, numbness, tingling, and fatigue. These would be classified as 'multiorgan' or complex functional somatic syndrome patients. The other half had few or no somatic symptoms outside the gastrointestinal tract and these would be regarded as organ-specific IBS.

As might be expected from the literature, the patients with the highest somatic symptoms score (eight or more extra-intestinal symptoms) were more disabled, more likely to have a concurrent psychiatric diagnosis and had incurred higher total costs before entering the trial. They improved greatly with treatment, however, whether it was antidepressant or psychotherapy. It was this group with the multiple somatic symptoms that showed greatest difference from treatment as usual in terms of improvement of health status (Figure 3.1 shows follow-up SF-36 physical component summary scores adjusted for age, sex, years of education, psychiatric disorder, abuse history and baseline SF-36 physical component score). This group with multiple somatic symptoms also showed greatest reduction in costs over the year following the end of treatment. These mean costs, adjusted for baseline costs, were £1092 (Standard Error (SE) 487), £1394

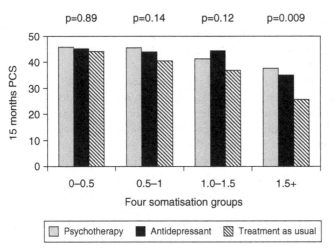

Figure 3.1 SF-36 physical component score (PCS) at one year after the end of treatment. Results are shown by treatment group for the four quartiles according to baseline somatisation score [125]. The group on the extreme right (1.5+) had multiple somatic symptoms.

(SE 443) and £2949 (SE 593) for the psychotherapy, antidepressant and treatment 'as usual' groups, respectively (p = 0.050 adjusted for age, sex, years of education, depression, panic and generalised anxiety disorders and abuse history and for baseline costs; see Figure 3.2).

This study suggests that those patients with severe IBS who do not respond to usual treatment, can still be divided into those with single-organ and multiorgan types. Both types respond to antidepressants or brief interpersonal psychotherapy but the change is greatest in the multiorgan type because they are more impaired and incur higher healthcare costs at baseline compared with single-organ type.

Conclusions

This chapter has reviewed the types of treatment, and their efficacy, used for patients with the different types of bodily distress syndromes (medically unexplained symptoms, somatoform disorders or functional somatic syndromes). It is clear that there is evidence of efficacy and effectiveness, though this tends to be stronger in some conditions than others. The evidence is stronger for some pharmacological treatments than for psychological treatments partly because of the universal use of placebo tablets and the lack of an attention-placebo in psychological treatment trials.

This book is concerned with improving the care of patients with somatoform and related disorders. From that standpoint, the improvement in symptoms and health status and reduction of costs that follows a psychological treatment is an advance. The crucial questions facing health service researchers in this area concern the therapeutic ingredients of treatments, their moderators and mediators, and their cost-effectiveness. Although there is very little research in this respect, we have shown that the disorders discussed in this book are expensive (Chapter 1) and some treatment trials lead to reduced healthcare costs as well as improved functioning.

With regards to therapeutic ingredients, it is clear that the so-called 'non-specific' aspects of treatment, such as time spent with the patient, the doctor's recognition of the reality of symptoms, and empathy and supportive approach, are important. There are some specific aspects of the doctor's behaviour, such as being responsive to the patient's worries about the symptoms, providing a clear and positive message regarding the diagnosis

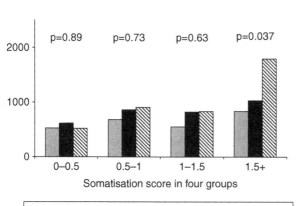

Figure 3.2 Total costs (adjusted geometric means) for one year after the end of treatment by treatment group for the four quartiles according to baseline somatisation score [125]. The group on the extreme right (1.5+) had multiple somatic symptoms.

and a specific management plan, can also be beneficial to patient care. In addition, specific relevant educational material, self-help manuals and a diary to better understand links between symptoms, behaviour and thoughts are important first-line treatments. There is reasonably sound evidence for the usefulness of these in the functional somatic syndromes. Establishing these in routine care would improve the management of medically unexplained symptoms and related syndromes considerably because of the large numbers of patients involved.

With regard to more intensive psychological treatments, the use of specialist cognitive interpersonal techniques needs to become much more widespread. There is some evidence that primary care physicians can learn these techniques but the best efficacy relates to mental health professionals delivering these treatments. The availability of these specialist treatments in general medical settings is inadequate in most centres. Although low-dose antidepressant prescribing is very widespread in primary and secondary medical care, the use of these drugs at therapeutic dose for depression, where appropriate, might be more useful.

Studies of predictors, moderators and mediators are in their early stages, requiring as they do, large trials to power them. We know already that treatment specificity is more helpful than blanket approaches – antidepressants are effective in fibromyalgia and IBS, but not in chronic fatigue syndrome. Similarly, the content of CBT varies according to the syndrome being addressed, suggesting mediators differ across the syndromes. Developing this approach should allow more focused interventions for subgroups of patients, which should improve effectiveness.

References

1. Henningsen P, Zipfel S, Herzog W. Management of functional somatic syndromes. *The Lancet* 2007; **369**(9565): 946–55.

2. Ruddy R, House A. Psychosocial interventions for conversion disorder. *Cochrane Database of Systematic Reviews* 2005; **4**: CD005331.

3. Kroenke K. Efficacy of treatment for somatoform disorders: a review of randomized controlled trials. *Psychosomatic Medicine* 2007; **69**(9): 881–8.

4. Goldberg D, Gask L, Odowd T. The treatment of somatization – teaching techniques of reattribution. *Journal of Psychosomatic Research* 1989; **33**(6): 689–95.

5. Gask L, Goldberg D, Porter R, Creed F. The treatment of somatization – evaluation of a teaching package with general-practice trainees. *Journal of Psychosomatic Research* 1989; **33**(6): 697–703.

6. van der Feltz Cornelis, Van Os TW, Harm WJ, Van Marwijk HW, Leentjens AF. Effect of psychiatric consultation models in primary care. A systematic review and meta-analysis of randomised controlled trials. *Journal of Psychosomatic Research* 2010; **68**: 521–33.

7. Raine R, Haines A, Sensky T, Hutchings A, Larkin K, Black N. Systematic review of mental health interventions for patients with common somatic symptoms: can research evidence from secondary care be extrapolated to primary care? *British Medical Journal* 2002; **325**(7372): 1082.

8. Allen LA, Woolfolk RL, Escobar JI, Gara MA, Hamer RM, Allen LA *et al.* Cognitive-behavioral therapy for somatization disorder: a randomized controlled trial. *Archives of Internal Medicine* 2006; **166**(14): 1512–18.

9. Kashner TM, Rost K, Cohen B, Anderson M, Smith GR. Enhancing the health of somatization disorder patients – effectiveness of short-term group-therapy. *Psychosomatics* 1995; **36**(5): 462–70.

10. Huibers MJ, Beurskens AJ, Bleijenberg G, van Schayck CP. The effectiveness of psychosocial interventions delivered by general practitioners. *Cochrane Database of Systematic Reviews* 2003; **2**: CD003494.

11. Blankenstein AH, van der Horst HE, Schilte AF, de Vries D, Zaat JO, Andre KJ *et al.* Development and feasibility of a modified reattribution model for somatising patients, applied by their own general practitioners. *Patient Education and Counseling* 2002; **47**(3): 229–35.

12. Lidbeck J. Group therapy for somatization disorders in general practice: Effectiveness of a short cognitive-behavioural treatment model. *Acta Psychiatrica Scandinavica* 1997; **96**(1): 14–24.

13. Larisch A, Schweickhardt A, Wirsching M, Fritzsche K. Psychosocial interventions for somatizing patients by the general

practitioner – A randomized controlled trial. *Journal of Psychosomatic Research* 2004; **57**(6): 507–14.

14. Volz HP, Moller HJ, Reimann I, Stoll KD. Opipramol for the treatment of somatoform disorders results from a placebo-controlled trial. *European Neuropsychopharmacology* 2000; **10**(3): 211–17.

15. Volz HP, Murck H, Kasper S, Moller HJ. St John's wort extract (LI 160) in somatoform disorders: results of a placebo-controlled trial. *Psychopharmacology* 2002; **164**(3): 294–300.

16. Kroenke K, Messina N, Benattia I, Graepel J, Musgnung J. Venlafaxine extended release in the short-term treatment of depressed and anxious primary care patients with multisomatoform disorder. *Journal of Clinical Psychiatry* 2006; **67**(1): 72–80.

17. Morriss R, Dowrick C, Salmon P, Peters S, Dunn G, Rogers A *et al.* Cluster randomised controlled trial of training practices in reattribution for medically unexplained symptoms. *British Journal of Psychiatry* 2007; **191**: 536–42.

18. Escobar JI, Gara MA, az-Martinez AM, Interian A, Warman M, Allen LA *et al.* Effectiveness of a time-limited cognitive behavior therapy – type intervention among primary care patients with medically unexplained symptoms. *Annals of Family Medicine* 2007; **5**: 328–35.

19. Sumathipala A, Siribaddana S, Abeysingha MR, De Silva P, Dewey M, Prince M *et al.* Cognitive-behavioural therapy v. structured care for medically unexplained symptoms: randomised controlled trial. *British Journal of Psychiatry* 2008; **193**(1): 51–9.

20. Aiarzaguena JM, Grandes G, Gaminde I, Salazar A, Sanchez A, Arino J. A randomized controlled clinical trial of a psychosocial and communication intervention carried out by GPs for patients with medically unexplained symptoms. *Psychological Medicine* 2007; **37**(2): 283–94.

21. Toft T, Rosendal M, Ørnbøl E, Olesen F, Frostholm L, Fink P. Training general practitioners in the treatment of functional

somatic symptoms: effects on patient health in a cluster-randomised controlled trial (the functional illness in primary care study). *Psychotherapy and Psychosomatics* 2010; **79**(4): 227–37.

22. Salmon P, Peters S, Stanley I. Patients' perceptions of medical explanations for somatisation disorders: qualitative analysis. *British Medical Journal* 1999; **318**(7180): 372–6.

23. Thomas KB. General-practice consultations – is there any point in being positive. *British Medical Journal* 1987; **294**(6581): 1200–2.

24. Morriss RK, Gask L, Ronalds C, Downes-Grainger E, Thompson H, Goldberg D. Clinical and patient satisfaction outcomes of a new treatment for somatized mental disorder taught to general practitioners. *British Journal of General Practice* 1999; **49**(441): 263–7.

25. Rosendal M, Bro F, Fink P, Christensen KS, Olesen F, Rosendal M *et al.* Diagnosis of somatisation: effect of an educational intervention in a cluster randomised controlled trial. *British Journal of General Practice* 2003; **53**(497): 917–22.

26. Gask L. Personal communication, 2011.

27. van der Feltz-Cornelis CM, van Oppen P, Ader HJ, van Dyck R, van der Feltz-Cornelis C, van Oppen P *et al.* Randomised controlled trial of a collaborative care model with psychiatric consultation for persistent medically unexplained symptoms in general practice. *Psychotherapy and Psychosomatics* 2006; **75**(5): 282–9.

28. Smith RC, Gardiner JC, Luo ZH, Schooley S, Lamerato L, Rost K. Primary care physicians treat somatization. *Journal of General Internal Medicine* 2009; **24**(7): 829–32.

29. Smith RC, Gardiner JC, Lyles JS, Sirbu C, Dwamena FC, Hodges A *et al.* Exploration of DSM-IV criteria in primary care patients with medically unexplained symptoms. *Psychosomatic Medicine* 2005; **67**(1): 123–9.

30. Smith RC, Lyles JS, Gardiner JC, Sirbu C, Hodges A, Collins C *et al.* Primary care clinicians treat patients with medically unexplained symptoms: A randomized

31. Rosendal M, Olesen F, Fink P. Management of medically unexplained symptoms. *British Medical Journal* 2005; **330**(7481): 4–5.

32. Salmon P, Dowrick CF, Ring A, Humphris GM. Voiced but unheard agendas: qualitative analysis of the psychosocial cues that patients with unexplained symptoms present to general practitioners. *British Journal of General Practice* 2004; **54**(500): 171–6.

33. Salmon P, Humphris GM, Ring A, Davies JC, Dowrick CF. Why do primary care physicians propose medical care to patients with medically unexplained symptoms? A new method of sequence analysis to test theories of patient pressure. *Psychosomatic Medicine* 2006; **68**(4): 570–7.

34. Salmon P, Humphris GM, Ring A, Davies JC, Dowrick CF. Primary care consultations about medically unexplained symptoms: patient presentations and doctor responses that influence the probability of somatic intervention. *Psychosomatic Medicine* 2007; **69**(6): 571–7.

35. Epstein RM, Hadee T, Carroll J, Meldrum SC, Lardner J, Shields CG. 'Could this be something serious?' – Reassurance, uncertainty, and empathy in response to patients' expressions of worry. *Journal of General Internal Medicine* 2007; **22**(12): 1731–9.

36. van Dulmen AM, Fennis JF, Mokkink HG, van der Velden HG, Bleijenberg G. Doctor-dependent changes in complaint-related cognitions and anxiety during medical consultations in functional abdominal complaints. *Psychological Medicine* 1995; **25**(5): 1011–18.

37. McDonald IG, Daly J, Jelinek VM, Panetta F, Gutman JM. Opening Pandora's box: The unpredictability of reassurance by a normal test result. *British Medical Journal* 1996; **313**(7053): 329–32.

38. Stephenson DT, Price JR. Medically unexplained physical symptoms in emergency medicine. *Emergency Medicine Journal* 2006; **23**(8): 595–600.

controlled trial. *Journal of General Internal Medicine* 2006; **21**(7): 671–7.

39. Lucock MP, Morley S, White C, Peake MD. Responses of consecutive patients to reassurance after gastroscopy: results of self administered questionnaire survey. *British Medical Journal* 1997; **315**(7108): 572–5.

40. Howard LM, Wessely S. Reappraising reassurance – The role of investigations. *Journal of Psychosomatic Research* 1996; **41**(4): 307–11.

41. Dowrick CFR. Normalisation of unexplained symptoms by general practitioners: a functional typology. *British Journal of General Practice* 2004; **54**(500): 165–70.

42. Petrie KJ, Muller JT, Schirmbeck F, Donkin L, Broadbent E, Ellis CJ *et al.* Effect of providing information about normal test results on patients' reassurance: randomised controlled trial. *British Medical Journal* 2007; **334**(7589): 352–4.

43. Thomson AB, Page LA. Psychotherapies for hypochondriasis. *Cochrane Database of Systematic Reviews* 2007; **4**: CD006520.

44. Barsky AJ, Ahern DK. Cognitive behavior therapy for hypochondriasis: a randomized controlled trial. *Journal of the American Medical Association* 2004; **291**(12): 1464–70.

45. Sumathipala A. What is the evidence for the efficacy of treatments for somatoform disorders? A critical review of previous intervention studies. *Psychosomatic Medicine* 2007; **69**(9): 889–900.

46. Kroenke K, Swindle R. Cognitive-behavioral therapy for somatization and symptom syndromes: a critical review of controlled clinical trials. *Psychotherapy and Psychosomatics* 2000; **69**(4): 205–15.

47. O'Malley PG, Jackson JL, Santoro J, Tomkins G, Balden E, Kroenke K. Antidepressant therapy for unexplained symptoms and symptom syndromes. *Journal of Family Practice* 1999; **48**(12): 980–90.

48. Jackson JL, O'Malley PG, Kroenke K. Antidepressants and cognitive-behavioral therapy for symptom syndromes. *CNS Spectrums* 2006; **11**(3): 212–22.

49. Moja PL, Cusi C, Sterzi RR, Canepari C. Selective serotonin re-uptake inhibitors (SSRIs) for preventing migraine and tension-type headaches. *Cochrane Database of Systematic Reviews* 2005; **3**: CD002919.

50. Rains JC, Penzien DB, McCrory DC, Gray RN. Behavioral headache treatment: History, review of the empirical literature, and methodological critique. *Headache* 2005; **45**: S92–S109.

51. Abbass A, Kisely S, Kroenke K. Short-term psychodynamic psychotherapy for somatic disorders systematic review and meta-analysis of clinical trials. *Psychotherapy and Psychosomatics* 2009; **78**(5): 265–74.

52. Smeets RJEM, Vlaeyen JWS, Kester AD, Knottnerus JA. Reduction of pain catastrophizing mediates the outcome of both physical and cognitive-behavioral treatment in chronic low back pain. *Journal of Pain* 2006; **7**(4): 261–71.

53. Spinhoven P, ter Kuile M, Kole-Snijders AMJ, Mansfeld MH, den Ouden DJ, Vlaeyen JWS. Catastrophizing and internal pain control as mediators of outcome in the multidisciplinary treatment of chronic low back pain. *European Journal of Pain* 2004; **8**(3): 211–19.

54. Busch AJ, Barber KAR, Overend TJ, Peloso PMJ, Schachter CL. Exercise for treating fibromyalgia syndrome. *Cochrane Database of Systematic Reviews* 2007; **4**: CD003786.

55. Staud R. Biology and therapy of fibromyalgia: pain in fibromyalgia syndrome. *Arthritis Research and Therapy* 2006; **8**(3): 208.

56. van Weering M, Vollenbroek-Hutten MMR, Kotte EM, Hermens HJ. Daily physical activities of patients with chronic pain or fatigue versus asymptomatic controls. A systematic review. *Clinical Rehabilitation* 2007; **21**(11): 1007–23.

57. Clark LV, White PD. The role of deconditioning and therapeutic exercise in chronic fatigue syndrome. *Journal of Mental Health* 2005; **14**: 237–52.

58. Prins JB, Bazelmans E, van der Werf S, van der Meer JWM, Bleijenberg G. Cognitive behaviour therapy for chronic fatigue syndrome: predictors of treatment outcome. *Psycho-Neuro-Endocrino-Immunology* 2002; **1241**: 131–5.

59. White PD. What causes chronic fatigue syndromes? *British Medical Journal* 2004; **329**(7472): 928–9.

60. van Houdenhove B, Luyten P. Customizing treatment of chronic fatigue syndrome and fibromyalgia: the role of perpetuating factors. *Psychosomatics* 2008; **49**(6): 470–7.

61. Surawy C, Hackmann A, Hawton K, Sharpe M. Chronic fatigue syndrome – a cognitive approach. *Behaviour Research and Therapy* 1995; **33**(5): 535–44.

62. Vercoulen JH, Bazelmans E, Swanink CM, Fennis JF, Galama JM, Jongen PJ *et al.* Physical activity in chronic fatigue syndrome: assessment and its role in fatigue. *Journal of Psychiatric Research* 1997; **31**(6): 661–73.

63. Lange M, Petermann F. Influence of depression on fibromyalgia. A systematic review. *Schmerz* 2010; **24**(4): 326–33.

64. Creed F, Ratcliffe J, Fernandes L, Palmer S, Rigby C, Tomenson B *et al.* Outcome in severe irritable bowel syndrome with and without accompanying depressive, panic and neurasthenic disorders. *British Journal of Psychiatry* 2005; **186**: 507–15.

65. Guthrie E, Creed F, Dawson D, Tomenson B. A controlled trial of psychological treatment for the irritable bowel syndrome. *Gastroenterology* 1991; **100**: 450–7.

66. Guthrie E. Brief psychotherapy with patients with refractory irritable bowel syndrome. *British Journal of Psychotherapy* 1991; **8**: 175–88.

67. National Institute for Health and Clinical Excellence. *Irritable Bowel Syndrome in Adults. Diagnosis and Management of Irritable Bowel Syndrome in Primary Care.* London: NICE; 2008.

68. Ford AC, Talley NJ, Schoenfeld PS, Quigley EMM, Moayyedi P. Efficacy of antidepressants and psychological therapies in irritable bowel syndrome: systematic review and meta-analysis. *Gut* 2009; **58**(3): 367–78.

69. Hauser W, Bernardy K, Uceyler N, Sommer C. Treatment of fibromyalgia syndrome with antidepressants: A meta-analysis. *Journal of the American Medical Association* 2009; **301**(2): 198–209.

70. Creed F. How do SSRIs help patients with irritable bowel syndrome? *Gut* 2006; **55**(8): 1065–7.

71. Spiller R, Aziz Q, Creed F, Emmanuel A, Houghton L, Hungin P *et al.* Clinical Services Committee of The British Society of Gastroenterology. Guidelines on the irritable bowel syndrome: mechanisms and practical management. *Gut* 2007; **56**(12): 1770–98.

72. Paiva ES, Jones KD. Rational treatment of fibromyalgia for a solo practitioner. *Best Practice and Research: Clinical Rheumatology* 2010; **24**(3): 341–52.

73. Carville SF, rendt-Nielsen S, Bliddal H, Blotman F, Branco JC, Buskila D *et al.* EULAR evidence-based recommendations for the management of fibromyalgia syndrome. *Annals of the Rheumatic Diseases* 2008; **67**(4): 536–41.

74. National Institute for Health and Clinical Excellence. *Chronic Fatigue Syndrome/ Myalgic Encephalomyelitis: Diagnosis and Management of CFS/ME in Adults and Children.* London: NICE; 2007.

75. Arnold LM, Clauw D, Wang F, Ahl J, Gaynor PJ, Wohlreich MM. Flexible dosed duloxetine in the treatment of fibromyalgia: A randomized, double-blind, placebo-controlled trial. *Journal of Rheumatology* 2010; **37**(12): 2578–86.

76. Arnold LM. Strategies for managing fibromyalgia. *American Journal of Medicine* 2009; **122**(Suppl 12): S31–S43.

77. Aaron LA, Herrell R, Ashton S, Belcourt M, Schmaling K, Goldberg J *et al.* Comorbid clinical conditions in chronic fatigue: a co-twin control study. *Journal of General Internal Medicine* 2001; **16**(1): 24–31.

78. Henningsen P, Zimmermann P. Medically unexplained physical symptoms, anxiety, and depression: a meta-analytic review. *Psychosomatic Medicine* 2003; **65**(4): 528–33.

79. Chambers D, Bagnall AM, Hempel S, Forbes C, Chambers D, Bagnall AM *et al.* Interventions for the treatment, management and rehabilitation of patients with chronic fatigue syndrome/myalgic

encephalomyelitis: an updated systematic review. *Journal of the Royal Society of Medicine* 2006; **99**(10): 506–20.

80. Edmonds M, McGuire H, Price J. Exercise therapy for chronic fatigue syndrome. *Cochrane Database of Systematic Reviews* 2004; **3**: CD003200.

81. Malouff JM, Thorsteinsson EB, Schutte NS. The efficacy of problem solving therapy in reducing mental and physical health problems: A meta-analysis. *Clinical Psychology Review* 2007; **27**(1): 46–57.

82. Price JR, Couper J. Cognitive behaviour therapy for adults with chronic fatigue syndrome. *Cochrane Database of Systematic Reviews* 2000; **2**: CD001027.

83. O'Dowd H, Gladwell P, Rogers CA, Hollinghurst S, Gregory A, O'Dowd H *et al.* Cognitive behavioural therapy in chronic fatigue syndrome: a randomised controlled trial of an outpatient group programme. *Health Technology Assessment* 2006; **10**(37): 1–121.

84. Knoop H, Bleijenberg G, Gielissen MFM, van der Meer JWM, White PD. Is a full recovery possible after cognitive behavioural therapy for chronic fatigue syndrome? *Psychotherapy and Psychosomatics* 2007; **76**(3): 171–6.

85. Deale A, Husain K, Chalder T, Wessely S. Long-term outcome of cognitive behavior therapy versus relaxation therapy for chronic fatigue syndrome: a 5-year follow-up study. *American Journal of Psychiatry* 2001; **158**(12): 2038–42.

86. Powell P, Bentall RP, Nye FJ, Edwards RHT. Patient education to encourage graded exercise in chronic fatigue syndrome – 2-year follow-up of randomised control led trial. *British Journal of Psychiatry* 2004; **184**: 142–6.

87. Stulemeijer M, De Jong LWAM, Fiselier TJW, Hoogveld SWB, Bleijenberg G. Cognitive behaviour therapy for adolescents with chronic fatigue syndrome: randomised controlled trial. *British Medical Journal* 2005; **330**(7481): 14–17.

88. Knoop H, Stulemeijer M, De Jong LWAM, Fiselier TJW, Bleijenberg G. Efficacy of cognitive behavioral therapy for adolescents with chronic fatigue syndrome: Long-term follow-up of a randomized, controlled trial. *Pediatrics* 2008; **121**(3): E619–E25.

89. Chalder T, Deary V, Husain K, Walwyn R. Family-focused cognitive behaviour therapy versus psycho-education for chronic fatigue syndrome in 11- to 18-year-olds: a randomized controlled treatment trial. *Psychological Medicine* 2010; **40**(8): 1269–79.

90. Heins MJ, Knoop H, Prins JB, Stulemeijer M, van der Meer JWM, Bleijenberg G. Possible detrimental effects of cognitive behaviour therapy for chronic fatigue syndrome. *Psychotherapy and Psychosomatics* 2010; **79**(4): 249–56.

91. White PD, Goldsmith KA, Johnson AL, Potts L, Walwyn R, DeCesare JC *et al.* and on behalf of the PACE trial management group. Comparison of adaptive pacing therapy, cognitive behaviour therapy, graded exercise therapy, and socialist medical care for chronic fatigue syndrome (PACE): a randomised trial. *The Lancet* 2011; **377**: 823–36.

92. Knoop H, Prins J, Moss-Morris R, Bleijenberg G. The central role of perception in the perpetuation of chronic fatigue syndrome. *Journal of Psychosomatic Research* 2010; **68**(5): 489–94.

93. Chalder T, Godfrey E, Ridsdale L, King M, Wessely S. Predictors of outcome in a fatigued population in primary care following a randomized controlled trial. *Psychological Medicine* 2003; **33**(2): 283–7.

94. Godfrey E, Chaider T, Ridsdale L, Seed P, Ogden J. Investigating the 'active ingredients' of cognitive behaviour therapy and counselling for patients with chronic fatigue in primary care: developing a new process measure to assess treatment fidelity and predict outcome. *British Journal of Clinical Psychology* 2007; **46**: 253–72.

95. Wiborg JF, Knoop H, Stulemeijer M, Prins JB, Bleijenberg G. How does cognitive behaviour therapy reduce fatigue in patients with chronic fatigue syndrome? The role of physical activity. *Psychological Medicine* 2010; **40**(8): 1281–7.

96. Fulcher KY, White PD. Strength and physiological response to exercise in patients with chronic fatigue syndrome. *Journal of Neurology Neurosurgery and Psychiatry* 2000; **69**(3): 302–7.

97. Moss-Morris R, Sharon C, Tobin R, Baldi JC. A randomized controlled graded exercise trial for chronic fatigue syndrome: Outcomes and mechanisms of change. *Journal of Health Psychology* 2005; **10**(2): 245–59.

98. Bentall RP, Powell P, Nye FJ, Edwards RHT. Predictors of response to treatment for chronic fatigue syndrome. *British Journal of Psychiatry* 2002; **181**: 248–52.

99. de Lange FP, Koers A, Kalkman JS, Bleijenberg G, Hagoort P, van der Meer JWM et al. Increase in prefrontal cortical volume following cognitive behavioural therapy in patients with chronic fatigue syndrome. *Brain* 2008; **131**: 2172–80.

100. Roberts ADL, Papadopoulos AS, Wessely S, Chalder T, Cleare AJ. Salivary cortisol output before and after cognitive behavioural therapy for chronic fatigue syndrome. *Journal of Affective Disorders* 2009; **115**(1–2): 280–6.

101. Tabas G, Beaves M, Wang J, Friday P, Mardini H, Arnold G. Paroxetine to treat irritable bowel syndrome not responding to high-fiber diet: a double-blind, placebo-controlled trial. *American Journal of Gastroenterology* 2004; **99**(5): 914–20.

102. Tack J, Broekaert D, Fischler B, Oudenhove LV, Gevers AM, Janssens J. A controlled crossover study of the selective serotonin reuptake inhibitor citalopram in irritable bowel syndrome. *Gut* 2006; **55**(8): 1095–103.

103. Drossman DA, Toner BB, Whitehead WE, Diamant NE, Dalton CB, Duncan S et al. Cognitive-behavioral therapy versus education and desipramine versus placebo for moderate to severe functional bowel disorders. *Gastroenterology* 2003; **125**(1): 19–31.

104. Vij JC, Jiloha RC, Kumar N. Effect of antidepressant drug (doxepin) on irritable bowel syndrome patients. *Indian Journal of Psychiatry* 1991; **33**: 243–6.

105. Robinson A, Lee V, Kennedy A, Middleton L, Rogers A, Thompson DG et al. A randomised controlled trial of self-help interventions in patients with a primary care diagnosis of irritable bowel syndrome. *Gut* 2006; **55**(5): 643–8.

106. Kennedy T, Jones R, Darnley S, Seed P, Wessely S, Chalder T et al. Cognitive behaviour therapy in addition to antispasmodic treatment for irritable bowel syndrome in primary care: randomised controlled trial. *British Medical Journal* 2005; **331**(7514): 435.

107. Creed F, Fernandes L, Guthrie E, Palmer S, Ratcliffe J, Read N et al. The cost-effectiveness of psychotherapy and paroxetine for severe irritable bowel syndrome. *Gastroenterology* 2003; **124**(2): 303–17.

108. Harris LR, Roberts L. Treatments for irritable bowel syndrome: patients' attitudes and acceptability. *BMC Complementary and Alternative Medicine* 2008; **8**: 65.

109. Häuser W, Thieme K, Turk DC. Guidelines on the management of fibromyalgia syndrome – a systematic review. *European Journal of Pain* 2010; **14**(1): 5–10.

110. Mease PJ, Choy EH. Pharmacotherapy of fibromyalgia. *Rheumatic Disease Clinics of North America* 2009; **35**(2): 359–72.

111. Bernardy K, Fuber N, Kollner V, Hauser W. Efficacy of cognitive-behavioral therapies in fibromyalgia syndrome – a systematic review and metaanalysis of randomized controlled trials. *Journal of Rheumatology* 2010; **37**: 1991–2005.

112. van Koulil S, Effting M, Kraaimaat FW, van Lankveld W, van Helmond T, Cats H et al. Cognitive-behavioural therapies and exercise programmes for patients with fibromyalgia: state of the art and future directions. *Annals of the Rheumatic Diseases* 2007; **66**(5): 571–81.

113. Thieme K, Gromnica-Ihle E, Flor H. Operant behavioral treatment of fibromyalgia: a controlled study. *Arthritis and Rheumatism* 2003; **49**(3): 314–20.

114. Hauser W, Klose P, Langhorst J, Moradi B, Steinbach M, Schiltenwolf M et al. Efficacy

of different types of aerobic exercise in fibromyalgia syndrome: a systematic review and meta-analysis of randomised controlled trials. *Arthritis Research and Therapy* 2010; **12**(3): R79.

115. Arnold LM, Rosen A, Pritchett YL, D'Souza DN, Goldstein DJ, Iyengar S *et al.* A randomized, double-blind, placebo-controlled trial of duloxetine in the treatment of women with fibromyalgia with or without major depressive disorder. *Pain* 2005; **119**(1–3): 5–15.

116. Arnold LM, Lu YL, Crofford LJ, Wohlreich M, Detke MJ, Iyengar S *et al.* A double-blind, multicenter trial comparing duloxetine with placebo in the treatment of fibromyalgia patients with or without major depressive disorder. *Arthritis and Rheumatism* 2004; **50**(9): 2974–84.

117. Russell IJ, Mease PJ, Smith TR, Kajdasz DK, Wohlreich MM, Detke MJ *et al.* Efficacy and safety of duloxetine for treatment of fibromyalgia in patients with or without major depressive disorder: results from a 6-month, randomized, double-blind, placebo-controlled, fixed-dose trial. *Pain* 2008; **136**(3): 432–44.

118. Rooks DS, Gautam S, Romeling M, Cross ML, Stratigakis D, Evans B *et al.* Group exercise, education, and combination self-management in women with fibromyalgia: a randomized trial. *Archives of Internal Medicine* 2007; **167**(20): 2192–200.

119. Kroenke K, Bair MJ, Damush TM, Wu JW, Hoke S, Sutherland J *et al.* Optimized antidepressant therapy and pain self-management in primary care patients with depression and musculoskeletal pain a randomized controlled trial. *Journal of the American Medical Association* 2009; **301**(20): 2099–110.

120. McCrone P, Knapp M, Kennedy T, Seed P, Jones R, Darnley S *et al.* Cost-effectiveness of cognitive behaviour therapy in addition to mebeverine for irritable bowel syndrome. *European Journal of Gastroenterology and Hepatology* 2008; **20**(4): 255–63.

121. Severens JL, Prins JB, van der Wilt GJ, van der Meer JWM, Bleijenberg G. Cost-effectiveness of cognitive behaviour therapy for patients with chronic fatigue syndrome. *QJM – Monthly Journal of the Association of Physicians* 2004; **97**(3): 153–61.

122. McCrone P, Ridsdale L, Darbishire L, Seed P, McCrone P, Ridsdale L *et al.* Cost-effectiveness of cognitive behavioural therapy, graded exercise and usual care for patients with chronic fatigue in primary care. *Psychological Medicine* 2004; **34**(6): 991–9.

123. Goossens ME, Rutten-van Molken MP, Leidl RM, Bos SG, Vlaeyen JW, Teeken-Gruben NJ. Cognitive-educational treatment of fibromyalgia: a randomized clinical trial. II. Economic evaluation. *Journal of Rheumatology* 1996; **23**(7): 1246–54.

124. Tummers M, Knoop H, Bleijenberg G. Effectiveness of stepped care for chronic fatigue syndrome: a randomized noninferiority trial. *Journal of Consulting and Clinical Psychology* 2010; **78**(5): 724–31.

125. Creed F, Tomenson B, Guthrie E, Ratcliffe J, Fernandes L, Read N *et al.* The relationship between somatisation and outcome in patients with severe irritable bowel syndrome. *Journal of Psychosomatic Research* 2008; **64**: 613–20.

Current state of management and organisation of care

4

Per Fink, Chris Burton, Jef De Bie, Wolfgang Söllner and
Kurt Fritzsche

Introduction

This chapter will consider first the unmet need for care among patients with bodily distress syndromes. As discussed in Chapter 2, the term 'bodily distress syndromes' encompasses patients referred to as having medically unexplained symptoms, somatoform disorders or functional somatic syndromes. The chapter then describes current models of care, including those in use in three European countries and specific clinical services for this group of patients. The last section provides a framework for recommending improved services.

Patients with bodily distress syndromes are cared for in many different ways by various medical specialties and health professionals. This is a result of the different modes of presentation, the lack of conceptual clarity about physical and mental disorders, and lack of diagnostic agreement between doctors about this group of patients.

As a result, across Europe and the USA, there is huge heterogeneity regarding how services operate and the types of patients they treat. Patterns of care have developed according to local traditions or dominant political factors, and also as a result of personal relationships and networks between different doctors. For instance, if a prominent cardiologist is interested in psychological issues, it could promote the development of a service for 'non-cardiac chest pain', or a gastroenterologist could promote a service for irritable bowel syndrome (IBS) [1]. In the UK, political pressure has led to the development of a nationwide service for chronic fatigue syndrome. In Germany, the psychosomatic movement has its roots in the environment that existed in the post-war era, but this psychosomatic service is unique to German-speaking countries. In most centres, however, there are no specific services for people with bodily distress and many patients with these symptoms feel that the health services have nothing to offer them once the investigations for possible organic disease have proved negative. In brief, the services for people with bodily distress across Europe and the USA are unsystematic, random and unsatisfactory. Before looking at how current care is organised and providing recommendations for the future organisation of care, we will examine the extent to which current health services actually meet the needs of the patients.

Do current models of care provide a satisfactory service? Unmet needs

The term 'unmet need' usually refers to a recognised, treatable disorder, which is not receiving adequate treatment and where the individuals, as a consequence, suffer impairment, or

Medically Unexplained Symptoms, Somatisation and Bodily Distress, ed. Francis Creed, Peter Henningsen and Per Fink. Published by Cambridge University Press. © Cambridge University Press 2011.

disability, because of the untreated disorder. There is evidence that bodily distress syndromes are treatable (see Chapter 3), yet many patients with bodily distress receive very little adequate treatment.

The evidence of unmet need among patients who have bodily distress syndromes comes from three sets of findings: evidence that specific appropriate treatment is not being offered, evidence of continuing symptoms with accompanying disability/high healthcare use, and patients' views on the availability of treatment.

Evidence that specific appropriate treatment is not being offered

Primary care

In primary and secondary care the proportion of patients with bodily distress is high. The numbers with recognised disorders, such as somatoform disorders and functional somatic syndromes has been described in Chapter 1. It is important to note, however, that not all patients presenting to doctors with bodily distress have unmet needs. Some have transient symptoms that resolve spontaneously so they do not have a treatment need [2].

A Danish primary care study examined whether patients with medically unexplained symptoms received adequate treatment. The study included 38 general practitioners (GPs) and 1785 patients [3]. For each patient, the GPs judged the current treatment to be: (i) adequate/best possible; (ii) inadequate as the GP needed more time in their own practice; or (iii) inadequate as the GP would have referred to a specialist if possible. GPs considered their own treatment as adequate for only half of the patients with medically unexplained symptoms (Table 4.1). This compared with 95.3% of the patients who had well-defined physical disease. Of patients with medically unexplained symptoms whose treatment was deemed to be inadequate, the GPs would have referred approximately half to a specialist, if possible. For the other half, the GPs felt they could have offered better treatment if they had more time to treat them in their own practice. Thus, to make treatment adequate for all patients with medically unexplained symptoms, GPs would need more time to treat them in primary care and a suitable specialist to whom the more severely affected patients could be referred. This study indicates clearly that the care of patients with bodily distress is lagging far behind the care offered to patients with physical diseases.

Another way to document the extent to which there is unmet need for patients with bodily distress can be found in the literature regarding depression. At least half of patients with depressive disorder seen in primary care present to their GP with numerous medically unexplained symptoms [4]. Such depression often goes unrecognised and untreated, and the risk of this happening is greater when the patient presents with numerous bodily symptoms [5;6]. Thus many patients with numerous bodily symptoms caused by depression go untreated and the bodily symptoms persist.

Secondary care – outpatients

In secondary-care clinics, bodily distress disorders are common and tend to be more persistent than in primary care (see Chapter 1). It has been documented that less than 10% of patients with medically unexplained symptoms receive specific treatment with antidepressants or psychological treatment [7;8;9;10]. Of patients attending specialist medical clinics with medically unexplained symptoms, anxiety and depression were documented in the case notes of one-third, yet only 4% were referred to psychiatrists and only 2% started on antidepressants [7]. In a similar, more recent study, psychosocial factors were recorded in over half of patients with medically unexplained symptoms, yet only 3% were referred to a psychiatrist, 7% were

Table 4.1 Unmet need for care in primary care patients [3]

Reason for encounter according to GP	Optimal		Inadequate[a]		Inadequate[b]	
	n	%	N	%	N	%
Physical disease	949	95.3	20	2.0	27	2.7
Probable physical disease	311	79.9	38	9.8	40	10.3
Medically unexplained symptoms	119	53.6	55	24.8	48	21.6
Mental disorder (with or without somatic symptoms)	51	56.7	13	14.4	26	28.9

[a] More time in practice needed.
[b] Wants to refer the patient to specialist but none available.
$\chi^2 = 318.9$, degrees of freedom = 8; $p<0.001$.

started on antidepressants and lifestyle advice given to 8% [8]. In a third study the neurologist considered that psychological or psychiatric treatment was appropriate in 40% of outpatients with medically unexplained symptoms, but one year later most complaints remained unresolved suggesting that effective treatment was not given [11;12].

A case-note study of patients with IBS attending a specialist clinic in the USA found that fewer subsequent clinic visits for irritable bowel syndrome (IBS) were associated with a positive patient–doctor interaction at the first consultation [13]. A positive interaction was one in which the doctor had taken and recorded a brief psychosocial history, investigated the reasons for seeking medical help and held a detailed discussion of diagnosis and treatment with the patient. These indicators of a positive interaction were present in fewer than a half of the doctor–patient encounters, however.

A pan-European study of unmet need in IBS identified those faced by patients and doctors [14]. From the patient's perspective the three unmet needs are: limited awareness and understanding of IBS as a medical condition; simple, non-invasive diagnostic procedures; and affordable, readily available treatments. The suggested remedies for these unmet needs were patient education schemes (see Chapter 8), an algorithm focusing on positive diagnosis and new treatment targeting the multiple symptoms of IBS. The last refers to the multiple somatic symptoms known as 'extraintestinal' symptoms of IBS, but which are better regarded as symptoms of bodily distress because of their associated treatment needs. This study recognised also the unmet needs from the doctors' perspective. These included better understanding of IBS, simple diagnostic procedures, treatment guidelines and effective, well-tolerated first-line treatments. The suggested remedies were: physician education, development of practice-based algorithm, pan-European treatment guidelines and new treatments targeting multiple IBS symptoms. The last referred to new drugs that act on the gastrointestinal tract rather than psychological treatments, which would be preferable (see Chapter 8).

A further insight into unmet needs in routine patient–doctor interactions can be gained from an intervention study in which physicians received minimal training and information on each patient's expectations of the consultation, their degree of illness worry and whether psychiatric disorder was present [15]. Consultations with patients who have bodily distress have gained a reputation for being regarded as 'difficult', but the proportion thus rated was halved after the intervention probably because the patients' unmet expectations of the consultation were reduced greatly. The doctors reported that addressing patients' symptom-related expectations did not take extra time. This study demonstrates, firstly, that prior to this intervention, patients had unmet needs in terms of unaddressed concerns, and, secondly, that it was quite easy to meet these needs.

Inpatients

Although the general impression is that patients with bodily distress are rarely admitted to medical wards nowadays, Danish studies have found mental illness and somatoform disorders to be the two most common psychiatric diagnoses among medical inpatients [9;10;16;17;18]. Of all those with psychiatric disorder, only 2.7% were referred to a consultation-liaison service, and 5.1% were already receiving psychiatric treatment [10]. The vast majority of patients with bodily distress and other psychiatric disorders remained untreated. Even when depressive disorders are detected and treated on a medical ward, the treatment may be discontinued at discharge – another source of unmet need [19].

The European Consultation Liaison Psychiatry Workgroup (ECLW) study collected data on 34 500 patients admitted to acute wards of general hospitals across Europe [20]. Although the prevalence of somatoform disorder in this cohort was 14%, only 61 patients (0.002%) were referred to a consultation-liaison psychiatry service with this diagnosis. A Danish study which included 294 consecutive internal medical inpatients found a prevalence of somatoform disorder of 17.6% [21]. Psychiatric consultations were few and most patients did not receive specific treatment for this disorder.

In a study on 198 new patients referred to a neurological unit as in- or outpatients, 16 cases of somatoform disorders were found by psychiatric research interview [9;16]. Of these, only three were referred to a psychologist or psychiatrist, and all three were already under treatment for a mental disorder by their GP before admission; none of the remainder was referred for psychiatric treatment. In a UK study, approximately half of the patients admitted to a neurology ward had medically unexplained symptoms (with or without concomitant organic disease) and for 60% of these, there was evidence of underlying psychiatric disorder [22]. The majority of these patients were not routinely referred to a psychiatrist, although some were prescribed antidepressants in low doses, which is likely to be ineffective for depressive disorder.

It can be concluded that the vast majority of in- and outpatients with bodily distress disorders in neurology, gastroenterology and general medical units do not receive appropriate treatment. They are rarely referred to a consultation-liaison psychiatric service and, if antidepressants are commenced, they may be discontinued at discharge. This represents unmet need.

Evidence of continuing symptoms with accompanying disability/ high healthcare use

Follow-up studies have shown that left untreated, bodily distress syndromes continue to be associated with disability and high healthcare costs. In a Dutch follow-up study of patients who had been investigated at a medical clinic and were found to have medically unexplained symptoms, 63% reported some improvement of their symptoms, but only 38% considered themselves to be in good health [23]. In a similar study of patients with medically unexplained symptoms attending hospital clinics in the UK, at 6-month follow-up 40% reported improvement in symptoms, although their health status was still impaired [24]. For the remaining 60%, their symptoms were the same or worse and their health status remained one standard deviation below the population norm. A smaller study of neurology outpatients showed that 54% remained the same or deteriorated during the eight months following a new outpatient appointment [12].

Factors known to be associated with continued high healthcare use among patients with bodily distress include continuing psychiatric disorder, persistent high number of bodily symptoms and high levels of health anxiety [18;25;26;27;28]. Some studies of single syndromes have indicated that depression may be responsible for a part of the disability associated with functional somatic syndromes (see Chapter 1) [29], whereas epidemiological studies including a broader range of patients have shown that psychiatric disorders and bodily distress result in an independent increase in healthcare use [18;27;30].

Follow-up studies have shown that primary-care patients with a moderate number of medically unexplained symptoms continue to have disability over a five-year period [31]. This is often associated with continuing depression. On the other hand, a follow-up study of health anxiety (hypochondriasis) showed persistent impairment during a two-year follow-up period with healthcare costs approximately 75% higher than those of patients with well-defined medical condition. The impairment and healthcare costs were independent of the presence of a depression or anxiety disorder [28].

Unmet needs are seen most clearly when treated and untreated patients with the same disorder are compared. In the study of severe IBS (see p. 27), patients with numerous somatic symptoms outside the gastrointestinal tract who received either psychotherapy or antidepressants improved in their health status score by 4–6 points on the Medical Outcome Survey Short Form (SF)-36 physical component summary score (equivalent to one standard deviation on this measure) [32]. By contrast, similar patients who received 'usual treatment' experienced a deterioration of their health status of approximately five points (right-hand column in Figure 4.1) and they continued to incur extremely high healthcare costs. The latter is a very clear description of unmet need; denied the psychotherapeutic or antidepressant treatment used by those in the other arms of the trial, these patients experienced worsening of their health-related quality of life.

Patient-centred approaches to unmet need

The most sophisticated approach to unmet need includes a dimension that is usually ignored – does the person who has unmet need want help from the medical or related professional [33;34]?

There is evidence that patients seeking help with medically unexplained symptoms in secondary-care medical units are not keen to entertain the idea of psychological treatment. In the neurology outpatients study mentioned above, the neurologist identified a need for psychological treatment in over half of patients with medically unexplained symptoms [11]. Fewer than a quarter of these patients saw the need for psychological treatment.

In another study, most patients with psychiatric disorders in a neurology unit (the majority of whom would have bodily distress), had not been asked by the neurologist about their mood. The majority were content about this because they felt it was inappropriate for the

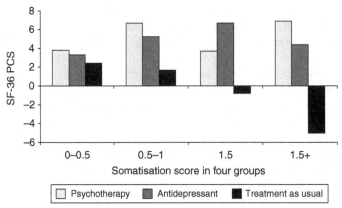

Figure 4.1 Change in health status in patients with severe irritable bowel syndrome between baseline and 15 months later. Increase in Medical Outcome Survey Short Form (SF)-36 physical component score (PCS; representing improved health status) shown as a positive score and vice versa. Patients treated with psychotherapy (light grey) or antidepressants (dark grey) generally showed improvement even if they were in the high somatisation group (1.5+). Patients in this group receiving treatment as usual experienced considerable deterioration in their health status.

neurologist to ask about psychological aspects of illness. The neurologist was perceived as a doctor who investigated only physical causes for their symptoms [35]. Additional reasons for patients not thinking that the neurologist should have asked about their mood included the neurologist's lack of time, the lack of privacy on the ward and the neurologist's tendency to use jargon and be evasive or vague when asked specific questions.

Unmet need based on patient perceptions is understudied in mental health [34], and rarely studied in bodily distress. One study of primary-care patients with persistent somatoform disorder found that approximately one-third did not wish for treatment so they could not be regarded as having unmet need [36]. Of the remainder, one-half were either in treatment or not considered to be suitable, so only one-third of the cohort required treatment and were prepared to receive it.

Two small studies have taken a patient-centred approach towards patients' goals of treatment. Affleck and colleagues studied women with fibromyalgia and found that only around 20% sought recovery, the remainder being equally split between seeking to live with their condition and to be accepted by others [37]. Nordin and colleagues interviewed patients with medically unexplained symptoms and their physicians [38]. The majority (62%) of patients hoped for support from the doctor and many (40%) reported that improvement in function and coping was their main goal of treatment [38].

A particular set of potential unmet needs relates to patients' views of treatment; there were several themes reported in one study of patients with IBS [39]. Patients disliked certain modalities, such as the fear of side effects from drugs or the pain of acupuncture, although some had said they wished for 'non-medical' treatment. Some were sceptical of the efficacy of certain treatments, including homeopathy and hypnotherapy. Quite a few patients considered that their condition was not severe enough to merit drugs or similar medical treatment. Many patients expressed a desire for more information but would be very persuaded if the clinician recommended a particular treatment. This description of patients' feelings about possible treatment suggests that many patients have an important unmet need for more information about possible treatments. This need is generally best met by the doctor explaining the treatment options clearly in an unbiased way.

Reasons for unmet needs

A number of psychiatric studies have explored why patients' needs are not met. Perceived stigma concerning use of psychiatric services is a very important factor that may inhibit many patients seeking such treatment. Good social support seems to reduce the perceived need for professional help.

Many medical specialists recognise the need for psychological or psychiatric treatment but complain that they do not have immediate access to a skilled mental health professional who could assess the patients and take them on for treatment if necessary. An appointment at a psychiatric clinic is often rejected by patients with bodily distress because of the stigma of attending a psychiatric unit, often expressed as 'I am not imagining the pain'. There is a lack of suitably skilled specialists in managing bodily distress working in general medical settings to whom medical specialists can refer patients with multiple somatic symptoms.

There is some evidence that the main problem lies in the doctor–patient interaction in the clinics. In secondary care, it has been documented that physicians are preoccupied by the search for a medical explanation for symptoms rather than attempting to make a positive diagnosis [40]. This leads to numerous technological investigations, whose repeated use may reinforce the patient's fear that organic disease is being missed. This reliance on technological investigations usually means that psychological problems are discussed only at the end of the diagnostic search. At this point the patient who is told that there is no explanation for the symptoms is likely to doubt the doctor's competence and seek an opinion from another doctor [41]. It seems to be the presence of numerous somatic symptoms, rather than the presence of anxiety and depression which leads some doctors to regard their interactions with these patients as frustrating [42]. It is likely that doctors' negative attitudes towards psychosocial aspects of patient care is a major contributing factor [43;44].

There is some indirect evidence that a positive doctor–patient interaction may lead to symptomatic improvement and reduced health service use. A reduction in number of visits by patients with IBS following a positive interaction with a gastroenterologist appears to result from less anxiety, reduced fear of cancer and less preoccupation with pain [45]. Thus a continued high rate of medical consultations may indicate continuing anxiety about illness – unmet need [46].

Many doctors do not have the skills and understanding to make the diagnosis of a bodily distress disorder accurately. The common misunderstanding that emotional or social stress is a necessary precondition for the diagnosis of bodily distress, and that behavioural and psychological treatment will work only in these cases, may also be a reason why patients are not diagnosed and treated.

Conclusion

Although studies of the measurement of unmet need for patients with bodily distress are limited, there is sufficient evidence that the majority of patients with persistent bodily distress have considerable unmet need. Efficacious treatment exists, but most patients do not receive such treatment – largely because it is not offered to them.

Current models of care

Service delivery for patients with bodily distress syndromes varies greatly across Europe. Patients with this type of disorder may be seen in general medical services where, as we have seen, the chances of getting good treatment are rather slim. There is a growing number of services that are being specifically established to deal with patients who have bodily distress syndromes, but these are still very much in the minority. These services recognise that bodily distress syndromes, at least when severe, are a group of disorders in their own right that require specific treatment, and not as a phenomenon secondary to another mental illness

Ideally, the management of these patients should be organised according to a stepped-care model with milder disorders treated in primary care and a hierarchy of services that match each level of severity with an appropriate intensity of treatment up to and including the possibility of collaborative care [47;48] (see Chapter 8). Existing services will be described, therefore, in terms of three tiers:

(1) non-specialised general medical services, where most patients with bodily distress syndromes are seen

(2) specialist services for individual functional somatic syndromes or diagnoses (e.g. chronic fatigue syndrome, fibromyalgia, somatoform disorders)

(3) specialist services for all types of bodily distress syndromes, i.e. including functional somatic syndromes and somatoform disorders. This type of specialised service is based on the view that the same treatment methods are effective regardless of the patient's label, and hence only a small adaptation of the therapy is needed for each patient.

The different models of service delivery for bodily distress syndromes are displayed in Figures 4.2, 4.3 and 4.4.

Traditional, non-specialised services (Model A, Figure 4.2)

Primary care

Most patients with bodily distress are seen in primary care. A few countries have developed a model of specialised treatment of bodily distress within primary care. The specialisation in primary care may appear inappropriate, but it is probably a natural consequence of the huge unmet need for care for this patient group and the fact that neither secondary mental health nor general medical services offer any specialist treatment appropriate for this group of patients. Only a minority of psychiatrists and psychologists have the appropriate skills or knowledge to diagnose and treat patients with bodily distress.

Some countries have introduced generic training for GPs which includes management of patients presenting with bodily distress. However, most of these training programmes focus on improving the GPs' general psychological and communication skills and do not focus specifically on bodily distress syndromes. For instance, in Germany the GPs are reimbursed for 'talk' therapy if they have trained in psychosocial treatment. In Denmark, more specific programmes for bodily distress have been established during recent years (see also Chapter 9). However, experience has shown that such training of GPs is not sufficient to provide adequate care for patients with bodily distress.

Models of collaborative care, in which the GPs are supported in their management by specialists at different levels, may be a way of improving care in primary care [49]. However, a precondition for this model is the existence of a local specialised service for bodily distress syndromes (psychiatrist, psychologist and/or nurses) with which the GP can collaborate, and this is only available in a few places worldwide.

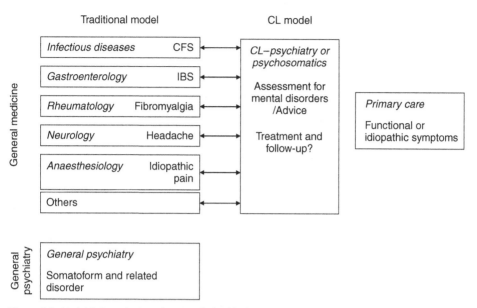

Figure 4.2 Model A: Organisation of services for bodily distress syndromes
CL, consultation-liaison; CFS, chronic fatigue syndrome; IBS, irritable bowel syndrome.

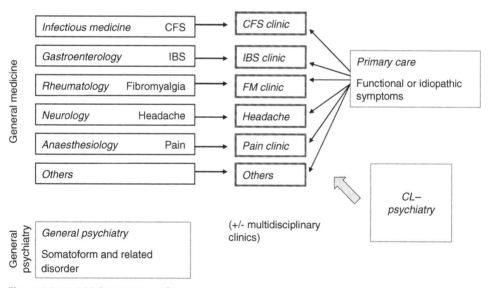

Figure 4.3 Model B: Syndrome-specific specialised clinics
CL, consultation-liaison; CFS, chronic fatigue syndrome; IBS, irritable bowel syndrome.

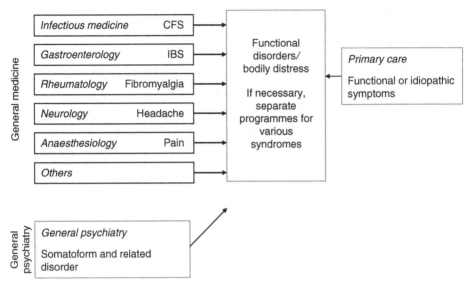

Figure 4.4 Model C: Specialised clinic for bodily distress syndromes
CL, consultation-liaison; CFS, chronic fatigue syndrome; IBS, irritable bowel syndrome.

Service delivery in secondary care

General mental health services

Patients with bodily distress syndromes are rarely seen in general psychiatric services, and only patients displaying prominent emotional symptoms or who have a concurrent mental disorder in addition to their bodily distress are seen. However, patients with health anxiety (hypochondriasis) may be included in programmes for anxiety.

Consultation-liaison psychiatry/psychosomatics approach

Consultation-liaison psychiatry or psychosomatics is the only medical or psychiatric subspecialty having bodily distress as a target group. For most consultation-liaison psychiatry services, however, bodily distress is only part of their service, and some services do not offer any specific care for this patient group. In the large European study of general hospital patients referred to 56 consultation-liaison psychiatric services, 19% of the patients were referred because of 'medically unexplained symptoms' [50]. Only eight of these fifty-six consultation-liaison services, however, had a marked preponderance of patients referred with bodily distress; six of these were psychosomatic services in Germany, in which approximately 65% of referrals were for medically unexplained symptoms. The psychosomatic services of Germany are better organised than most others to meet the needs of patients with bodily distress syndromes.

An early survey of a consultation-liaison psychiatry service in the USA found that 38% of referrals were for somatisation [51]. A more recent large survey of patients referred to an American consultation-liaison service found that approximately 10% of referrals from the medical inpatient units had bodily distress syndromes; this compared with 15.5% of patients seen in a psychosomatic outpatient clinic and 4% of referrals to the community psychiatry service [52]. By contrast, a smaller UK study reported that bodily distress disorders accounted for 28% of referrals to a consultation-liaison psychiatry service from medical inpatient wards, 45% of referrals to the consultation-liaison psychiatry outpatient clinic and 14% of referrals direct from primary care [53]. Three other UK consultation-liaison psychiatry services reported that the proportion of patients referred with medically unexplained symptoms was 30%, 12% and 9% in the three services, respectively [41].

General medicine

Patients with bodily distress syndromes are often seen in various medical specialties (IBS in gastroenterology clinics, fibromyalgia in rheumatology clinics, chronic fatigue in endocrine or neurology clinics, etc.). In most cases, the patients are investigated for possible organic disease and referred back to primary care without any specific treatment having been commenced. If the patients also have emotional symptoms, a referral to psychiatry may be tried, but, as mentioned above, often these patients are also neglected by general psychiatry, especially as general psychiatry services are primarily focused on psychotic disorders [54;55].

Some medical specialists have responded to the large number of patients attending their clinics with these disorders by developing, within their own service, a special interest facility for treating 'their own' functional somatic syndrome, such as rheumatologists treating fibromyalgia or gastroenterologists treating IBS (Figure 4.3). The care is mostly monodisciplinary and not coordinated between specialists, so patients with numerous somatic symptoms are at high risk of moving between the different clinics. For example, abdominal symptoms lead to a referral to the gastroenterology clinic, musculoskeletal pains to rheumatology and fatigue to neurology. In a few centres, the management occurs in collaboration with a consultation-liaison psychiatrist or a health psychologist. An example is the collaboration of neuro-otology and consultation-liaison psychiatry in Sweden in the treatment of chronic dizziness [56].

Although this model seems to be poorly coordinated and meeting the needs only of a narrow patient group, this model is the most common in most countries. For patients with a single functional somatic syndrome it may work quite well, however, especially as it is sometimes linked to a helpful patient group concerned with that particular disorder (e.g. IBS network (www.thegutrust.org) or fibromyalgia support (www.fibromyalgia-uk.org). The organisation of care in this model is unsystematic and dependent on local initiatives and personal interests, although some of the established programmes may function very well.

Syndrome-specific specialised clinics (Model B, Figure 4.3)

Many countries have developed specialist services for various functional somatic syndromes. The most common example is pain clinics, which are found in most countries. Some of these clinics focus not on functional or idiopathic pain but on pain caused by well-defined disease, such as cancer and neurogenic pain, but others are primarily treating patients with functional or idiopathic pain or a mixture of patients.

Except for pain clinics, the type of specialist clinics for various functional somatic syndromes varies greatly between countries. In the UK and Netherlands, there are well-developed services for chronic fatigue syndrome (e.g. see www.manchestercfsme.nhs.uk/). In Belgium and Norway, huge networks of clinics for chronic fatigue syndrome are being set up under the central initiative of the governments. In other countries, chronic fatigue syndrome clinics do not exist at all, for instance in the other Nordic countries and Germany. In some countries there are other specialist clinics, e.g. for multiple chemical sensitivity and fibromyalgia in Denmark. These types of clinic are often not established by doctors, according to their patients' needs, but by official authorities who have been persuaded to establish a special service for a particular group. Politicians may be under pressure from patient organisations and/or the media, which may highlight an individual case of suffering. An example of this is the clinics established for patients with amalgam poisoning in Sweden during the 1990s, which were subsequently closed because of the disappointing results. More recently, clinics for multiple chemical sensitivity have been established in many countries under pressure from patient organisations.

The specialised clinics for individual functional somatic syndromes are often organised and run by medical specialists from the specialty of the organ in question. This may be the only way such clinics can be funded, but the monodisciplinary nature of such clinics is a drawback. Pain clinics may be headed by various medical specialists, most commonly by anaesthetists, but GPs, psychiatrists, psychologists and neurologists are also involved in assessing and treating patients in these clinics. There seems to be general agreement that the multidisciplinary team model is most suitable for patients with severe bodily distress syndromes and functional somatic syndromes as the same treatment seems to be effective across various functional somatic syndromes [47]. Establishing different clinics, one for each functional somatic syndrome, is therefore wasteful of resources and probably limits the number of disciplines involved. As a natural consequence of this, some specialised clinics are expanding to include other functional somatic syndromes but often they remain within the domain of a single medical subspecialty and the treatment is dominated by pharmacological methods of treatment [57]. A disadvantage of these syndrome-specific clinics is that they sanction the separate, specialty-dominated view of the functional somatic syndromes and perpetuate fragmented care instead of moving towards a more generic model.

Specialised units for bodily distress syndromes (Model C, Figure 4.4)

Several different types of care have evolved at a few centres around Europe in an attempt to improve the quality of care offered to the broader group of patients with bodily distress. One new approach is based on the identification of bodily distress syndrome as a diagnosis in its own right, and which encompasses the functional somatic syndromes and somatoform disorders but with different subtypes, reflecting severity. This approach is supported by studies that have indicated a huge overlap in symptoms and illness pictures between patients who have received different diagnostic labels. Furthermore, the same treatment methods, such as cognitive behavioural therapy (CBT), antidepressants and physical activation, have proven to be effective for the patients regardless of their diagnosis, whereas somatic treatment has shown no effect [47]. As there seem to be more similarities than differences between the patients, it therefore appears rational to treat them within the same service. Larger groups of therapists with different areas of expertise can offer a wider range of therapies within the academic setting. This may also prevent simultaneous treatment by different services or sequential treatment in different clinics, and it would make referrals much easier for GPs with only one point of entry into secondary care. Additionally, it seems to be a herculean task to establish services for each functional syndrome and even single symptoms because of the high number of functional somatic syndromes that have been suggested.

These specialised units are designed for patients with the complicated functional somatic syndromes, or multiorgan bodily distress syndromes. It is unclear whether such units can meet the full demand for the intensive multidisciplinary treatment required by such patients – perhaps they should be strictly limited to the treatment of these complex patients. Some might also have the capacity for patients with single-organ functional somatic syndromes, who can also benefit from a management programme such as CBT tailored to their particular problem (see Chapter 3). It would be preferable if a separate, but linked, service could cater for single-organ bodily distress syndromes, in which the effective drugs for these conditions could be used in tandem with psychological treatments. The specialised units for patients with complicated or multiorgan bodily distress syndromes do not usually use drugs as part of their treatment regimen.

The following descriptions of relevant services in Belgium and Germany highlight the different types of service which might address the needs of patients with severe bodily distress disorders. The German psychosomatic model applies currently to German-speaking countries only. The situation in Belgium is more typical of most European countries.

Relevant services in Belgium and Germany
Services in Belgium

In Belgium, there exists no such thing as a psychosomatic clinic. Patients with mild to moderate bodily distress syndromes are mostly treated on an outpatient basis, by their GP or the medical specialist to whom the patient self-refers or to whom she or he is referred by their GP. The care is mostly monodisciplinary, fragmented and not coordinated. The non-structured organisation of healthcare in Belgium encourages patients to go from one specialist to another, which is associated with repeated investigations for possible organic disease and high healthcare costs.

The needs of patients who are more severely disabled by a bodily distress syndrome and/or who have comorbid psychiatric conditions are not met. Their care is mostly neglected by mainstream medicine (somatic and psychiatric) and spread out over several clinics, dependent on local initiatives and personal interests. The national health insurance does not give incentives for the development of more integrated care models and pathways. There are two exceptions, however: the government has initiated the development of expert centres for chronic fatigue syndrome and multidisciplinary pain clinics. Local initiatives have been started to provide care for those patients whose needs were not met by the existing healthcare organisation. Several general hospitals have started to develop more medical rehabilitation programmes, led by specialists in physical medicine/rehabilitation medicine (graded exercise therapy (GET)). The following initiatives are particularly relevant to people with more severe bodily distress syndromes.

Expert centres for chronic fatigue syndrome and pain clinics

Since 2002, Belgium's national health insurance (RIZIV/INAMI) has funded five expert centres ('referentiecentra') for the diagnosis and treatment of chronic fatigue syndrome. They are situated within five university hospitals (tertiary care), four for adults and one for children. They are multidisciplinary (psychiatrists, psychologists, physiotherapists) and are run by doctors in internal medicine. They focus mainly on the diagnosis of chronic fatigue syndrome and have a basic day-clinic treatment programme with the focus on GET, pacing and CBT. In 2006, an audit of their functioning was, however, quite disappointing. The main points of criticism were: the disappointingly low number of patients who went back to work and the myopic view focused on chronic fatigue syndrome alone and not on other medically unexplained symptoms. At this moment, the RIZIV/INAMI has asked a working committee to develop a new plan that should guarantee that both primary and secondary care (university-affiliated hospitals) become more involved in the care of these patients. Several issues have already come to light during this review, such as the tension between a clinic solely for chronic fatigue syndrome versus a clinic that includes other functional somatic syndromes, and developing new guidelines concerning the nature, severity and duration of which disorders should be referred to which clinics for what kind of treatment.

Patients with chronic pain can consult pain clinics. These are run by anaesthetists and are developed locally within most general hospitals. Nine of these centres have been given additional resources by RIZIV/INAMI and serve as reference centres for chronic pain. They are funded to provide multidisciplinary assessment and treatment with input from nurses, physiotherapists, psychologists and psychiatrists.

Local initiatives

Given the unmet needs of patients with severe bodily distress disorders, four Flemish hospitals have started to offer more integrated treatment modalities. Three provide a day treatment programme and one offers an inpatient treatment programme. It is important to note that the programmes are open to all forms of severe bodily distress syndromes and that the use of specific diagnostic labels or specific somatic syndromes (chronic fatigue syndrome, fibromyalgia, etc.) does not limit participation in these programmes unlike the 'official' chronic fatigue syndrome centres. All initiatives were borne out of a perceived need for patients with severe bodily distress syndromes in local psychiatric services. Other (general medical) local health services could not provide the care needed for these patients. Unfortunately, no formal research or audit data have been obtained in these centres.

The *psychiatric day clinic* programmes have been developed from pre-existing consultation-liaison psychiatry services in general hospitals. They combine evidence-based treatment modalities such as GET and CBT with psychodynamic forms of therapy and mind-body therapy (focusing for instance on mentalisation). In Bruges, a more specific psychotherapeutic approach (short-term or problem-focused psychotherapy) is used in combination with evidence-based treatments. Both in Bruges and in Duffel, strong working relations and involvement with physical medicine/rehabilitation medicine have been developed.

In 2004, a modified *inpatient programme* was started for 10 patients in a psychiatric hospital at Sint-Truiden. The target group is patients with somatoform disorders combined with other severe mental health problems (major depressive disorders, anxiety disorders, substance abuse, dissociative disorder, personality disorders) who cannot be managed in outpatient clinics or consultation-liaison settings or whose needs cannot be met in a classic psychiatric outpatient clinic. Most patients have a history of traumatic childhood experiences.

Initially, patients participate in a programme that is CBT orientated, with a focus on GET and pacing. The programme is tailored to the needs of the individual patient and in the course of their treatment other psychotherapeutic sessions are added, directed at substance abuse, depression, anxiety, childhood traumas, etc. The psychiatric clinic has several psychologists with different psychotherapeutic backgrounds, who are able to join the team providing treatment for these complex cases. Family and individual therapy is often necessary. The focus of the treatment is on the consequences of their illness, the perpetuating factors, acceptance of physical constraints, modifying illness behaviours and treating comorbid psychiatric conditions.

The stepped-care programme starts with an observation period of three weeks and continues with treatment periods of six weeks. In the course of their treatment, patients can switch from being inpatients to day patients (on the same ward). There is no fixed duration of hospitalisation. On average, patients are hospitalised for six months.

The German psychosomatic model

The origins of psychosomatic medicine in Germany are more deeply rooted in internal medicine and psychoanalysis than in psychiatry. Indeed, psychosomatic medicine has often been in conflict with, or even in opposition to, psychiatry, not least because of a fundamental difference in methods: in Germany, psychiatry was mostly dismissive of psychotherapy up until 20 years ago, whereas this has always been the main therapeutic method in psychosomatic medicine.

Since the 1970s, independent departments of psychosomatic medicine and psychotherapy have been firmly established, separate from psychiatric and psychological institutions, with their own inpatient and outpatient facilities as well as teaching and research objectives. In 2007, 151 departments of psychosomatic medicine existed throughout Germany (compared with 408 departments of psychiatry and 133 departments of child and adolescent psychiatry) and about 50 000 patients were treated in psychosomatic medicine departments. Most university hospitals have such a department, but they also exist in other public and in private settings. It has to be said, however, that some of the large departments for psychosomatic medicine do not particularly specialise in treating patients with bodily distress syndromes, but primarily care for patients with affective disorders, burn-out syndromes, etc.

Psychosomatic medicine in Germany is based on two conceptual traditions. An integrative tradition, mainly based in internal medicine, stressed a biopsychosocial model long before this term was coined in the 1970s; it was good for reaching a diagnosis and the general rules of 'Umgang', i.e. at doctor–patient communication and for patients with bodily distress, but it was not necessarily good at specialised therapy. The latter was the main emphasis of the psychogenic tradition, which was firmly based on psychoanalysis and its applications. However, as discussed in other chapters, for several reasons this approach is problematic in the field of bodily distress syndromes, because, among other aspects, it alienates many patients. Modern psychosomatic medicine in Germany tries to combine and develop both traditions, applying specialised therapy against the background of a biopsychosocial model of aetiology in settings that are optimally independent and equidistant between classical somatic and psychological medicine.

Germany offers three levels of psychosocial medical services for management of patients with bodily distress syndromes.

Level 1: Management of bodily distress by GPs – psychosomatic basic care

A curriculum of 80 hours, combining theory, communication training and Balint group work, was introduced into primary care routine in 1987 and was a milestone in improving psychosocial care. This led to a growing interest in psychosomatic care by primary care physicians. In 1992, psychosomatic basic care was defined as an educational standard for all clinical disciplines and, since 1994, standard requirements for the training were established. Primary care physicians and gynaecologists have to complete at least 40 hours of the curriculum during their specialisation, but most physicians follow the full curriculum under their own motivation. More than 60 000 of the 360 000 German GPs have completed courses in psychosomatic basic care. Having completed the training in psychosomatic basic care, these GPs may later be reimbursed, in their practice, for certain longer consultations with their patients, but the amount of money paid for this is very small. Even with training in psychosomatic basic care, many patients with bodily distress prove difficult to manage in primary care. Therefore, collaborative groups of primary-care physicians and psychotherapists have been established in some places to develop and provide more specific treatments for somatising patients. The treatment manual [58] developed by these groups utilises training and interventions based on the reattribution model and the TERM model [59;60] adapted to the German primary-care setting.

Level 2: Collaborative models of management of medically unexplained symptoms: specialists cooperating with physicians in primary care or in general hospitals

At a second level, outpatient psychotherapy is provided by thousands of psychologists and doctors in their private practices. Psychodynamic and cognitive behavioural psychotherapy are mostly covered by health insurance, for up to more than 100 sessions. However, there are two problems at this level of care for patients with bodily distress syndromes: first, only some patients with bodily distress syndromes are willing to go to psychotherapy for help with their problems, and second, many psychotherapists lack sufficient specialised skills for managing patients with these syndromes; they prefer prototypical psychologically minded patients who come for help, e.g. with relationship problems, etc.

As a consequence, models of collaborative care of non-psychiatric/psychosomatic physicians with specialists in psychosomatic medicine (PSM) or psychologists have been developed and tested in different medical settings. For example, brief CBT or a single session of treatment has been made available in the framework of a consultation-liaison service to departments of internal medicine, neurology, gynaecology and the emergency department of a general hospital. Patients with bodily distress syndromes are also treated in interdisciplinary pain clinics or day hospitals [61]. Through these initiatives, many patients engage in specialised psychosomatic treatment.

Level 3: Specialised psychosomatic/psychotherapeutic treatment of patients with bodily distress syndromes

At the third level, German healthcare is offering psychosomatic outpatient or inpatient treatment for patients with severe bodily distress. Psychosomatic medicine is well developed in Germany. A total of 2996 physicians with a specialisation in psychosomatic medicine were recorded to have been working in their own practice, and a further 726 psychosomatic medicine specialists in a hospital department or in rehabilitation.

There have been a number of randomised controlled trials of interventions for bodily distress syndromes in Germany. These are summarised in Table 4.2.

Outpatient treatment by psychosomaticists or physicians/psychologists with advanced training in psychotherapy is well established in Germany and it is not difficult to receive such treatment (treatment costs are fully paid by health insurances in most cases after a positive expert review). These services have not been evaluated and there is still a challenge of engaging patients with bodily distress syndromes in this kind of therapy because many have a purely somatic perception of their complaints and fear the stigmatisation of becoming a psychiatric or psychological patient. A high proportion of patients do not follow recommendations for psychotherapy or drop out from therapy.

For patients with chronic and severe somatoform disorder, intensive inpatient psychosomatic treatment seems to have a positive effect on symptom severity, use of healthcare system, and direct and indirect illness-related costs. In such a setting, multimodal treatment

Table 4.2 Studies on management of medically unexplained symptoms/somatisation in Germany

	Setting	Design	Intervention	N	Primary outcome (instruments)	Secondary outcome (instruments)	Follow-up	Results (intervention vs. control group)
Larisch et al., 2004 [62]	GP	RCT	12-hour training of GPs	42 GPs, 127 patients with MUS	Severity of MUS (SOMS), quality of life, illness-related healthcare costs	Anxiety, depression (HADS), general psychopathology (GHQ), QoL (SF-36), healthcare utilisation	3, 6 and 12 months	Severity of MUS ↓ after 6 months (p = 0.029), higher utilisation of psychotherapy after 12 months (16.3% vs. 8.8%), stronger reduction of doctor visits at 6 months 54.2% vs. 26.6% (n.s.), reduction of supplementary direct healthcare costs in the intervention group by 38.2% per patient/quarter

Table 4.2 (cont.)

	Setting	Design	Intervention	N	Primary outcome (instruments)	Secondary outcome (instruments)	Follow-up	Results (intervention vs. control group)
Rief et al., 2006 [63]	GP	RCT	One-day training of GPs	26/200 GPs 289 patients with multiple MUS	Healthcare utilisation (structured interview); satisfaction with training (5-point Likert scale)	Severity of MUS (SOMS, WI), depression (BDI), anxiety (BAI)	6 months	No. of doctor visits ↓ (p = 0.003, ES = 0.45)
Martin et al., 2007 [64]	Collaborative	RCT	One-session intervention by psychologist	25/70 GPs, 140 patients with multiple MUS	Healthcare utilisation (structured interview); severity of MUS (BSI-SOM, SOMS-7, WI)	General psychopathology (BSI-GSI), depression (BDI)	6 months	No. of GP visits ↓ (p = 0.031, small ES), somatisation severity score ↓ (p = 0.018, medium ES)
Schweickhardt et al., 2007 [65]	Collaborative, consultation-liaison service	RCT	3–5-session intervention PSM C-L service	91 consecutive patients in dept. of internal medicine and neurology	Motivation for and use of psychotherapy (psychotherapy motivation questoinnaire)	Severity of MUS (SOMS-7), emotional distress (HADS, GHQ), QoL (SF-12)	3 and 6 months	Better motivation for psychotherapy (p = 0.001); higher use of psychotherapy after 3 months (42 vs. 20%, p = 0.045) but not after 6 months

| Bleichhart et al., 2004 [66] | In-patient psychosomatic hospital | Three-arm RCT: Group A: specialised treatment for somatisation Group B: standard inpatient treatment Group C: waiting list control group | Multimodal based on CBT | 225 patients with somatisation disorder (group A: n = 107; group B: n = 84; group C: n = 34) | Number of somatoform symptoms (IDCL) and severity of MUS (SOMS) | General psychopathology (SCL-90-R), anxiety and depression (HADS), QoL (EuroQoL), healthcare utilisation (visits to doctors) | 12 months | Both intervention groups showed a significant (p<0.01) reduction of somatoform symptoms (ES_A = 1.22; ES_B = 1.07), anxiety (ES_A = 0.43; ES_B = 0.45), and depression ($ES_{A,B}$ = 0.50) and an increase in QoL (ES_A = 0.63; ES_B = 0.33), whereas the control group showed only a trend for lower anxiety (p = 0.055). |

Table 4.2 (cont.)

	Setting	Design	Intervention	N	Primary outcome (instruments)	Secondary outcome (instruments)	Follow-up	Results (intervention vs. control group)
Nickel et al., 2006 [67]	In-patient psychosomatic hospital	RCT: Group A: Body-oriented specialised treatment for somatoform disorder Group B: standard inpatient treatment with gymnastic exercises	Multimodal based on bioenergetic exercises	128 Turkish immigrants with somatoform disorder	Severity of MUS (SCL-90-somatisation subscale)	General psychopathology (SCL-90-R), anger expression (STAXI)	No follow-up data	Group A showed significantly larger reduction of somatoform symptoms (p = 0,01), anxiety (p = 0.04), depression (p = 0.03) and anger suppression (p<0.01) at discharge (high effect sizes in both groups).

BAI, Beck Anxiety Inventory; BDI, Beck Depression Inventory; BSI, Brief Symptom Index; BSI-GSI, Global Symptom Index; BSI-SOM, Somatisation Subscale of the BSI; CBT, cognitive behavioural therapy; C-L, consultation-liaison; ES, effect size; GHQ, General Health Questionnaire; GP, general practitioner; HADS, Hospital Anxiety and Depression Scale; IDCL, International Diagnostic Checklists; MUS, medically unexplained symptoms; QoL, Quality of life; PSM, psychosomatic; RCT, randomised controlled trial; SCL-90-R, Symptom Check List 90 revised; SF, Short Form; SOMS, Screening for Somatoform Disorders; STAXI, State Trait Anger Inventory; WI, Whiteley Index.

approaches combining several types of psychotherapy (single, group, body psychotherapy, etc.) with physiotherapy, and standard somatic diagnostics and care are used, where necessary. Usually, this type of treatment is well accepted by patients because it does not in itself imply psychogenesis of the problem that led to treatment. Inpatient services have not been fully evaluated, however, partly because there is a clear selection bias in patients with bodily distress syndromes receiving inpatient treatment. Such patients have to apply for inpatient treatment themselves. These applications are reviewed by an expert and only patients with long-standing, severe symptoms are authorised to receive inpatient treatment from their health insurance. Given the high prevalence of bodily distress syndromes it seems that only a minority of patients with such disorders receive inpatient treatment; it is estimated that only about 10% of all patients undergoing inpatient/day hospital psychosomatic treatment in Germany have a primary diagnosis of a somatoform disorder [68].

Recommended model of care

The basic structure of services within a healthcare system for bodily distress syndromes and related conditions should be the same as those for other disorders or diseases, i.e. appropriate treatment is provided in primary care with referral of more severely affected patients to specialised services for bodily distress syndromes at general hospitals or specialist clinics. There should be a highly specialised service at university hospitals, which carries responsibility for training and research. The specialised service for bodily distress syndromes may be part of a comprehensive consultation-liaison psychiatry or psychosomatic service outside of university hospitals but the necessary specific assessment and treatment skills should be available to those patients who require them. There are also some clear differences, however, between service delivery for bodily distress syndromes and other services.

Assumptions (and challenges)

The recommendation for a specific service for bodily distress disorders is built on the assumption that bodily distress syndrome and related conditions are regarded as distinct disorders in their own right, which are disabling and expensive to the healthcare system and merit a proper service. At present, bodily distress is too often dismissed as a trivial problem of patients worrying too much about bodily sensations or merely symptoms of depression or anxiety disorders. The former notion leads to inadequate care in medical clinics; the latter leads to the low priority that the disorders are given in psychiatric services.

A major challenge is that bodily distress syndromes lie in the hinterland between psychiatry and general medicine. The classic way of attempting to classify bodily distress syndromes into a purely psychiatric or non-psychiatric condition does not make sense; similarly, the management of the patients cannot be pushed into one or the other. Unfortunately the healthcare system of most European countries is based on this body–mind dichotomy, and challenging this dichotomy can cause major problems for healthcare administrative and management systems. The most immediate problem faced by those trying to develop such a service is the question of who will fund the service for bodily distress syndromes. Neither general medicine nor psychiatry regard this as truly their responsibility. To establish something that does not fit into the established organisational structure may meet considerable resistance.

Furthermore, if one is trying to establish a single, well-coordinated service, it makes no sense to use multiple diagnostic labels for patients with multiple symptoms. As indicated in the Chapters 2 and 8, patients whose primary symptoms lie in one organ system also have symptoms in other systems. Therefore the appropriate treatment is not symptom- or organ-specific but is more generic to reduce the psychological processes that lead to symptoms in any organ system. Thus treatment for bodily distress syndromes should be available to patients, no matter which department of the hospital they consult first. We therefore recommend a common specialised service for bodily distress such as model C, displayed in Figure 4.4.

Staff

The recommended form of service for bodily distress syndromes requires a multidisciplinary team that includes both psychological/psychiatric and medical-surgical expertise, because there is often a need for general or specialist medical assessment and treatment as well as psychiatric/psychological assessment and treatment. Sometimes there needs to be active treatment from both medical and psychiatric/psychological areas of expertise. As patients with severe bodily distress syndromes are chronically ill with a high risk of being excluded from the labour market, social medicine and rehabilitation expertise is also needed, together with expertise in physical training. The number of experts needed from various specialties could be quite large, so a realistic way of organising this would be that the specialists/counsellors have a partial attachment to a clinic, but are otherwise employed elsewhere. Each discipline relies on input from other specialists – for example, psychologists may experience difficulties when working with patients with bodily distress since medical knowledge is often required, yet psychologists may be the most valuable members of the team when it comes to treatment, provided they have the backup of psychiatrists and general medical doctors.

As there is a spectrum of severity of bodily distress syndromes, their management has to be organised accordingly in a stepped-care model (see Chapter 8). To try to prevent patients with a mild bodily distress problem developing a chronic disorder, GPs and other doctors should be trained in the diagnosis and treatment of bodily distress. By establishing collaborative care, the GPs may further develop their skills so they are able to manage more severe bodily distress syndromes, while the most severely ill patients would still need specialised treatment by a multidisciplinary team.

Location of a specialist clinic

Owing to the multidisciplinary approach and the need for general medical services, specialist clinics for bodily distress syndromes are best located at general hospitals. Most patients find it disconcerting to be asked to attend a psychiatric hospital or clinic for their mainly physical ailment; in reality, many will not attend a psychiatric clinic. As patients with bodily distress syndromes are at high risk of multiple investigations and ineffective symptomatic treatments within the general medical setting, it is important that the treatment unit for bodily distress syndromes is located in close proximity to general and specialist medical departments with easy referral and communication between the two.

Besides making sure that patients with bodily distress syndromes receive appropriate care, university hospital clinics have an important additional function in making sure that such specialist treatment it is made available to all patients who need it. They must resist pressure to limit the treatment to those who belong to certain subcategories, e.g. patients primarily presenting with pain or patients with chronic fatigue syndrome. As with any set of disorders, specialised university hospital clinics should provide facilities for research and teaching.

Administration/affiliation

It is beyond doubt that such clinics are best located at general hospitals in order to promote collaboration with other medical specialties as well as patient acceptance, but it will depend on local factors whether a clinic is organised under psychiatry or the non-psychiatric specialties. The model of pain clinics may be an example.

In some countries, it is natural to organise the clinics together with or as a part of consultation-liaison psychiatry/psychosomatic medicine. However, US experience shows that this may not be ideal. In the USA, a well-organised subspecialty of psychosomatic medicine has been established but there are no clinics that specifically care for patients with bodily distress [69]. The lack of specialised clinics means that the field is not developed, in terms of research, training or clinical services.

The German model of psychosomatic medicine seems attractive as it includes doctors with many different backgrounds who are specialised in psychosomatic medicine and includes specialised units with inpatient facilities. However, it is important to ensure that the psychosomatic services take full responsibility for patients with bodily distress syndromes, as there appears to be a tendency at some clinics to maintain a focus on psychological complications of well-defined medical conditions and ignore bodily distress syndromes. Furthermore, although the German psychosomatic model is working well in Germany and German-speaking countries, it has been developed on the basis of the German tradition and history and it may not be realistic to export it to other countries.

Strategies

The best way of developing a good clinical service for patients with bodily distress syndromes may be to establish the area as a specialty of its own, as is the case for psychosomatic medicine in Germany. An alternative is to develop it as a subspecialty of psychiatry, and to organise care, as in other specialties, with highly specialised university clinics and less specialised services in non-university hospitals. In most parts of the world, however, this may not be a realistic first goal. A certain amount of pragmatism may be necessary, making use of political pressure and fashions and developing clinics by evolution. Thus the strategy has to be adapted to the local possibilities. For instance, in the UK, there are specialised clinics only for chronic fatigue syndrome. One strategy might be to start with such clinics and then establish programmes for other bodily distress syndromes as the comparable need for care in other functional somatic syndromes is recognised. These issues of a recommended model of care are developed further in Chapter 10.

Conclusion

There is clear evidence of unmet need for care in relation to bodily distress syndromes. Psychosomatic medicine services in German-speaking countries bridge the general medical and mental health service divide to provide a service appropriate for patients with these disorders but the service may still not attract all those who could benefit from it.

In a few other places, such as Aarhus, Denmark, there is a specialised service for severe disorders and well-established training for general practitioners. In other countries, it appears that there are examples of one of these components in isolation (e.g. training of GPs) but no full service. A few countries have specialised services for individual functional somatic syndromes, such as chronic fatigue syndrome, but these do not offer any service to the majority of people with moderate to severe bodily distress syndromes. The overall picture is one of a lack of services for such people.

References

1. Herrman-Lingen C. Steps towards integrated psychosomatic medicine – the example of psycho-cardiology. *Journal of Psychosomatic Research* 2011; **42**: 17–41.

2. Verhaak PF, Meijer SA, Visser AP, Wolters G. Persistent presentation of medically unexplained symptoms in general practice. *Journal of Family Practice* 2006; **23**: 414–20.

3. Fink P, Rosendal M. Unmet need for care for the somatizing and mentally ill patients in primary care. In: 55th Annual Meeting Academy of Psychosomatic Medicine, poster and oral presentation abstracts; 2008: 44. Available at: www.apm.org/ann-mtg/2008/APM-proceedings-2008.pdf (accessed 27 March 2011).

4. Simon GE, VonKorff M, Piccinelli M, Fullerton C, Ormel J. An international study of the relation between somatic symptoms and depression. *New England Journal of Medicine* 1999; **341**: 1329–35.

5. Wittchen HU, Pittrow D. Prevalence, recognition and management of depression in primary care in Germany: the Depression 2000 study. *Human Psychopharmacology* 2002; **17**(Suppl 1): S1–11.

6. Goldberg D. Detection and assessment of emotional disorders in a primary care setting. *International Journal of Mental Health and Addiction* 1979; **8**: 30–48.

7. Hamilton J, Campos R, Creed F. Anxiety, depression and management of medically unexplained symptoms in medical clinics. *Journal of the Royal College of Physicians, London* 1996; **30**: 18–20.

8. Mangwana S, Burlinson S, Creed F. Medically unexplained symptoms presenting at secondary care – a comparison of white Europeans and people of South Asian ethnicity. *International Journal of Psychiatry in Medicine* 2009; **39**: 33–44.

9. Fink P, Hansen MS, Sondergaard L, Frydenberg M. Mental illness in new neurological patients. *Journal of Neurology, Neurosurgery and Psychiatry* 2003; **74**: 817–19.

10. Hansen MS, Fink P, Frydenberg M, Oxhoj M, Sondergaard L, Munk-Jørgensen P. Mental disorders among internal medical inpatients: prevalence, detection, and treatment status. *Journal of Psychosomatic Research* 2001; **50**: 199–204.

11. Carson AJ, Ringbauer B, MacKenzie L, Warlow C, Sharpe M. Neurological disease, emotional disorder, and disability: they are related: a study of 300 consecutive new referrals to a neurology outpatient department. *Journal of Neurology, Neurosurgery and Psychiatry* 2000; **68**: 202–6.

12. Carson AJ, Best S, Postma K, Stone J, Warlow C, Sharpe M. The outcome of neurology outpatients with medically unexplained symptoms: a prospective cohort study. *Journal of Neurology, Neurosurgery and Psychiatry* 2003; **74**: 897–900.

13. Owens DM, Nelson DK, Talley NJ. The irritable bowel syndrome: long-term prognosis and the physician–patient interaction. *Annals of Internal Medicine* 1995; **122**: 107–12.

14. Quigley EM, Bytzer P, Jones R, Mearin F. Irritable bowel syndrome: the burden and unmet needs in Europe. *Digestive and Liver Disease* 2006; **38**: 717–23.

15. Jackson JL, Kroenke K, Chamberlin J. Effects of physician awareness of symptom-related expectations and mental disorders. A controlled trial. *Archives of Family Medicine* 1999; **8**: 135–42.

16. Fink P, Hansen MS, Sondergaard L. Somatoform disorders among first-time referrals to a neurology service. *Psychosomatics* 2005; **46**: 540–48.

17. Fink P, Hansen MS, Oxhoj ML. The prevalence of somatoform disorders among internal medical inpatients. *Journal of Psychosomatic Research* 2004; **56**: 413–18.

18. Hansen MS, Fink P, Frydenberg M, Oxhoj ML. Use of health services, mental illness, and self-rated disability and health in medical inpatients. *Psychosomatic Medicine* 2002; **64**: 668–75.

19. Gater RA, Goldberg DP, Evanson JM, Lowson K, McGrath G, Tantam D *et al.*

Detection and treatment of psychiatric illness in a general medical ward: a modified cost-benefit analysis. *Journal of Psychosomatic Research* 1998; **45**: 437–48.

20. de Jonge P, Huyse FJ, Herzog T, Lobo A, Malt U, Opmeer BC et al. Referral pattern of neurological patients to psychiatric Consultation-Liaison Services in 33 European hospitals. *General Hospital Psychiatry* 2001; **23**: 152–7.

21. Hansen MS, Fink P, Frydenberg M, de Jonge P, Huyse FJ. Complexity of care and mental illness in medical patients. *General Hospital Psychiatry* 2001; **23**: 319–25.

22. Creed F, Firth D, Timol M, Metcalfe R, Pollock S. Somatization and illness behaviour in a neurology ward. *Journal of Psychosomatic Research* 1990; **34**: 427–37.

23. Kooiman CG, Bolk JH, Rooijmans HG, Trijsburg RW. Alexithymia does not predict the persistence of medically unexplained physical symptoms. *Psychosomatic Medicine* 2004; **66**: 224–32.

24. Jackson J, Fiddler M, Kapur N, Wells A, Tomenson B, Creed F. Number of bodily symptoms predicts outcome more accurately than health anxiety in patients attending neurology, cardiology, and gastroenterology clinics. *Journal of Psychosomatic Research* 2006; **60**: 357–63.

25. Barsky AJ, Wyshak G, Klerman LG. Medical and psychiatric Determinants of outpatients medical utilization. *Medical Care* 1986; **24**(6): 548–68.

26. Hansen MS, Fink P, Frydenberg M. Follow-up on mental illness in medical inpatients: health care use and self-rated health and physical fitness. *Psychosomatics* 2004; **45**: 302–10.

27. Hansen MS, Fink P, Sondergaard L, Frydenberg M. Mental illness and health care use: a study among new neurological patients. *General Hospital Psychiatry* 2005; **27**: 119–24.

28. Fink P, Ørnbøl E, Christensen KS. The outcome of health anxiety in primary care. A two-year follow-up study on health care costs and self-rated health. *PLoS ONE* 2010; **5**: e9873.

29. Creed F, Guthrie E, Ratcliffe J, Fernandes L, Rigby C, Tomenson B et al. Does psychological treatment help only those patients with severe irritable bowel syndrome who also have a concurrent psychiatric disorder? *Australia and New Zealand Journal of Psychiatry* 2005; **39**: 807–15.

30. Kapur N, Hunt I, Lunt M, McBeth J, Creed F, Macfarlane G. Psychosocial and illness related predictors of consultation rates in primary care – a cohort study. *Psychological Medicine* 2004; **34**: 719–28.

31. Jackson JL, Kroenke K. Prevalence, impact, and prognosis of multisomatoform disorder in primary care: a 5-year follow-up study. *Psychosomatic Medicine* 2008; **70**: 430–4.

32. Creed F, Tomenson B, Guthrie E, Ratcliffe J, Fernandes L, Read N et al. The relationship between somatisation and outcome in patients with severe irritable bowel syndrome. *Journal of Psychosomatic Research* 2008; **64**: 613–20.

33. Andrews G, Carter GL. What people say about their general practitioners' treatment of anxiety and depression. *Medical Journal of Australia* 2001; **175**(Suppl): S48–S51.

34. Prins MA, Verhaak PF, Bensing JM, van der Meer MK. Health beliefs and perceived need for mental health care of anxiety and depression – the patients' perspective explored. *Clinical Psychology Review* 2008; **28**: 1038–58.

35. Bridges KW, Goldberg DP. Psychiatric illness in inpatients with neurological disorders: patients' views on discussion of emotional problems with neurologists. *British Medical Journal* 1984; **15**(289): 656–8.

36. Arnold IA, De Waal MW, Eekhof JA, van Hemert AM. Somatoform disorder in primary care: course and the need for cognitive-behavioral treatment. *Psychosomatics* 2006; **47**: 498–503.

37. Affleck G, Tennen H, Zautra A, Urrows S, Abeles M, Karoly P. Women's pursuit of personal goals in daily life with fibromyalgia: a value-expectancy analysis. *Journal of Consulting and Clinical Psychology* 2001; **69**: 587–96.

38. Nordin TA, Hartz AJ, Noyes R, Jr, Anderson MC, Rosenbaum ME, James PA et al. Empirically identified goals for the management of unexplained symptoms. *Journal of Family Practice* 2006; **38**: 476–82.

39. Harris LR, Roberts L. Treatments for irritable bowel syndrome: patients' attitudes and acceptability. *BMC Complementary and Alternative Medicine* 2008; **8**: 65.

40. Nimnuan C, Hotopf M, Wessely S. Medically unexplained symptoms: how often and why are they missed? *QJM – Monthly Journal of the Association of Physicians* 2000; **93**: 21–8.

41. Royal College of Physicians and Royal College of Psychiatrists. *The Psychological Care of Medical Patients. Recognition of Need and Service Provision*. London: Royal College of Physicians and Royal College of Psychiatrists, 1995.

42. Lin EH, Katon W, Von Korff M, Bush T, Lipscomb P, Russo J et al. Frustrating patients: physician and patient perspectives among distressed high users of medical services. *Journal of General Internal Medicine* 1991; **6**: 241–6.

43. Jackson JL, Kroenke K. Difficult patient encounters in the ambulatory clinic: clinical predictors and outcomes. *Archives of Internal Medicine* 1999; **159**: 1069–75.

44. Sharpe M, Mayou R, Seagroatt V, Surawy C, Warwick H, Bulstrode C et al. Why do doctors find some patients difficult to help? *QJM – Monthly Journal of the Association of Physicians* 1994; **87**: 187–93.

45. van Dulmen AM, Fennis JF, Mokkink HG, van der Velden HG, Bleijenberg G. Doctor-dependent changes in complaint-related cognitions and anxiety during medical consultations in functional abdominal complaints. *Psychological Medicine* 1995; **25**: 1011–18.

46. Lucock MP, Morley S, White C, Peake MD. Responses of consecutive patients to reassurance after gastroscopy: results of self administered questionnaire survey. *British Medical Journal* 1997; **315**: 572–5.

47. Henningsen P, Zipfel S, Herzog W. Management of functional somatic syndromes. *The Lancet* 2007; **369**: 946–55.

48. Fink P, Rosendal M. Recent developments in the understanding and management of functional somatic symptoms in primary care. *Current Opinion in Psychiatry* 2008; **21**: 182–8.

49. van der Feltz-Cornelis CM, van Oppen P, Ader HJ, Van Dyck R. Randomised controlled trial of a collaborative care model with psychiatric consultation for persistent medically unexplained symptoms in general practice. *Psychotherapy and Psychosomatics* 2006; **75**: 282–9.

50. Huyse FJ, Herzog T, Lobo A, Malt UF, Opmeer BC, Stein B et al. Consultation-liaison psychiatric service delivery: results from a European study. *General Hospital Psychiatry* 2001; **23**: 124–32.

51. Katon W, Ries RK, Kleinman A. A prospective DSM-III study of 100 consecutive somatization patients. *Comprehensive Psychiatry* 1984; **25**: 305–14.

52. Rundell JR, Amundsen K, Rummans TL, Tennen G. Toward defining the scope of psychosomatic medicine practice: psychosomatic medicine in an outpatient, tertiary-care practice setting. *Psychosomatics* 2008; **49**: 487–93.

53. Creed F, Guthrie E, Black D, Tranmer M. Psychiatric referrals within the general hospital: comparison with referrals to general practitioners. *British Journal of Psychiatry* 1993; **162**: 204–11.

54. Bass C, Peveler R, House A. Somatoform disorders: severe psychiatric illnesses neglected by psychiatrists. *British Journal of Psychiatry* 2001; **179**: 11–14.

55. Creed F. Should general psychiatry ignore somatization and hypochondriasis? *World Psychiatry* 2006; **5**: 146–50.

56. Staab JP. Chronic dizziness: the interface between psychiatry and neuro-otology. *Current Opinion in Neurology* 2006; **19**: 41–8.

57. Hauser W, Thieme K, Turk DC. Guidelines on the management of fibromyalgia syndrome – a systematic review. *European Journal of Pain* 2010; **14**: 5–10.

58. Fritzsche K, Larisch A. Treating patients with functional somatic symptoms. A treatment guide for use in general practice.

Scandinavian Journal of Primary Health Care 2003; **21**: 132–5.

59. Goldberg D, Gask L, O'Dowd T. The treatment of somatization: teaching techniques of reattribution. *Journal of Psychosomatic Research* 1989; **33**: 689–95.

60. Fink P, Rosendal M, Toft T. Assessment and treatment of functional disorders in general practice: The extended reattribution and management model – an advanced educational program for nonpsychiatric doctors. *Psychosomatics* 2002; **43**: 93–131.

61. Arnold B, Brinkschmidt T, Casser HR, Gralow I, Irnich D, Klimczyk K et al. Multimodal pain therapy: principles and indications. *Schmerz* 2009; **23**: 112–20.

62. Larisch A, Schweickhardt A, Wirsching M, Fritzsche K. Psychosocial interventions for somatizing patients by the general practitioner: a randomized controlled trial. *Journal of Psychosomatic Research* 2004; **57**: 507–14.

63. Rief W, Martin A, Rauh E, Zech T, Bender A. Evaluation of general practitioners' training: how to manage patients with unexplained physical symptoms. *Psychosomatics* 2006; **47**: 304–11.

64. Martin A, Rauh E, Fichter M, Rief W. A one-session treatment for patients suffering from medically unexplained symptoms in primary care: a randomized clinical trial. *Psychosomatics* 2007; **48**: 294–303.

65. Schweickhardt A, Larisch A, Wirsching M, Fritzsche K. Short-term psychotherapeutic interventions for somatizing patients in the general hospital: a randomized controlled study. *Psychotherapy and Psychosomatics* 2007; **76**: 339–46.

66. Bleichhardt G, Timmer B, Rief W. Cognitive-behavioural therapy for patients with multiple somatoform symptoms – a randomised controlled trial in tertiary care. *Journal of Psychosomatic Research* 2004; **56**: 449–54.

67. Nickel M, Cangoez B, Bachler E, Muehlbacher M, Lojewski N, Mueller-Rabe N et al. Bioenergetic exercises in inpatient treatment of Turkish immigrants with chronic somatoform disorders: A randomized, controlled study. *Journal of Psychosomatic Research* 2006; **61**: 507–13.

68. Tritt K, von Heymann F, Loew T, Benker B, Bleichner F, Buchmüller R et al. Patients of a psychotherapeutic inpatient setting: patient description and effectiveness of treatment. *Psychotherapie* 2003; **8**: 245–51.

69. Lyketsos CG. Training in psychosomatic medicine: a psychiatric subspecialty recognized in the United States by the American Board of Medical Specialties. *Journal of Psychosomatic Research* (in press).

Chapter

5

Barriers to improving treatment

Peter Henningsen, Christian Fazekas and
Michael Sharpe

Introduction

If we are to improve care for patients with bodily distress syndromes, the barriers that currently stand in the way of effective management must be addressed. Many of these barriers are simple but nonetheless fundamental. In this chapter we will consider these barriers, first as problems in the context in which patient care is provided (terminology and understanding; policy planning and organisation), then as problems in the individual doctor–patient encounter (the patient's role, the doctor's role and the doctor–patient relationship) that takes place within that context.

The context of care

First, what are the barriers in the system in which care is provided? In other words, what are the problems in the general context of care for patients with bodily distress?

Problems in terminology and understanding

One of the most important barriers to the improved treatment of these patients is the confusing and ambiguous terminology that is currently used for the problem, which in turn reflects conceptual confusion. Psychiatry refers to such patients as having somatoform disorders or somatisation, with the implicit assumption that these terms indicate psychological conditions. Medicine refers to them with a plethora of names, such as fibromyalgia and irritable bowel syndrome, according to medical specialty, with the assumption that they reflect disordered physiological functioning [1]. The terms and concepts used to describe and understand bodily distress syndromes differ not only between psychiatry and medicine but also between specialist and primary care and between countries. The resulting confusion has produced a fragmentation of approach that has acted as a serious barrier to the recognition of the size and importance of the problem, and to the development of coherent and shared approaches to care. Many aspects of this sorry state of affairs are dealt with in other chapters of this book, so we will only briefly allude to them here.

Medically unexplained, somatoform, somatisation, functional, bodily distress ... the list goes on. It is easy to understand how differences in professional perspectives and interests underlie these variations in terminology and classification. However, it is not so easy to come up with an alternative that would be acceptable to all the different groups of medical specialists [2].

Medically Unexplained Symptoms, Somatisation and Bodily Distress, ed. Francis Creed, Peter Henningsen and Per Fink. Published by Cambridge University Press. © Cambridge University Press 2011.

New terms are being currently developed for *Diagnostic and Statistical Manual of Mental Disorders* (DSM)-V, such as 'complex somatic symptom disorder' [3]. It seems doubtful that these will solve the problem of terminological confusion, since the new terminology and classification emanates only from within psychiatry, whereas the problem of bodily distress requires cooperation between psychiatry, specialist medicine and primary care. It is as if different specialists and general practitioners (GPs) all had their own different terms for stroke.

A related problem is to create terms that are also acceptable to the patients. Many of our current terms are regarded as offensive by patients who see them as a dismissal of the reality of their somatic concerns [4]. Ideally, we need a more flexible term that acknowledges the reality of somatic symptoms but also allows for the role of psychological factors [5]. However, again, we lack a consensus on how to achieve this acceptability to patients, or even whether it is necessary.

These problems with terminology also affect data collection. They result in different coding practices, especially in primary care. Whereas somatic and mental health specialists will usually prefer the diagnoses either of specific functional somatic syndromes or of the appropriate coding for psychiatric disorders, primary care physicians have three options: to code as a *physical symptom* (e.g. muscle pain), as a *physical syndrome* (e.g. fibromyalgia) or as a *psychiatric diagnosis* (e.g. somatoform disorder). In the case of a woman with typical widespread muscular pain and disturbed sleep, this may be fairly straightforward, and it is reasonable to view the syndrome term as overlapping, with both the physical symptoms and the psychiatric label. However, it becomes more difficult when there is no intermediate syndrome: for instance a patient may have abdominal pain, dizziness and headache. Here somatoform disorder may well be the correct diagnosis, but it is much more likely that if anything was coded it would simply be one or more of the physical symptoms. Even where there is a syndrome code, this may not be applied by the GP until used by a specialist. Robust diagnostic criteria such as the Rome criteria for irritable bowel syndrome are not in common use by primary care physicians, who may be reluctant to formally make these diagnoses to the level of certainty based on their clinical databases. Whether newer developments, such as an amendment to the International Classification of Primary Care classification [6], will make it easier to bridge the gap between individual symptoms and the broader concepts of bodily distress remains to be determined. What is clear is that the lack of systematic data on bodily distress syndromes means that healthcare planners and politicians are not confronted with the scale and importance of this problem.

Problems in policy, planning and service organisation

One thing is clear – the effective management of patients with bodily distress syndromes requires a combination of medical and psychiatric/psychological management [7]. However, the health policies and the planning of medical and psychiatric/psychological services have become totally separated in many countries. Consequently, the delivery of integrated care at a specialist level is almost impossible to implement; patients seen in a general medical setting are largely denied psychological or psychiatric treatments. The doctors who work in these separate services often work in different hospitals and rarely see each other. Consequently, they have few opportunities even to influence each others' thinking or to discuss the care of individual patients. The patients have to decide whether they want to be referred to a medical specialist or to a 'mental health service'. The latter may seem inappropriate to a person with somatic complaints as well as unnecessarily stigmatising.

Existing health policies not only fail to address the barriers to managing patients with bodily distress more effectively, but may also contribute to them. For example, a policy of reimbursing hospitals and GPs for technical diagnostic tests and treatments, but not for high quality communication skills and effective symptomatic treatment and rehabilitation, will exacerbate the difficulties in achieving rational management of bodily distress. Social and insurance policies may also exacerbate the problem. For example, the need to have a 'physical' cause for symptoms is often reinforced by the requirement of workplace and insurance companies which grant greater benefits for symptoms if physical causes can be identified.

There have been many attempts to bridge this unhelpful division between medical and psychiatric/psychological services. One approach is to improve the psychological aspects of the management of patients within primary medical care. It is often assumed that primary care is the best place for psychological and medical care to be integrated, but this is often not true in practice. Although efforts have been made to improve this situation by training and supporting GPs in the care of patients with bodily distress [8], these patients often need specialist medical assessment and psychiatric/psychological management. In specialist care there is a long tradition of bridging or so-called 'liaison' psychiatry services [9] – now called psychosomatic medicine in the USA [10]. These developments have been important in improving our understanding of how we could manage patients with bodily distress more effectively, but to date they have been inadequate to address the problem effectively.

There are a few examples of well integrated services where a patient's mental and physical state can be investigated and treated with equal vigour. The departments of psychosomatic medicine in Germany offer this possibility. In some European countries, the worldwide web is being used to help patients and physicians find these options [11]. Nevertheless, there is a broad lack of such specialist management, and it remains unclear which medical specialty is ultimately responsible for these patients, who may end up lost in a medical 'no man's land'.

Summary
The context of care is dualistic in thinking, language and service organisation. It is within this unfavourable context that the individual doctor–patient encounter occurs.

The individual doctor–patient encounter
The dualistic context of medical care provides a frame work for dualistic encounters between doctors and patients. Traditionally, doctors have regarded patients with bodily distress as 'difficult to treat' [12;13] or 'difficult and frustrating' [14;15;16]. In other words, these patients are not 'simply difficult' to treat in the sense that they are challenging and stimulating for doctors who want to prove their expertise; rather they are 'difficult difficult' patients, who evoke the negative emotional reactions of frustration and helplessness in their doctors ('heart-sink patients') and seem to undermine rather than stimulate the expertise of the doctor.

Until recently, these difficulties were attributed solely to the idea that doctors and patients had different views about the aetiology and treatment of bodily distress: the patient with bodily distress presented bodily, rather than emotional, symptoms and (erroneously) insisted that the symptoms had a physical cause, thereby forcing the doctor to do tests. Meanwhile the doctor (correctly) attributed the symptoms to 'somatised' emotional distress and tried to avoid medicalising them with investigations [15]. This understanding led to the recommendation that doctors could achieve better management by persuading the patient to reattribute his or her physical symptoms to a psychological cause, and then treating it. But is this really the whole story? New evidence suggests that it is not, and that more complex processes are at work.

The patient's role in the problem

It has been assumed that patients with bodily distress pressure their doctors into providing diagnoses and treatments that conform to their subjective explanatory medical model but which, from an objective point of view, are not appropriate. These factors do undoubtedly operate in many cases. However, recent studies tell us that the situation may not be as simple as this view implies. Many patients with bodily distress actually come to the consultation with complex ideas about the cause of their symptoms; that is, they can acknowledge several different possible causes at the same time, frequently including psychological ones [17;18]. So, a fixed physical attribution may not be the problem; at least not initially. But, although they can see their symptoms in this complex way, they frequently decide simply not to disclose the psychological and social factors when talking to the doctor with the result that the interaction with the doctor is limited in scope. Why do they do this? They may have a negative attitude towards psychological illness and treatments [19]; they may fear that bringing the doctor's attention to psychological factors will distract the doctor from an adequate search for physical disease [20]; or they may simply not trust doctors with the discussion of emotional aspects of their problems [20].

However, research suggests that just because patients do not disclose psychological factors does not mean that they do not want their doctors to respond psychologically. Patients with bodily distress actually seek more emotional support from their doctors than patients with symptoms attributable to disease [21;22;23]. They can be observed to provide many cues to this desire for emotional support, even more than they do for their desire for an explanation or medical intervention [24]. However, these cues are frequently not picked up by their doctors and the dialogue remains stuck in a somatic idiom.

The doctor's role in the problem

The major problem for the doctor seems to be not only eliciting psychological causes for symptoms when the patient is reluctant to disclose them explicitly, but also one of overcoming his or her own insecurity in dealing with the patient's need for emotional support. Studies have repeatedly found a discrepancy between being able to recognise potential psychological factors on the one hand, and feeling capable of dealing adequately with these factors on the other [13;15;20;25]. Doctors do not seem to know how to negotiate and act on a shared understanding with the patient about the nature of the problem of bodily distress [26]. Interestingly, the agreement of a shared explanatory model, of a 'common reality', seems to be more important to many patients than getting a cure for their complaints [27;28]. It is important to note, however, that this subjective feeling of insecurity does not necessarily mean that the doctor does not address the patient's psychological and social needs. Even physicians who declined training in the treatment of patients with bodily distress may work in an intuitive, but nevertheless, elaborated psychological fashion with these patients. This has led researchers to conclude that one barrier to better care of patients with bodily distress was not the patient's but rather the doctor's own devaluation of their own demonstrable psychological expertise [26].

This insecurity among medical doctors about the management of psychological issues (and not only the well-known insecurity associated with the fear of missing disease) appears to lead doctors to stick defensively to what they are confident doing, i.e. suggesting disease-focused investigations and treatment, even if it is clear that this is not the best way to proceed. For example, it was noted that after having taken part in reattribution training, doctors suggested potential psychosocial explanations for symptoms to patients more frequently than doctors who did not take part in the training – but at the same time they still proposed disease-focused treatments, thereby sending mixed messages to the patients [29]. In fact, doctors suggest disease-focused investigation and treatment more frequently than their patients with bodily distress [30;31]. They also, typically, do not pick up the cues to emotional needs that patients regularly provide [21;22;23]. And, the longer the consultation the greater the probability that a disease-focused intervention will be offered [28], suggesting that doctors use this strategy as a method to end the consultation. These medical interventions are prescribed regardless of the patients' attributions regarding their medical condition and their demands for treatment.

The doctor–patient relationship

The early models which viewed physical symptoms as a culturally acceptable way of seeking help for mental distress [32] have evolved to ones that see patients as actually having a complex understanding of their symptoms, which is unhelpfully shaped by their interaction with the doctor [33].

How does this happen? Salmon [28] suggests the following model for the dynamics of consultations with patients with bodily distress: patients emphasize physical symptoms and the doctors respond to these with attempts to say that, as they are not evidence of disease, they are not serious. They also ignore the patients' hints about the role of psychological and social factors. This dismissal of both the patients' symptoms and their emotional needs provokes the patients to intensify and magnify their account of the reality and medical importance of their physical complaints in order to claim their physicians' commitment and understanding. In response to these intensified accounts, physicians resort to implementing disease-focused management strategies.

Why does this happen? As Kenny [25] argues, both doctors and patients are struggling defensively to maintain their identity and integrity in the face of a perceived threat to these. This leads to physicians resorting to disease-focused interventions even when they favour a more psychological approach and to patients continuing to stick to a physical cause for their complaints even though their real needs are mainly emotional [23].

Does this more complex understanding of what might be going wrong tell us how to intervene? Evidence is now accumulating that simply striving to persuade the patient to reattribute the cause of their symptoms to psychological factors does not make them better [20]. Sobering results of trials employing the so-called reattribution model (and variants thereof, see Chapter 3 for the evidence) and 'particularly' new insights into the dynamics of doctor–patient interactions through qualitative studies in primary care suggest a more sophisticated approach is required. In this new approach we must pay more attention to the role of doctors' behaviour in generating and maintaining bodily distress. In short, it may not be primarily a question of changing the incorrect perceptions of the patient, but rather a question of changing the 'somatising' behaviour of the doctors, if we are to improve an often maladaptive interaction between doctor and patient.

Summary

Within the problematic context of a fundamentally dualistic healthcare system, medical doctors in both primary and secondary care find patients with bodily distress difficult to help. That is because patients with bodily distress have needs that do not fit well with either the doctors' training or the services available for doctors to refer to. Consequently, a patient who comes with a relatively open mind about his or her somatic symptoms may get sent down the route of disease-focused care; a first step on the journey to developing chronic disabling bodily distress.

Overcoming the barriers

There is a huge gap between the great clinical and societal significance of bodily distress syndromes on the one hand and the limited efforts to understand and better treat them on the other. We need to achieve greater recognition of the problem and to offer practical solutions. A clear understanding of the barriers to effective care is an important beginning to this process. How can these barriers to effective care of bodily distress syndromes be overcome? The analysis outlined above suggests that we need to shift from a simplistic perspective of difficult patients to one of a difficult health service. Change will be required not only in the organisation of services but also in the training of those working in them.

Doctors train and work in the context of dualistic health services. Much of the discomfort and insecurity felt by many medical doctors in their consultations with patients who have bodily distress reflects a lack of appropriate and specific training. We need training in how to think about symptoms non-dualistically, and how to respond appropriately and with confidence to patients' emotional needs. This may be as true of general psychiatrists as it is of internists, surgeons and GPs. While many medical schools now offer special courses in doctor–patient communication, the intimate link between better communication and more appropriate action, i.e. the communicative aspects of ordering and interpreting of investigations or of prescription of treatments, is rarely taught adequately. We need to provide training in these 'communication plus' skills [34] if we are to overcome this barrier to the management of patients with bodily distress syndromes.

Conclusion

In this chapter, we have briefly reviewed barriers to improved treatment of patients with bodily distress. It is evident that the barriers directly related to the individual doctor–patient encounter as well as the more general ones of the problematic status of this significant health problem require the knowledge and skills of both medicine and psychiatry/psychology. As long as our understanding, terminology, assessment and treatment of bodily distress continues to be dominated by dualistic, either/or alternatives instead of an integrated, personalised biopsychosocial model, we will continue to create, instead of overcoming, barriers to the better care of a large proportion of our patients.

References

1. Wessely S, Nimnuan C, Sharpe M. Functional somatic syndromes: one or many? *The Lancet* 1999; **354**(9182): 936–39.

2. Creed F, Guthrie E, Fink P, Henningsen P, Rief W, Sharpe M et al. Is there a better term than 'medically unexplained symptoms'? *Journal of Psychosomatic Research* 2010; **68**: 5–8.

3. Dimsdale J, Creed F; DSM-V Workgroup on Somatic Symptom Disorders. The proposed diagnosis of somatic symptom disorders in DSM-V to replace somatoform disorders in DSM-IV – a preliminary report. *Journal of Psychosomatic Research* 2009; **66**: 473–6.

4. Stone J, Wojcik W, Durrance D, Carson A, Lewis S, MacKenzie L et al. What should we say to patients with symptoms unexplained by disease? The 'number needed to offend'. *British Medical Journal* 2002; **325**(7378): 1449–50.

5. Sharpe M, Carson AJ. 'Unexplained' somatic symptoms, functional syndromes, and somatization: do we need a paradigm shift? *Annals of Internal Medicine* 2001; **134**(Suppl 9): 926–30.

6. Rosendal M, Olesen F, Fink P, Toft T, Sokolowski I, Bro F. A randomized controlled trial of brief training in the assessment and treatment of somatization in primary care: effects on patient outcome. *General Hospital Psychiatry* 2007; **29**: 364–73.

7. Kroenke K. Efficacy of treatment for somatoform disorders: a review of randomized controlled trials. *Psychosomatic Medicine* 2007; **69**(9): 881–8.

8. Goldberg RJ, Novack DH, Gask L. The recognition and management of somatization. What is needed in primary care training. *Psychosomatics* 1992; **33**(1): 55–61.

9. Mayou RA. The history of general hospital psychiatry. *British Journal of Psychiatry* 1989; **155**: 764–76.

10. Gitlin DF, Levenson JL, Lyketsos CG. Psychosomatic medicine: a new psychiatric subspecialty. *Academic Psychiatry* 2004; **28**(1): 4–11.

11. Fazekas C, Stelzig M, Moser G, Matzer F, Schüßler G, Harnoncourt K et al. Austrian network for psychometric medicine: background, development and participation. [in German] *Psychosomatic Medicine and Psychotherapy* 2007; **53**: 397–403.

12. Carson AJ, Stone J, Warlow C, Sharpe M. Patients whom neurologists find difficult to help. *Journal of Neurology, Neurosurgery and Psychiatry* 2004; **75**: 1776–8.

13. Sharpe M, Mayou R, Seagroatt V, Surawy C, Warwick H, Bulstrode C et al. Why do doctors find some patients difficult to help? *QJM – Quarterly Journal of Medicine* 1994; **87**: 187–93.

14. Chew-Graham C, May C. Chronic low back pain in general practice: the challenge of the consultation. *Journal of Family Practice* 1999; **16**: 46–9.

15. Wileman L, May C, Chew-Graham CA. Medically unexplained symptoms and the problem of power in the primary care consultation: a qualitative study. *Journal of Family Practice* 2002; **19**: 178–82.

16. Woivalin T, Krantz G, Mäntyranta T, Ringsberg KC. Medically unexplained symptoms: perceptions of physicians in primary health care. *Journal of Family Practice* 2004; **21**: 199–203.

17. Henningsen P, Jakobsen T, Schiltenwolf M, Weiss MG. Somatization revisited: diagnosis and perceived causes of common mental disorders. *Journal of Nervous and Mental Disease* 2005; **193**: 85–92.

18. Hiller W, Cebulla M, Korn HJ, Leibbrand R, Röers B, Nilges P. Causal symptom attributions in somatoform disorder and chronic pain. *Journal of Psychosomatic Research* 2010; **68**: 9–19.

19. Fritzsche K, Sandholzer H, Werner J, Brucks U, Cierpka M, Deter HCH et al. Psychotherapeutic and psychosocial treatments in primary care. [in German]. *Psychotherapie Psychosomatik Medizinische Psychologie* 2000; **50**: 240–6.

20. Peters S, Rogers A, Salmon P, Gask L, Dowrick C, Towey M et al. What do patients choose to tell their doctors? Qualitative analysis of potential

barriers to reattributing medically unexplained symptoms. *Journal of General Internal Medicine* 2009; **24**: 443–9.

21. Dowrick CHF, Ring A, Humphris GM, Salmon P, Normalisation of unexplained symptoms by general practitioners: a functional typology. *British Journal of General Practice* 2004; **54**: 165–70.

22. Salmon P, Dowrick CF, Ring A, Humphris GM. Voiced but unheard agendas: qualitative analysis of the psychosocial cues that patients with unexplained symptoms present to general practitioners. *British Journal of General Practice* 2004; **54**: 171–6.

23. Salmon P, Ring A, Dowrick CHF, Humphris GM. What do general practice patients want when they present medically unexplained symptoms, and why do their doctors feel pressurized? *Journal of Psychosomatic Research* 2005; **59**: 255–62.

24. Salmon P, Ring A, Humphris GM, Davies JC, Dowrick CF. Primary care consultations about medically unexplained symptoms: how do patients indicate what they want? *Journal of General Internal Medicine* 2009; **24**: 450–6.

25. Kenny DT. Constructions of chronic pain in doctor–patient relationships: bridging the communication chasm. *Patient Education and Counseling* 2004; **52**: 297–305.

26. Salmon P, Peters S, Clifford R, Iredale W, Gask L, Rogers A et al. Why do general practitioners decline training to improve management of medically unexplained symptoms? *Society of General Internal Medicine* 2007; **22**: 565–71.

27. Glenton C. Chronic back pain sufferers – striving for the sick role. *Social Science and Medicine* 2003; **57**: 2243–52.

28. Salmon P, Wissow L, Carrol J, Ring A, Humphris GM, Davies JC et al. Doctors' responses to patients with medically unexplained symptoms who seek emotional support: criticism or confrontation? *General Hospital Psychiatry* 2007; **294**: 454–60.

29. Morriss R, Gask L, Dowrick C, Dunn G, Peters S, Ring A et al. Randomized trial of reattribution on psychosocial talk between doctors and patients with medically unexplained symptoms. *Psychological Medicine* 2010; **40**: 325–33.

30. Ring A, Dowrick C, Humphris G, Salmon P. Do patients with unexplained physical symptoms pressurise general practitioners for somatic treatment? A qualitative study. *British Medical Journal* 2004; **328**: 1057.

31. Ring A, Dowrick CF, Humphris GM, Davies J, Salmon P. The somatising effect of clinical consultation: what patients and doctors say and do not say when patients present medically unexplained physical symptoms. *Social Science and Medicine* 2005; **61**: 1505–15.

32. Bridges KW, Goldberg DP. Somatic presentation of DSM III psychiatric disorders in primary care. *Journal of Psychosomatic Research* 1985; **29**: 563–9.

33. Salmon P, Humphris GM, Ring A, Davies JC, Dowrick CF. Primary care consultations about medically unexplained symptoms: patient presentations and doctor responses that influence the probability of somatic intervention. *Psychosomatic Medicine* 2007; **69**(6): 571–7.

34. Fazekas C, Matzer F, Greimel ER, Moser G, Stelzig M, Langewitz W et al. Psychosomatic medicine in primary care: influence of training. *Wiener Klinische Wochenschrift* 2009; **121**: 446–53.

Chapter

6

Gender, lifespan and cultural aspects

Constanze Hausteiner-Wiehle, Gudrun Schneider,
Sing Lee, Athula Sumathipala and Francis Creed

Gender aspects

It is well established in the literature that women experience and report more somatic symptoms than men and the prevalence of bodily distress syndromes, i.e. medically unexplained symptoms, functional somatic syndromes and somatoform disorders, is higher in women than in men [1]. In this chapter, we will demonstrate that there are several biological, psychological and social factors that could contribute to gender differences in these disorders, even if the evidence is still incomplete with respect to some questions. It has become clear that these differences stem not only from social injustices, or from biological variation between male and female individuals ('sex'), but also from socioculturally coined masculine and feminine stereotypes ('gender') which are not necessarily bound to the biological sex. The chapter aims to demonstrate that a gender perspective can provide valuable insights for better management of bodily distress syndromes – and of symptoms in general.

Previous reviews have examined various possibilities to explain why women report more somatic symptoms than men. The reasons mentioned by Barsky *et al.* included innate, biological differences in pain perception such that women have greater sensitivity to bodily sensations than men [1]. Furthermore, women describe and report somatic symptoms differently from men, and symptom reporting by women is more culturally approved than by men. In addition, women seek medical care for symptoms more readily than men [1]. Psychiatric disorders such as anxiety and depression, which are associated with increased pain are more common in women than in men, and women have higher rates of childhood trauma than men [1].

Gijsbers van Weijk and Kolk provided a rather similar list of reasons in their gender-specific *general* symptom perception model [2]. This included an excess of somatic information in women, as a result of the female reproductive role, the disadvantageous social position of women associated with either a relative lack or a relative excess of external information, a female tendency to selectively attend to bodily cues, a female preference for a somatic attributional style, a stronger female disposition to somatise, or merely a greater willingness to report the symptoms they perceive to others [2].

Epidemiology

Across the world, women report more symptoms than men, not only in clinical but also in healthy study samples. They report more psychological, more medically 'explained', and

---

Medically Unexplained Symptoms, Somatisation and Bodily Distress, ed. Francis Creed, Peter Henningsen and Per Fink. Published by Cambridge University Press. © Cambridge University Press 2011.

more 'unexplained', somatic symptoms [1;2;3]. Accordingly, women have a higher overall morbidity than men, despite their higher life expectancy [4;5]. Studies investigating the prevalence of bodily distress syndromes almost unanimously find a female preponderance of about 70%; the frequent overlap of different functional somatic syndromes seems also to be more common in women [6;7;8;9].

Often, men and women report different symptoms. In fibromyalgia, for example, women report significantly more fatigue, gastrointestinal symptoms, generalized pain and tender points than do men [10;11]. In irritable bowel syndrome, women report different gastrointestinal and also extraintestinal symptoms than do men [12;13]. Whether female gender poses a risk marker for symptom chronicity, however, is contentious [14].

Healthcare use

Women show more *healthcare utilisation*, including prescription drugs in response to various health problems, and the female preponderance for 'medically unexplained' symptoms is much higher in clinical than in population studies [9;12]. Verbrugge hypothesised that women are more likely to label symptoms as physical illness, adopt the sick role and utilise the healthcare system for several reasons [4]. *Men* may tolerate physical discomfort better, be less interested in and concerned about their health, have less knowledge about signs and symptoms, feel it is not masculine to be ill or wish to ignore the implications of symptoms for their activities [4;15]. *Women* may experience social pressures and dispensations about the sick role, believe in the expedience of bed rest, activity restrictions and medical care, they may be more dependent and help-seeking for all kinds of problems. Women are less likely to deny troubles, and have more trust in authorities. Furthermore, they may have more flexible time schedules and more frequently see a regular physician, they may be more compliant and more willing to take follow-up actions [4]. It has been speculated that the high utilisation behaviour of women may be influenced by the need to repeat encounters to receive desired or necessary care which they would otherwise be denied [16].

Symptom perception and symptom processing

Of particular relevance to bodily distress syndromes is perceptual sensitivity, which differs between men and women. For example, pain perception and pain sensitivity appear to be influenced by sex hormones, gender-specific somatosensation and central nervous system (CNS) processing [3]. Women score higher on somatosensory amplification measures, and their sensitivity to pain, taste, smell, foods and medications varies depending on their menstrual phase [3;9;17;18].

A recent review of gender differences in pain perception and processing concluded that there is sufficient evidence for greater pain sensitivity among women compared with men for most pain modalities, but that the evidence regarding sex differences in laboratory measures of endogenous pain modulation, pain-related cerebral activation and responses to pharmacological and non-pharmacological pain treatments is mixed [3]. Most authors ascribe gender differences in symptom perception and processing not only to biological but also to psychosocial (e.g. gender role expectations or coping styles) mechanisms [3;9].

Body schemes, symptom attribution and illness beliefs

Gender aspects of body image in bodily distress syndromes have received relatively little relevant attention. For comparison, in body dysmorphic disorder (BDD), men are more likely to be concerned about their genitals, body build and thinning hair/balding; women are more likely to be concerned about their skin, stomach, weight, breasts/chest, buttocks, thighs, legs, hips, toes and excessive body/facial hair, and are excessively concerned with more body areas [19].

As to causal illness beliefs, it has been suggested that patients with 'medically unexplained' symptoms tend towards somatic rather than psychological illness attributions [2]. In two qualitative studies, women with chronic fatigue syndrome (CFS) and pain agreed to both psychosocial (way of living, workload, self-blaming) and organic (fragile immune system, virus infection, damage, strain) explanations [20;21]. Women in the general population or unselected primary care samples also tend towards psychosocial or multifactorial symptom explanations, whereas men are more likely to utilise somatic attribution styles [9;22]. Reviewing the psychological basis of symptom reporting, Pennebaker concluded that women are more likely to base their symptom reports on (stressful) external, i.e. situational cues than are men [9;23]. Accordingly, 'modern' worries about pollution, radiation, etc. are more common in women than in men [24;25]. Kaptein and colleagues were able to relate these concerns to the use of health services [25].

Specific health-related beliefs and behaviours that determine a *man's* attitude to his bodily symptoms include the denial of weakness or vulnerability, the appearance of being strong and robust, dismissal of any need for help, a ceaseless interest in sex, the display of aggressive behaviour and physical dominance [26]. There are strongly held cultural beliefs that men are more powerful and less vulnerable than women, that men's bodies are structurally more efficient than and superior to women's bodies, that asking for help and caring for one's health are feminine, and that the most powerful men are those for whom health and safety are irrelevant [26]. An analysis of narratives of 14 men with fibromyalgia syndrome found several different themes: feeling afraid of being looked upon as being a whiner; feeling like a guinea pig; experiencing the body as an obstruction; being a different man; striving to endure; feeling there would be no recovery; and not only feeling hopeful after having been referred to a specialist clinic, but also feeling neglected as an uninteresting patient [27]. Some of these themes are also reported by women with fibromyalgia: possible loss of freedom, a threat to integrity and a struggle to achieve relief and understanding [28].

Personality, emotion, coping styles, and gendered roles

The tendency to experience negative emotional states is referred to as 'neuroticism', one of the 'Big Five' personality traits. It appears to be more prominent in patients with 'medically unexplained' symptoms, it is associated with a heightened vigilance towards bodily symptoms and is more frequent, across different cultures, in women [9;29;30]. On the other hand, several studies found that women experience and express more emotions in general, i.e. not only distress, embarrassment, fear, guilt and sadness, but also more happiness, than men [17]. These differences are less obvious in children, so that the question has been raised whether environmental factors such as lifetime experiences, gender stereotypes and role expectations play the central role in the association between female gender, neuroticism and bodily complaints [9;17].

Symptom and illness experience is influenced by one's cognitive style, such as coping strategies. There is some evidence for gender differences in coping in general. Due to higher scores of rumination and helplessness, women score higher than men on pain catastrophising measures [3;9]. Girls were found to utilise interpersonal coping more than boys and, consistently, women were found to use social support and close friends more often than men – these differences in coping repertoires have been partly explained by a higher expression of (learned) illness behaviour and the sick role [4;9;31;32].

Probably, most of these gender differences in health-related cognitions, emotions and behaviours depend on gender role expectations rather than female sex. For example, emotional expressiveness is more likely to be reinforced in girls and women, and complaining of symptoms violates gender role norms for boys and men (the 'boys don't cry' doctrine) [2;9]. Toner and Akman emphasised the problematic socialisation of women to be compliant, understanding, never overtly angry and to please others instead of giving priority to themselves, in order to maintain safe, intimate relationships [12]. This behaviour may contribute to women's higher rates of utilisation of healthcare, because as patients they may be complying with their doctor's suggestions even when they are not in agreement with the treatment plan [12].

Psychosocial distress and psychiatric morbidity

The close association between anxiety and depression and bodily distress is well recognised (see Chapter 1). It is also recognised that women experience depression and anxiety about twice as often as men, and many studies have found higher rates of anxiety and depression in women presenting with 'medically unexplained' symptoms [3;9;33;34]. The gender-specific risk factors for anxiety and depression that disproportionally affect women include: gender-based violence, socioeconomic disadvantage, low income and income inequality, low or subordinate social status or rank, and unremitting responsibility for the care of others [33]. Although it might appear that a higher burden of psychosocial distress could sufficiently explain women's higher rates of bodily distress syndromes, this seems not to be the case: gender appears to influence symptom reporting in patients whether or not there is psychiatric comorbidity [1].

Illness consequences

Few studies have investigated gender-specific illness consequences such as disability, lower self-rated health and a lower health-related quality of life. Several studies have reported more illness consequences in men with 'medically unexplained' symptoms, others more in women, and yet others have found only small differences between the two. It has also been speculated though that, due to different coping mechanisms and role expectations, women may accept illness-related lifestyle disruptions more readily than men [9;35].

Stress and trauma

Social stress and prior trauma are associated with bodily distress syndromes (see Chapter 1). A meta-analytic review of gender differences in major and minor life events concluded that women report both greater exposure to and appraisal of stressful events than did men, but that the results were stronger for indicators of subjective stress appraisal than for the more objective indicators of stress exposure [36]. Regarding the nature of the stressor, women more often reported interpersonal (e.g. in the family) or workplace stressors [36;37]. Verbrugge pointed out that for women, too much but also too little social involvement causes distress [9;38].

Girls are generally more likely than boys to be victims of sexual abuse in childhood, and as adults, women are still more likely than men to be sexually and physically abused [9;39],

Several studies point towards a higher rate of trauma in female than male patients with bodily distress syndromes, but there are also studies reporting comparable rates in both sexes [9;12].

Genetics

A different *genetic pattern* in men and women could influence symptom generation as well as symptom perception or symptom interpretation. So far, there are no data indicating gender-specific genetic patterns in bodily distress, but there appear to be some genetic linkages for neuroticism [40]. It has been suggested that somatisation disorder and antisocial personality disorder might be gender-linked expressions of a common hereditary diathesis [41].

Physiology

None of the studies investigating physiological parameters in men *and* women with bodily distress syndromes have described gender differences [42], although, in general, men and women react differently to stressors, express different biomarkers of stress and immunity, and experience a different spectrum of diseases, e.g. autoimmune diseases [3;9;31]. There are also gender differences in the reaction to certain drugs, such as alosetron for irritable bowel syndrome [18] and analgesics [3].

Patient–doctor relationships and gendered communication

Medical encounters of patients with bodily distress syndromes have been described as difficult and frustrating for both patient and physician, but there are few data concerning gender differences in patient–doctor communication [43]. It has been shown that many more women than men (41% versus 27%, respectively) change physicians due to communication problems [15]. An analysis of gynaecological consultations revealed that it is not physician gender but gender-related specific communicative skill that predicted patient satisfaction and compliance [44].

Compared with their male colleagues, female physicians [15;43;45;46]:

- spend more time interviewing patients of both genders
- are more affective
- engage in significantly more active partnership behaviours, positive talk, psychosocial counselling, psychosocial questioning and emotionally focused talk
- more frequently use gender-specific communication strategies to explore the patient's perspective, whereas male physicians are said to be more imposing and presumptuous.

Male and female patients differ in the way they elaborate their complaints: women refer more to persons (family, friends, colleagues) than do men and include affective information along with physical symptoms [15;45]. A study about communicating fatigue in general practice reported that male fatigued patients tended to expect more biomedical communication than women; male as well as female physicians accommodated their verbal behaviour to fatigued patients by giving more psychosocial information and more counselling, but were not more affective towards fatigued than towards non-fatigued patients [46].

There are differences in the way that physicians respond to female and male patients, but this appears largely to be a consequence of the patient's behaviour [15]. Physicians ask women fewer questions and are more likely to reject their symptom explanations [15]. In one UK survey, more women than men felt that physicians talked down to them (25%

versus 12%, respectively) and told them their problems were 'in their heads' (17% versus 7%, respectively) [15]. All in all, however, it has been reported that over the past 30 years, gender differences in medical encounters have decreased [47].

Gender differences in diagnostic and treatment actions

The establishment of a diagnosis has been described as 'a gendered process', resulting from human interpretation of signs and symptoms within a sociopolitical context [48]. This may be an extreme view but there is evidence that physicians tend to interpret non-specific symptoms in women more readily as 'psychological' than in men, leading, for example, to a delayed diagnosis of autoimmune disorders in women [9;49]. Greer and colleagues showed that primary care physicians were more likely to believe that the presenting symptoms represented a psychological problem when patients were female, older or endorsing psychological symptom attributions [22]. This may lead to *mis*diagnoses in women but not in men [15]. With regard to abdominal pain, the diagnosis of functional gastrointestinal disorder was predominantly made after exclusion of an organic disease (more diagnostic procedures and specific therapies) more often in men than in women, despite similar final diagnoses for both genders [50]. There are several more vignette studies confirming the observation that either women wrongfully receive *too few* organic work-ups and labels – or men wrongfully receive *too many* [3;51].

Stigma and legitimacy

Societies that do not generally accept bodily distress syndromes as 'disease' often make patients struggle for the legitimacy of their symptoms, but this appears to apply for men and women alike [9;32]. Similarly, the difficulties faced by patients concerning bodily distress syndromes, such as stigma, scepticism and distrust from others regarding the credibility of their pain, are experienced by both men and women. On the other hand, positive experiences have been reported from a women-only group treatment for musculoskeletal pain ('recovery through recognition'), where recognition of their symptoms had enhanced their strength, confidence and competence [52].

Treatment response

Men and women respond differently to pharmacotherapy and also to non-pharmacological treatments. The findings, however, are conflicting and more research is needed [3]. For example, one review found that conventional physiotherapy was more effective for men, whereas intensive dynamic back exercises produced better pain reduction among women; women but not men with back pain undergoing cognitive behavioural treatment exhibited improved health-related quality of life; and women in active treatment showed reduced likelihood of permanent disability than women in the standard care control group, but no such effect emerged for men [3]. In contrast to these results, other studies found equal treatment gains for women and men after active rehabilitation for chronic low back pain [3]. A recent study reported that men benefitted less than women from a multidisciplinary treatment approach to fibromyalgia syndrome [53].

Conclusions

There are many differences between men and women which extend far beyond the higher prevalence of bodily distress syndromes in women. Since men and women differ in many biological, psychological and social characteristics, the care of patients with these disorders should be planned within this context. Doctors should be well aware that gender issues can affect the way that patients present symptoms as well as the way that doctors respond to them. It has been shown, for example, that physicians become less likely to propose somatic interventions after psychosocial presentations, which are more typical in women [15;45;54]. Further, Toner and Akman explicitly criticised the common misinterpretations of women patients as needy and demanding [12]. They stated that, for many women, the expression of distress and their demand for treatment may represent very rare occurrences in their lives that should rather be reframed as a healthy expression of good self-care and assertion [12]. Not surprisingly, patients feel satisfied and empowered by doctors who explain their symptoms in a tangible way, free of blame and which provide opportunities for self-management [55].

Thus, the consideration of gender issues (from pain perception to role expectations) is an important aspect of a more patient-centred, personalised approach to patients with bodily distress [9]. To improve care, doctors should be especially mindful of gender issues in the patient–doctor interaction, the process of making a diagnosis, treatment needs and response.

Older age

Early reports suggested that somatoform disorders were less common in the elderly than in younger age groups and this was attributed either to a decline in neuroticism with age or with difficulties in diagnosis [56]. The latter includes the fact that DSM-IV somatisation disorder requires symptoms commencing before the age of 30, and there are difficulties of accurate recall of symptoms over time [57]. Probably more difficulty is caused by the criterion of 'medically unexplained' symptoms in older people when physical illnesses are so much more common than at younger ages. Differentiating between 'medically unexplained' symptoms and those caused by organic disease is a special challenge when there is a high somatic comorbidity as is often the case in older people [58;59]. Recent research suggests that the problems of somatoform disorders are similar in older people to those at younger ages, but the problem of recognition may be greater if the diagnosis depends on 'medically unexplained' symptoms.

Epidemiology of somatic symptoms in older people

In a population-based study, Ladwig and colleagues reported that the total number of somatic symptoms increased with age until the 55–59 years age group [60]. For participants aged 60 years or over there was a slight decrease in the number of symptoms reported and the female predominance was less pronounced in this age group. A similar pattern was found for healthcare utilisation, with a steady increase in both sexes from the age of 35 years onwards. These results suggest that somatic symptom reporting increases from 20 years to 55 years and this probably reflects increasing physical illnesses as one gets older. Over 59 years, however, the slight decrease may be accounted for by older people complaining less about symptoms as the number physical illnesses tends to increase at this age.

A more recent publication from the same dataset showed that in both sexes a high number of reported somatic symptoms in the *absence* of a chronic physical illness was associated with a marked increase in healthcare use in participants over 64 years of age [61]. So it appears that the association between high healthcare use and numerous somatic symptoms in the absence of physical illness holds in older people just as in younger populations.

Another large population-based study in Germany reported that the prevalence of any somatoform disorders, diagnosed according to the *Diagnostic and Statistical Manual of Mental Disorders* (DSM)-IV criteria (14.9%), was similar in women aged 50–65 years and women aged 18–34 years (also 14.9%) [62]. Among men, however, somatoform disorders were significantly higher in the 50–65 years age group compared with the 18–34 years group (8.6% versus 5.7%: odds ratio 1.6; 95% CI 1.1–2.4). Thus although there is an increasing prevalence of somatoform disorders among men as they age, the female predominance of the disorder remains through the lifespan.

A detailed analysis of somatic symptom reporting in general population studies found that medically *explained* symptoms increase with age but medically *unexplained* symptoms (often measured on a lifetime basis) remain at a similar level across the lifespan [63]. The latter is important here – 'medically unexplained' symptoms and somatoform disorders are common in older people and they are more common in females than males.

The prevalence of chronic fatigue in a population-based sample in UK was highest in the 25–44 years age group but the prevalence remained high in the age groups 55–64 years and 65–74 years [64]. The odds ratio (95% CI) for the prevalence of chronic fatigue in the two older age groups compared with the 16–24 years age group was 2.53 (1.81–3.53) and 2.31 (1.65–3.24), respectively. This study showed that the prevalence of chronic fatigue increased with the number of physical illnesses but the association between these was unaffected by age, suggesting that in old age the high prevalence of chronic fatigue cannot be attributed solely to the presence of numerous physical illnesses. An Australian study showed that the prevalence of chronic fatigue in primary care attenders over 60 years of age was 27.4%, and the independent correlates were female sex, psychological disorder and physical illness [65]. At follow-up after one year, there was no tendency for fatigued patients to develop psychological disorder or vice versa, indicating that much fatigue was independent of psychological disorder. These data suggest that the relationship between fatigue, psychological disorder and physical illness is similar to that in younger age groups and this is supported by other studies described below.

A factor analytic study of symptoms reported by patients over 60 years of age attending primary care (n = 10 662) identified two factors pertaining to musculoskeletal symptoms and fatigue [66]. These were independent of the other two factors that emerged from the analysis, namely mood and cognitive symptoms. The authors argued that the independence of the musculoskeletal symptoms and fatigue from psychological symptoms is similar to that found in younger people and that it is incorrect to assume that somatic symptoms in older people are a reflection of underlying depression or anxiety.

Another study of adults aged 60 years or older (n = 3 498) attending primary care found that the most commonly reported symptoms were musculoskeletal pain (65%), fatigue (55%), back pain (45%) and shortness of breath (41%) [67]. It was apparent, not surprisingly, that the individual symptoms were associated with the expected physical conditions (e.g. musculoskeletal pain with arthritis, shortness of breath with chronic obstructive pulmonary disease) but, even after adjustment for chronic conditions the total score of physical symptoms (range 0–12) was a significant independent predictor of hospitalisation and death over the subsequent year. For example, 16% of the sample had a total symptom count in the top quartile. This group with a high total somatic symptom count showed an increased chance of subsequent hospitalisation (odds ratio 1.4 (1.0–1.9)) and death (OR 3.0 (1.42–6.4) even after controlling for age, sex, race, chronic medical conditions, perceived health, depression and anxiety [67]. In a more recent study of cancer patients with depression and/or pain, the number of somatic symptoms was associated with health status but not healthcare use [68]. The mean age of this cohort was 59 years (range 23–96 years) and number of somatic symptoms was weakly negatively correlated with age. In multivariate analysis, age was not associated with health status; the number of somatic symptoms and depression were the only significant correlates of disability. All of these epidemiological findings suggest strongly that the epidemiology of bodily distress syndromes is similar in older people to that reported in younger people.

In one of the few prospective studies of somatisation in primary care attenders over 65 years of age, it was found that the number of somatic symptoms regarded as bothersome was constant over a one-year period [69]. The proportion of people with a somatic attributional style also remained constant over one year but hypochondriacal neurosis waned from 5% to 1.6% during this time. In this study the high number of somatic symptoms was associated with female sex, low socioeconomic status, depression, physical illness and lack of social support. In a multivariate analysis to predict all contacts with the general practitioner, somatic symptom score and lack of social support were the only predictors; depression and physical illness were not included in the final model as significant predictors. In this study, the general practitioners rated a quarter of physical symptoms as having both physical and psychological origins and 13% were regarded as being primarily psychological in origin.

Diagnosing bodily distress syndromes in older people

Assessing whether symptoms are 'medically unexplained' presents some problems in older people. It requires a careful differential evaluation of the aetiology of symptoms, consideration of the relationship between subjective physical complaints and the objective medical situation. Given the large number of people who do not seek medical care for similar symptoms, the level of distress caused by the symptoms and other complex factors that drive the patient to seek medical care have to be taken into account.

Differentiating between 'medically unexplained' symptoms and symptoms caused by recognised physical illnesses is a special challenge when there is a high somatic comorbidity as may be the case in the elderly and in settings of medical disease [58;59]. Therefore using self-assessment screening instruments for 'medically unexplained' symptoms might be problematic in the elderly.

While for younger adults, validity and reliability of clinical diagnoses of somatoform disorders based on a comprehensive clinical work-up of every patient (semi-structured interviews, physical examination, routine laboratory tests, radiological examination and careful evaluation of available records) have been presented in the literature, this has not been specifically shown for elderly patients. Such a comprehensive work-up promises more valid results for diagnosing 'medically unexplained' symptoms in the elderly than employment of self-assessment screening instruments.

Bodily distress and factors associated with general perception of health

Epidemiological studies have shown that whereas the number of medical diseases and functional impairment increases with age, depressive mood, subjective well-being and subjective assessment of health in the elderly show no clear association with age [70;71;72]. In a representative Berlin city population aged over 70 years, there was a tendency to a more positive assessment of subjective health than indicated by objective health measures, increasingly so in the higher age groups [71].

Subjective assessment of health was correlated with subjectively experienced body complaints in a German general population sample aged over 60 years [73]. This study found an increasing number of bodily complaints with higher age in women and in older people with depressed mood, but the partner situation had no influence on the amount of body complaints, whereas in outpatients of an urban primary care practice 'medically unexplained' symptoms were more frequent in patients living alone [74]. Another finding in this sample was that in patients with 'medically unexplained' symptoms the rate of any current psychiatric disorder was twice that in the remainder [74]. Rather similar findings have been recorded in older patients: personality characteristics, depressive mood and social network were related to the total somatic symptom report, and trait negative affect provides valid information about older individuals' perceptions of their somatic states [75;76].

In a sample of patients in a general hospital, there were two groups who reported multiple somatic symptoms [77]. The first group (8.8% of the whole sample) reported multiple somatic symptoms, but they reported a positive attitude to life and relatively little impairment. The other group (14.9% of the sample) reported many somatic symptoms, negative evaluation of self, low life satisfaction, few social contacts and dissatisfaction with their most important close relationship. This group also showed the highest level of impairment as a result of psychological disorder.

Self-perception of health in older people does not appear to have a strong association with objective health parameters. The three independent predictors of self-perception of health have been reported as number of somatic complaints, sense of coherence and depression [78]. Subjectively experienced body complaints show a stronger association with self-assessment scales measuring life satisfaction and perception of age-related changes, as well as with the expert rating of somatisation. In cluster analysis of these data from older people in hospital there was a discrepancy between medical findings and subjective physical complaints in two clusters (altogether 23% of the sample) (77;79;80;81). On the whole, these results suggest that in the elderly (as in younger adults), the level of *subjective* body complaints is determined by subjective rather than by objective health measures and by other factors (personality, depressive mood, social factors), thus being an indicator for bodily distress syndromes in elderly inpatients.

Management of bodily distress syndromes in the elderly

Most studies on prevalence and management of medically unexplained symptoms in primary and secondary care settings focus on younger age groups and exclude subjects older than 65 years or, if they include them, they do not present the results differentiating for age groups and seem to apply the same procedures to younger and older adults. A Cochrane review on 'psychosocial interventions by general practitioners' identified three randomised controlled trials concerning bodily distress, but only adults up to 65 years of age were included [82]. Data on specific psychiatric or psychotherapeutic interventions for bodily distress syndromes in the elderly are also scarce. Studies have excluded elderly individuals or do not differentiate for age groups, or include only few individuals [83]. Interestingly, in a study by Arnold *et al.*, of 104 patients with a mean age of 47 years, with medically unexplained symptoms according to the general practitioner seven patients with a mean age of 60 years accepted cognitive-behavioural psychotherapy, indicating higher acceptance in the older patients [84].

Therefore the current evidence is insufficient to provide *specific* recommendations for management of bodily distress syndromes in older people in primary or secondary care or psychiatric or psychotherapeutic settings. Most data suggest that the problem of numerous somatic symptoms in older people is very similar to that found in younger people, so it is appropriate to assume that the same forms of treatment should be used in older people as in younger people. Much more research on these issues in older people is needed.

Cultural aspects

It has long been recognised that the presentation of bodily symptoms can be profoundly influenced by culture or ethnicity. This section will review some of the different aspects of this phenomenon. It starts with the principal concern for many years, namely the preoccupation with the notion that in non-Western cultures, or low income countries, distress was more likely to be expressed in terms of somatic symptoms rather than in psychological ones. Research over the last three decades has shown, however, that this phenomenon of 'somatisation' is universal, even though its expression may vary considerably across cultures and ethnic groups [85]. The literature concerning medically unexplained symptoms in different ethnic groups will be briefly reviewed. This will be followed by some comments on treatment seeking in different countries, which are pertinent to improving services in European countries for people of ethnic minority groups who present with bodily distress syndromes.

Somatic presentation of distress

'Culture-bound' syndromes

Somatic symptoms have been described in many cultures but their universality has only been recognised relatively recently. Many 'culture-bound syndromes' have been described; these are defined in DSM-IV as 'locality-specific, folk, diagnostic categories that frame coherent meanings for certain troubling sets of experiences'; they are specific to a particular community'[86]. The Indian and Sri Lankan 'dhat' syndrome, for example, comprises vague somatic symptoms of fatigue, weakness, anxiety, loss of appetite, guilt and sexual dysfunction attributed to loss of semen in nocturnal emissions, through urine and masturbation [87]. The syndrome may mystify doctors who are unaware of this syndrome, but it becomes understandable if seen in a cultural context.

According to South Asian cultural beliefs, a great deal of food is required to create a drop of blood and a considerable quantity of blood is required to form a drop of flesh. This is concentrated and converted to marrow and much marrow is required to create a drop of semen. Thus, seen against this background, the loss of semen represents a considerable threat to an individual's health. This may be regarded by the sufferer as either a psychological or physical problem; the latter view has been reported to be more common in lower socioeconomic groups [87]. A similar syndrome relating to loss of semen occurs in Chinese culture, as it is thought that semen (jing) contains the essence of qi, which, when lost, leads to weakness. A recent review of this phenomenon suggested that semen-loss anxiety is more widespread than generally realised [87]. It had been reported in Western cultures during the eighteenth and nineteenth centuries. The review argued that dhat syndrome is not culture-bound and it is certainly not an exclusive exotic neurosis of the Orient [87]. It can be seen as a cultural explanation of somatic symptoms. Such symptoms are common and universal but they are understood according to local explanatory models, which provide particular attributions of somatic symptoms.

Another example of a culture-bound syndrome in DSM-IV is 'brain fag', which has been described among students in Nigeria who experience stress when they have to leave their families to gain education, combined with heavy expectations upon them to succeed [88]. The symptoms include sensation of heaviness, heat or burning in the head and crawling sensations in the body, which become worse when studying for longer hours. A recent study found that these somatic symptoms were reported by over a third of apprentices in a Nigerian setting and a similar proportion experienced marked fatigue during their work [89]. Only a small proportion reported that the somatic symptoms were specifically associated with the learning process, which is regarded as a hallmark of the syndrome [89]. The symptoms have been associated with rural schools, schools serving more socially deprived areas and limited prior use of English, the language of tuition in many schools or colleges. Similarly, the Korean syndrome 'hwa-byung' includes feelings of heaviness, burning or a mass in the epigastric region, headaches, muscular aches and pains, dry mouth, insomnia, palpitations, and indigestion [85;90]. These somatic symptoms are understood to be due to the suppression of feelings of anger and resentment that form a sort of mass in the chest; patients can usually identify readily interpersonal and social problems that give rise to the anger, which is suppressed and leads to the somatic symptoms.

The review of dhat syndrome re-assessed the nosology of culture-bound syndromes using this as a particular example [87]. Syndromes such as those described above are heterogeneous and are best seen as psychological or psychosomatic symptoms that have been given a particular attribution according to cultural influences. They cannot always be forced into recognised DSM-IV diagnostic categories, but the appropriate diagnosis often becomes clearer if the full cultural context is appreciated.

These symptoms can cause difficulties in the patient–doctor relationship if the doctor does not recognise them and does not understand the cultural context in which they arise. The cultural context may determine both the nature of the symptoms, some of which may be alien to European or American doctors, and the explanation given by the patient for the symptoms. There is evidence that multiple somatic symptoms occur in all populations but the local labels given to this phenomenon and their interpretations differ much more than the exact somatic symptoms. It is necessary that a detailed review be performed of the individual's cultural background and the role of the cultural context in the expression and evaluation of symptoms. This should be done by a health professional who has an appropriate understanding and appreciation of the patient's culture.

Universality of 'medically unexplained' symptoms

A recent study from Sri Lanka recruited patients who had consulted a physician repeatedly with 'medically unexplained' symptoms [91]. The most common symptoms in this population are shown in Table 6.1. These are similar to those reported by patients in Europe and USA (listed in Chapter 1). Despite the similarity of the symptoms, however, some of the explanations would be unfamiliar to doctors in Europe or USA: 'A poison has got into my body'; 'I have swallowed a metal pin in 1950'; 'Because I breastfed my child while another child was watching'; 'Brother got paralysed at the age of 37 years and I think about it'; 'Because of chewing betel'; 'Because of the *Vatha*' (Ayurvedic concept referring to wind or gas); 'Due to too much heat in the body'.

Culture-bound syndromes mostly originated decades ago from careful clinical descriptions of a limited number of patients made by former generations of cultural psychiatrists and medical anthropologists. Under the influence of global nosology and rise in mental

Table 6.1 Common somatic symptoms in Sri Lankan patients recruited to a trial of cognitive behavioural therapy for medically unexplained symptoms [91]

Symptom	Per cent
Low backache	54
Chest pain	40
Pain in the limbs	38
Abdominal pain	22
Headache	34
Pain in the joints	31
Numbness in various body parts	29
Fatigue	28
Bloating of the abdomen	21
Faintish feeling	13
Loss of appetite	10
Burning sensation over various body parts	12
Sleep disturbance	7
Pain along the spine	4
Pain in other parts of the body not listed above	38

health literacy of both the public and healthcare practitioners, it is noteworthy that the once popular labels may no longer be fashionable. For example, a change in diagnostic habits has been reported recently in China. It had been thought previously that neurasthenia (*shenjing shuairuo*) was much more common in China than in Western cultures, but the use of this diagnosis has waned in recent years [92]. Doctors in China are now much more likely to diagnose depressive disorder and it is likely that they previously diagnosed depressed people as having neurasthenia. The reasons for this include the dominance of the DSM diagnostic system, the power of pharmaceutical companies and the prominence of depressive disorder in rigorous public health efforts that followed the global burden of disease study [93].

The fact that culture may influence the presentation and label of a set of somatic symptoms is not confined to Asian or low income countries. In fact over 30 years ago, Murphy observed that 'Transcultural psychiatry should begin at home' [94]. Examples of this are found in 'burn-out' and chronic fatigue syndrome, which are two syndromes found more commonly in Western countries than elsewhere. These appear to be separate syndromes, but share the symptoms of fatigue, muscle pains, nausea, headaches, flu-like symptoms and depressed mood. A recent review suggests that they have grown up in different 'cultural' settings – chronic fatigue in medical settings and burn-out in psychological ones [95]. Both disorders are attributed to external causes – either a medical illness or work – which leaves the sufferer free of any blame or responsibility for the disorder. The same is true of allergies, sick building syndrome and multiple chemical sensitivity. New syndromes appear and disappear, in fact, this is relabelling of the same symptoms [96].

Chronic fatigue syndrome is recognised more widely in UK than some other countries. A recent study has shown that Brazilian patients and doctors are less likely than their UK counterparts to recognise this as a diagnosis; patients are also less likely to regard disabling fatigue as a physical disease and more likely to regard it as a psychological disorder compared with UK patients [97;98]. The reasons that chronic fatigue syndrome is more widely recognised in UK than some other European countries include the prevailing beliefs held by health professionals and patients regarding causation, in particular the relative importance of psychological or somatic causes. These appear to be powerfully reinforced by patient support groups. The system of social benefits is also likely to be a powerful determinant [99].

There are few data that enable us to determine the relationship between culturally specific syndromes and diagnoses according to Western diagnostic systems. The following two examples illustrate some discrepancies. A study in Zimbabwe found there was only moderate agreement between the classification of patients with common mental disorders using an Euro-American classification system (the Clinical Interview Schedule, CIS, devised in UK) and the local care providers' judgement as to which patients were mentally ill [100]. It seemed that the local care providers were failing to diagnose common mental disorders (measured using CIS) in some patients, in line with much other research. On the other hand, the local care providers diagnosed as mentally ill a group of women with chronic physical illness, little education and a spiritual view of the cause of their symptoms. A third group of patients, who described the local phenomenon of 'kufungisisa' (thinking too much), was associated with common mental disorder (diagnosed using the CIS), giving some validity to this diagnosis.

In Hong Kong, a primary-care sample of patients who had chronic fatigue reported as their most frequent symptoms: pains, insomnia, headache, worries, fatigue and unhappiness [101]. These symptoms did not readily fit the categories of somatoform disorder because the concept of 'medically unexplained' requires a separation of mind and body, which is alien to the Chinese. Nor did they fit readily the diagnosis of chronic fatigue (syndrome), which requires the central feature of disabling fatigue. A more appropriate diagnosis, well recognised in Chinese society and widely used by Chinese clinicians until a couple of decades ago, was *shenjing shuairuo* (weakness of nerves), which requires three of the following symptoms: fatigue, pain, dysphoria, mental agitation and sleep symptoms. This reflects also the holistic view of Chinese medicine. Patients with this disorder identified psychosocial problems as the cause of their disorder and could talk about psychological distress in addition to the somatic symptoms. Concurrent anxiety and depression were common, and were associated with greater fatigue and more pronounced impairment, exactly as has been described in European and American populations (see Chapter 1).

Although population-based studies of somatic symptoms are largely lacking in non-Western communities, it appears that the somatic expression of distress is ubiquitous and there are different explanatory models in different cultures. It is important that health professionals working in European countries are familiar with these culturally specific ideas, otherwise they may be mystified by the symptoms presented by patients of ethnic minority status.

Medically unexplained symptoms in different ethnic groups

Assessing the cultural influences on the expression of distress is not easy. Systematic study of this phenomenon requires using the same measure in different cultural groups but this is problematic because standardised measures have usually been developed and validated only in a single culture, raising doubts about their validity in another culture. The Canadian study that follows used self-report of symptoms, which had been deemed 'medically unexplained' by a doctor; this is the method used by Western instruments to measure such symptoms.

A population-based study of five different ethnic groups living in Canada (anglophone and francophone Canadian-born and immigrants from the Caribbean, Vietnam and the Philippines) found no overall difference between these groups in the proportion who reported 'medically unexplained' somatic symptoms [102]. The only independent correlate of 'medically unexplained' symptoms was psychological distress; no socio-demographic factor was independently associated. It was found, however, that more Vietnamese men reported a 'medically unexplained' symptom than Vietnamese women, which was unexpected. The authors felt this was due to the high level of trauma experienced by these Vietnamese men. The immigrant groups used general medical care at the same rate as Canadian-born groups, but were significantly less likely to use specialised mental health services [85].

Early population-based studies in the USA, which used a standardised American research measure, suggested that the rare DSM-III diagnosis of somatisation disorder was more common in African-American women than white women, and even more common among Hispanic Americans [103;104]. It has been suggested subsequently that these differences might be explained by disparities in educational status between the groups rather than cultural differences [85]. More recently, Asian immigrants to the USA have been found to report *fewer* somatic symptoms than other ethnic groups and they also used general medical and mental health services less [105]. This might have been due to less anxiety disorder in this ethnic group. It is not clear whether educational level is truly a determinant of the predomination of somatic over psychological symptoms of distress. In an early study in India, contrary to popular belief, it was found that the literate people were more likely than the illiterate to report somatic symptoms of distress [106]. In Western cultures, the tendency to present somatic symptoms is not necessarily associated with educational level [107;108].

A worldwide World Health Organization (WHO) study examined patients attending primary care in 14 countries and took considerable care to try to assess psychiatric disorder using the same measure across different cultures while trying to take account of language and cultural differences across cultures [109]. It found that, after adjustment for age, sex, educational level and coexisting medical conditions, there was no significant difference between centres in the proportion of patients with depressive disorder who also met the criteria for multi-somatoform disorder [110]. The study found that the number of somatic symptoms was closely related to the level of depression, and this was similar across all centres. This positive correlation between somatic and affective distress speaks against the previously held notion that distress in non-Western people was merely transformed into a somatic form or that these people are less 'psychological-minded' than their Western counterparts.

On another measure, the proportion of depressed patients who presented only somatic symptoms, there was a difference across centres; this presentation was *least* likely at centres where there was an ongoing patient–physician relationship, scheduled appointments, detailed medical records and an emphasis on the privacy of the visit [110]. The presentation of purely somatic symptoms was more common where appointments were not scheduled and there was no ongoing patient–physician relationship. This finding suggests that presentation of somatic symptoms may be related to the nature of the healthcare system, which may influence the mode of help-seeking behaviour [85].

In the WHO study, the diagnoses of somatisation disorder, hypochondriasis and neurasthenia were not clearly associated with the prevalence of depression nor the geographical

Table 6.2 World Health Organization study: prevalence (%) of somatisation, hypochondriasis and neurasthenia among primary-care attenders by centre, arranged according to prevalence of current depression [109]

	Somatisation	Hypochondriasis	Neurasthenia	Depression
Santiago	**17.7**	**3.8**	**10.5**	29.5
Manchester	0.4	0.5	**9.7**	16.9
Groningen	**2.8**	**1.0**	**10.5**	15.9
Rio de Janeiro	**8.5**	**1.1**	4.5	15.8
Paris	1.7	0.1	**9.3**	13.7
Ankara	1.9	0.2	4.1	11.6
Mainz	**3.0**	**1.2**	7.7	11.2
Bangalore	1.8	0.2	2.7	9.1
Athens	1.3	0.2	4.6	6.4
Seattle	1.7	0.6	2.1	6.3
Berlin	1.3	0.4	**7.4**	6.1
Verona	0.1	0.3	2.1	4.7
Ibadan	0.4	**1.9**	1.1	4.2
Shanghai	1.5	0.4	2.0	4.0
Nagasaki	0.1	0.4	3.4	2.6
Total	2.7	0.8	5.4	10.4

area or state of economic development of the countries concerned (Table 6.2). The only slight association that can be observed in Table 6.2 is that neurasthenia tends to be a disorder seen mostly in high income countries. The authors of this study pointed out that in different cultures there are different concepts, as we have observed above, which underlie psychological symptoms. For example, 'burn-out' in the USA, 'postviral fatigue' in Europe and North America, 'kidney weakness' in China, '*jibyo*' in Japan, are common culturally accepted explanations for symptoms. These are different labels for essentially the same symptoms. Such constructs may influence the way in which symptoms are perceived and selected for presentation to doctors. Conversely, local practitioners might selectively attend to and elicit patients' symptoms in particular clinical settings.

Bodily distress syndromes in single ethnic groups

There are fewer methodological difficulties when representative samples of people of the same culture are studied. Among Chinese people living in the USA, those who recorded a high score on a self-administered somatic symptoms questionnaire were more likely than the remainder to be female, older, have few years of education and report anxiety, depression and financial strain [111]. These findings are similar to those found in indigenous white populations. The number of years spent in the USA since immigration and level of acculturation were not associated with number of somatic symptoms. The most frequently reported symptoms were almost identical to those documented in European and American populations: headaches, lower back pains, muscle soreness, body feeling weak, body numbness/tingling [112;113].

Irritable bowel syndrome is as common in Asian populations as it is in the USA and Europe where this syndrome has been studied widely. Its characteristics are very similar in Asian countries to those seen in Western cultures, with the possible exception that the sex difference is less pronounced [114;115]. The disorder is associated with anxiety and depression in Asian cultures, just as in the West, and this could contribute to the lack of a sex difference in those countries [116;117;118;119]. Such studies suggest that within a single culture, the factors associated with numerous somatic symptoms are similar to those that have been recorded in Western cultures. An additional factor concerns the local healthcare system: these vary greatly between different countries and may have considerable impact on how symptoms are presented to those who provide care.

Treatment seeking

As well as influencing symptoms, society and culture will also have a strong effect on pathways to help-seeking and healthcare; economic, political and human resources are also important in this respect. For example, in Western countries there is a predominance of females among clinic attenders with bodily distress syndromes, whereas in Pakistan men present more frequently to doctors, even though for the disorders which are more common in women; this reflects the cultural and economic influences on medical help-seeking [117]. In UK, primary-care studies have shown that people of an ethnic minority group, such as those of South Asian origin, present to primary care with more somatic symptoms than white Europeans, but this could be a reflection of more severe depression [120].

In a population-based UK study, depressed people of Pakistani origin consulted their general practitioner more than twice as often as their depressed white European counterparts, a finding that could not be explained by more severe depression [121]. It was observed also that these medical consultations were twice as likely to be primarily for bodily symptoms in participants of Pakistani origin compared with white Europeans, yet the number of consultations for anxiety or depression was identical in the two groups. Thus in a situation where access to medical care is open and free, depressed people of Pakistani origin were making the same number of consultations as white Europeans for psychological symptoms but they made additional consultations for bodily symptoms. These findings could not be accounted for by an excess of physical illness in people of Pakistani origin as such illness was equally prevalent in the two ethnic groups [121]. There was also no difference between the ethnic groups in the number of somatic symptoms reported on a self-administered questionnaire. This study was accompanied by a qualitative study aimed at determining any differences between the two ethnic groups concerning the language and representation of mental distress and whether this may be part of the explanation for different patterns of help seeking and health outcomes [122].

Overall, it was found that the language used to describe depression and the accompanying somatic metaphors were similar in the two groups [122]. There were some differences, however: people of Pakistani origin in general used the idea of 'too much thinking', which rarely featured in the descriptions given by white Europeans. The somatic symptoms of heavy headedness, numbness, and emptiness were also found primarily among the people of Pakistani origin. The link between mental distress and pain was made most often by the least educated, older women of Pakistani origin. This study is instructive as it suggests a marked difference between the appreciation of somatic symptoms within the context of depression, which is similar across the ethnic groups, and the medical help-seeking behaviour. Depressed people of Pakistani origin were turning to doctors much more frequently for somatic symptoms than depressed white Europeans, a finding which has not been fully explained.

A study of American and Thai children came to similar conclusions [123]. In population-based samples, depressive and somatic symptoms were equally prevalent in the American and Thai children. Among clinic attenders, however, somatic symptoms were more prominent in the Thai children compared with the American children. This difference held even after controlling for level of psychopathology. The authors concluded that the experience of somatic and psychological symptoms was similar in the two ethnic groups but that when it came to seeing a doctor, somatic symptoms were given preference by the Thai, but not American families. It is clear that the healthcare system and practitioners tend to influence the clinical presentation when people with distress seek medical help.

Among Chinese people living in the USA, it has been found that somatisation or somatoform disorders are closely associated with increased medical help-seeking. In a multivariate analysis that controlled for confounders, somatoform disorders, not anxiety or depressive disorders, were independently associated with medical help-seeking. It appears that there is something specific about seeking medical help for somatic symptoms [124]. It is unclear if this is so for Chinese people living in Chinese communities.

The UK study of people of Pakistani origin showed a marked difference regarding treatment of depression in the two ethnic groups. In spite of the higher consultation rate among depressed women of Pakistani origin, they were only half as likely as their depressed white counterparts to be prescribed antidepressant medication (22.5% versus 50%, respectively). The difference was even greater for the proportion receiving psychological therapy (6.1% versus 24.5%, respectively). There was no difference between the ethnic groups for the treatment received by men. Interestingly, alternative sources of help, including from a hakim/homoeopath, did not differ significantly between the two ethnic groups. It is not clear which aspect of the doctor–patient interaction leads to this finding (whether the doctor fails to recognise the depression and/or the patient is not assertive or is reluctant to take antidepressants), but it is an important failing of the health system that people in need fail to receive appropriate treatment.

Treatment seeking in low- and middle-income countries

There are now an increasing number of studies from low- and middle-income countries suggesting rather similar patterns of morbidity and treatment seeking for somatic symptoms as those previously documented in European and American studies. For example, the presentation of medically unexplained symptoms at general medical clinics in Karachi is similar to the pattern seen in European and American clinics; the proportion of women with these symptoms is higher than men and there is a close association with anxiety and depression [125].

Randomised controlled treatment trials for 'medically unexplained' symptoms have been performed in Sri Lanka [126;127]. These have been high-quality studies and are discussed in some detail in Chapter 3. Essentially the pattern of symptoms among patients thus classified and their response to treatment is similar to that seen in Western countries. Moreover, it is worth noting that when patients' explanatory models are elicited and used in the clinical negotiation process, Western-style therapies such as cognitive behavioural therapy are likely to be just as applicable to non-Western patients, even if the latter hold certain local attributions of illness that are not commonly encountered in the West [128].

The culturally sensitive treatments being developed for depression among Chinese Americans and Pakistani people in UK are likely to be highly appropriate for members of these ethnic minority groups in Western countries who have multiple somatic symptoms

[129;130]. These approaches recommend that therapists elicit patient's illness beliefs, understand and acknowledge multiple explanatory models, and understand depressive symptoms within the context of the patient's physical health and social system [131]. It is not clear whether low- and middle-income countries are becoming more industrialised and Westernised, so a similar pattern of symptoms and treatment seeking is now observed, or whether research techniques have improved, e.g. by including more representative samples, so that symptoms and treatment response are being documented in a way which allows the similarity to become evident.

Implications for delivering services in European countries

The main aim of this book is to identify ways in which services for patients with bodily distress syndromes can be improved. It is tempting to suggest specialist services for people of ethnic minorities living in Europe, but there are several reasons against this. Firstly, it implies that most doctors cannot be trained to identify and manage satisfactorily bodily distress syndromes in people of ethnic minorities in Europe. It is true that doctors who have an intimate knowledge of the culture of people of ethnic minorities are at an advantage, but it is unlikely that an exact match of cultural background of doctors and patients can ever be achieved. It is more important that all doctors routinely ask patients who present with bodily distress about their views concerning the cause of the symptoms. Additional help from an interpreter or a person with appropriate cultural knowledge can be sought if necessary. Improving the cultural competence of all doctors in Europe is desirable and could be effective in helping them to improve their management of people with a different cultural background from their own. This holds for medical conditions, not just bodily distress syndromes. In the case of the latter, however, understanding fully the patient's view of their symptoms could play a part in reducing investigations for organic disease.

It would be expensive to set up specialist services for people of ethnic minorities. This means they are less likely to be developed. It also means that other doctors, who are not culturally competent, can continue to refrain from developing these essential skills. This would be undesirable as understanding symptoms from the patient's viewpoint is an essential skill which is necessary both to manage somatic symptoms and to cope with cultural differences between doctors and patients. Separate specialist services do not help people from ethnic minorities to integrate fully and make proper use of all health services.

References

1. Barsky AJ, Peekna HM, Borus JF. Somatic symptom reporting in women and men. *Journal of General Internal Medicine* 2001; **16**: 266–75.

2. Gijsbers Van Wijk CM, Kolk AM. Sex differences in physical symptoms: The contribution of symptom perception theory. *Social Science and Medicine* 1997; **45**: 231–46.

3. Fillingim RB, King CD, Ribeiro-Dasilva MC, Rahim-Williams B, Riley JL 3rd. Sex, gender, and pain: a review of recent clinical and experimental findings. *Journal of Pain* 2009; **10**: 447–85.

4. Verbrugge L. Gender and health: An update on hypotheses and evidence. *Journal of Health and Social Behaviour* 1985; **26**: 156–82.

5. World Health Organization. Department of Gender and Women's Health. *Gender, Health and Aging*. Geneva: World Health Organization; 2003.

6. Ladwig KH, Marten-Mittag B, Erazo N, Gündel H. Identifying somatization disorder in a population-based health examination survey: psychosocial burden and gender differences. *Psychosomatics* 2001; **42**: 511–18.

7. Aggarwal VR, McBeth J, Zakrzewska JM, Lunt M, Macfarlane GJ. The epidemiology of chronic syndromes that are frequently unexplained: do they have common associated factors? *International Journal of Epidemiology* 2006; **35**: 468–76.

8. Kanaan RA, Lepine JP, Wessely SC. The association or otherwise of the functional somatic syndromes. *Psychosomatic Medicine* 2007; **69**: 855–9.

9. Johnson S. *Medically Unexplained Illness. Gender and Biopsychosocial Implications.* Washington: American Psychological Association; 2008.

10. Wolfe F, Ross K, Anderson J, Russell IJ. Aspects of fibromyalgia in the general population: sex, pain threshold, and fibromyalgia symptoms. *Journal of Rheumatology* 1995; **22**: 151–6.

11. Yunus MB, Inanici F, Aldag JC, Mangold RF. Fibromyalgia in men: comparison of clinical features with women. *Journal of Rheumatology* 2000; **27**: 485–90.

12. Toner BB, Akman D. Gender role and irritable bowel syndrome: literature review and hypothesis. *American Journal of Gastroenterology* 2000; **95**: 11–16.

13. Heitkemper MM, Cain KC, Jarrett ME, Burr RL, Hertig V, Bond EF. Gender differences in gastrointestinal, psychological, and somatic symptoms in irritable bowel syndrome. *Digestive Diseases and Sciences* 2009; **54**: 1542–9.

14. olde Hartman TC, Borghuis MS, Lucassen PL, van de Laar FA, Speckens AE, van Weel C. Medically unexplained symptoms, somatisation disorder and hypochondriasis: course and prognosis. A systematic review. *Journal of Psychosomatic Research* 2009; **66**: 363–77.

15. Elderkin-Thompson V, Waitzkin H. Differences in clinical communication by gender. *Journal of General Internal Medicine* 1999; **14**: 112–21.

16. Galdas PM, Cheater F, Marshall P. Men and health help-seeking behaviour: literature review. *Journal of Advanced Nursing* 2005; **49**: 616–23.

17. Else-Quest NM, Hyde JS, Goldsmith HH, van Hulle CA. Gender differences in temperament: a meta-analysis. *Psychological Bulletin* 2006; **132**: 33–72.

18. Ouyang A, Wrzos HF. Contribution of gender to pathophysiology and clinical presentation of IBS: should management be different in women? *American Journal of Gastroenterology* 2006; **101**: S602–9.

19. Phillips KA, Menard W, Fay C. Gender similarities and differences in 200 individuals with body dysmorphic disorder. *Comprehensive Psychiatry* 2006; **47**: 77–87.

20. Soderlund A, Malterud K. Why did I get chronic fatigue syndrome? A qualitative interview study of causal attributions in women patients. *Scandinavian Journal of Primary Health Care* 2005; **23**: 242–7.

21. Johansson EE, Hamberg K, Westman G, Lindgren G. The meanings of pain: an exploration of women's descriptions of symptoms. *Social Science and Medicine* 1999; **48**: 1791–802.

22. Greer J, Halgin R, Harvey E. Global versus specific symptom attributions: predicting the recognition and treatment of psychological distress in primary care. *Journal of Psychosomatic Research* 2004; **57**: 521–7.

23. Pennebaker JW. Psychological bases of symptom reporting: perceptual and emotional aspects of chemical sensitivity. *Toxicology and Industrial Health* 1994; **10**: 497–511.

24. Petrie KJ, Broadbent EA, Kley N, Moss-Morris R, Horne R, Rief W. Worries about modernity predict symptom complaints after environmental pesticide spraying. *Psychosomatic Medicine* 2005; **67**: 778–82.

25. Kaptein AA, Helder DI, Kleijn WC, Rief W, Moss-Morris R, Petrie KJ. Modern health worries in medical students. *Journal of Psychosomatic Research* 2005; **58**: 453–7.

26. Courtenay WH. Constructions of masculinity and their influence on men's well-being: a theory of gender and health. *Social Science and Medicine* 2000; **50**: 1385–401.

27. Paulson M, Danielson E, Söderberg S. Struggling for a tolerable existence: the meaning of men's lived experiences of living with pain of fibromyalgia type. *Qualitative Health Research* 2002; **12**: 238–49.

28. Söderberg S, Lundman B, Norberg A. Struggling for dignity: the meaning of women's experiences of living with fibromyalgia. *Qualitative Health Research* 1999; **9**: 575–87.

29. Rosmalen JG, Neeleman J, Gans RO, de Jonge P. The association between neuroticism and self-reported common somatic symptoms in a population cohort. *Journal of Psychosomatic Research* 2007; **62**: 305–11.

30. Schmitt DP, Realo A, Voracek M, Allik J. Why can't a man be more like a woman? Sex differences in Big Five personality traits across 55 cultures. *Journal of Personality and Social Psychology* 2008; **94**: 168–82.

31. Baum A, Grunberg NE. Gender, stress, and health. *Health Psychology* 1991; **10**: 80–5.

32. Nettleton S. 'I just want permission to be ill': towards a sociology of medically unexplained symptoms. *Social Science and Medicine* 2006; **62**: 1167–78.

33. World Health Organization. *Gender and Women's Mental Health. Gender Disparities in Mental Health: The Facts.* Geneva: World Health Organization; 2010. Available at: www.who.int/mental_health/prevention/genderwomen/ (Accessed 28 March, 2010).

34. World Health Organization, Mental Health Determinants and Populations, Department of Mental Health and Substance Dependence. *Women's Mental Health: An Evidence-Based Review.* Geneva: World Health Organization; 2000.

35. Dancey CP, Hutton-Young SA, Moye S, Devins GM. Perceived stigma, illness intrusiveness and quality of life in men and women with irritable bowel syndrome. *Psychology, Health and Medicine* 2002; **7**: 382–95.

36. Davis MC, Matthews KA, Twamley EW. Is life more difficult on Mars or Venus? A meta-analytic review of sex differences in major and minor life events. *Annals of Behavioral Medicine* 1999; **21**: 83–97.

37. World Health Organization, European Ministerial Conference. Mental Health and working life. In: *Mental health: facing the challenges, building solutions.* Helsinki: World Health Organization; 2005: 59–65.

38. Verbrugge L. The twain meet: Empirical explanation of sex differences in health and mortality. *Journal of Health and Social Behavior* 1989; **30**: 282–304.

39. Russo NF, Pirlott A. Gender-based violence: concepts, methods, and findings. *Annals of the New York Academy of Sciences* 2006; **1087**: 178–205.

40. Gillespie NA, Zhu G, Evans DM, Medland SE, Wright MJ, Martin NG. A genome-wide scan for Eysenckian personality dimensions in adolescent twin sibships: psychoticism, extraversion, neuroticism, and lie. *Journal of Personality* 2008; **76**: 1415–46.

41. Lilienfeld SO. The association between antisocial personality and somatization disorder: a review and integration of theoretical models. *Clinical Psychology Review* 1992; **12**: 641–62

42. Rief W, Barsky AJ. Psychobiological perspectives on somatoform disorders. *Psychoneuroendocrinology* 2005; **30**: 996–1002.

43. Roter DL, Hall JA, Aoki Y. Physician gender effects in medical communication: a meta-analytic review. *Journal of the American Medical Association* 2002; **288**: 756–64.

44. Christen RN, Alder J, Bitzer J. Gender differences in physicians' communicative skills and their influence on patient satisfaction in gynaecological outpatient consultations. *Social Science and Medicine* 2008; **66**: 1474–83.

45. Meeuwesen L, Schaap C, van der Staak C. Verbal analysis of doctor–patient communication. *Social Science and Medicine* 1991; **32**: 1143–50.

46. Meeuwesen L, Bensing J, van den Brink-Muinen A. Communicating fatigue in general practice and the role of gender. *Patient Education and Counseling* 2002; **48**: 233–42.

47. Bensing JM, Tromp F, van Dulmen S, van den Brink-Muinen A, Verheul W, Schellevis FG. Shifts in doctor–patient communication between 1986 and 2002: a study of videotaped general practice consultations with hypertension patients. *BMC Family Practice* 2006; **7**: 62.

48. Malterud K. The (gendered) construction of diagnosis interpretation of medical signs in women patients. *Theoretical Medicine and Bioethics* 1999; **20**: 275–86.

49. Chrisler JC, O'Hea EL. Gender, culture, and autoimmune disorders. In: Eisler RM, ed. *Handbook of Gender, Culture, and Health*. Mahwah (New Jersey): Erlbaum; 2000: 321–42.

50. Healy B. The Yentl syndrome. *New England Journal of Medicine* 1991; **325**: 274–6.

51. Armitage KJ, Schneiderman LJ, Bass RA. Response of physicians to medical complaints in men and women. *Journal of the American Medical Association* 1979; **241**(20): 2186–7.

52. Werner A, Steihaug S, Malterud K. Encountering the continuing challenges for women with chronic pain: recovery through recognition. *Qualitative Health Research* 2003; **13**: 491–509.

53. Hooten WM, Townsend CO, Decker PA. Gender differences among patients with fibromyalgia undergoing multidisciplinary pain rehabilitation. *Pain Medicine* 2007; **8**: 624–32.

54. Salmon P, Humphris GM, Ring A, *et al.* Why do primary care physicians propose medical care to patients with medically unexplained symptoms? A new method of sequence analysis to test theories of patient pressure. *Psychosomatic Medicine* 2006; **68**: 570–7.

55. Salmon P, Peters S, Stanley I. Patients' perceptions of medical explanations for somatisation disorders: qualitative analysis. *British Medical Journal* 1999; **318**(7180): 372–6.

56. Wijeratne C, Hickie I. Somatic distress syndromes in later life: the need for paradigm change. *Psychological Medicine* 2001; **31**(4): 571–6.

57. Simon GE, Gureje O. Stability of somatization disorder and somatization symptoms among primary care patients. *Archives of General Psychiatry* 1999; **56**(1): 90–5.

58. Schneider G, Heuft G, Senf W, Schepank H. Adaptation of the impairment-score (IS) for gerontopsychosomatics and psychotherapy

in old age. *Zeitschrift fur Psychosomatische Medizin und Psychoanalyse* 1997; **43**(3): 261–79.

59. Fava GA, Mangelli L, Ruini C. Assessment of psychological distress in the setting of medical disease. *Psychotherapy and Psychosomatics* 2001; **70**(4): 171–5.

60. Ladwig KH, Marten-Mittag B, Formanek B, Dammann G. Gender differences of symptom reporting and medical health care utilization in the German population. *European Journal of Epidemiology* 2000; **16**: 511–18.

61. Ladwig KH, Marten-Mittag B, Lacruz ME, Henningsen P, Creed F; MONICA KORA Investigators. Screening for multiple somatic complaints in a population-based survey: does excessive symptom reporting capture the concept of somatic symptom disorders? Findings from the MONICA-KORA Cohort Study. *Journal of Psychosomatic Research* 2010; **68**(5): 427–37.

62. Klose M, Jacobi F. Can gender differences in the prevalence of mental disorders be explained by sociodemographic factors? *Archives of Women's Mental Health* 2004; **7**(2): 133–48.

63. Tomenson B, Creed F, on behalf of the DSM-V population project group. Can we diagnose somatoform disorders using all bodily symptoms rather than 'medically unexplained' symptoms? In: XIII annual meeting of the European Association for Consultation-Liaison Psychiatry and Psychosomatics (EACLPP) XXVIII European Conference on Psychosomatic Research (ECPR): a selection of abstracts submitted Innsbruck, June 30 – July 3, 2010. *Journal of Psychosomatic Research* 2010; **68**(6): 605–79.

64. Watanabe N, Stewart R, Jenkins R, Bhugra DK, Furukawa TA, Watanabe N *et al.* The epidemiology of chronic fatigue, physical illness, and symptoms of common mental disorders: a cross-sectional survey from the second British National Survey of Psychiatric Morbidity. *Journal of Psychosomatic Research* 2008; **64**(4): 357–62.

65. Wijeratne C, Hickie I, Brodaty H. The characteristics of fatigue in an older primary

care sample. *Journal of Psychosomatic Research* 2007; **62**(2): 153–8.

66. Wijeratne C, Hickie I, Davenport T. Is there an independent somatic symptom dimension in older people? *Journal of Psychosomatic Research* 2006; **61**(2): 197–204.

67. Sha MC, Callahan CM, Counsell SR, Westmoreland GR, Stump TE, Kroenke K. Physical symptoms as a predictor of health care use and mortality among older adults. *American Journal of Medicine* 2005; **118**(3): 301–6.

68. Kroenke K, Zhong X, Theobald D, Wu JW, Tu WZ, Carpenter JS. Somatic symptoms in patients with cancer experiencing pain or depression prevalence, disability, and health care use. *Archives of Internal Medicine* 2010; **170**(18): 1686–94.

69. Sheehan B, Bass C, Briggs R, Jacoby R. Somatization among older primary care attenders. *Psychological Medicine* 2003; **33**(5): 867–77.

70. Harwood RH, Prince MJ, Mann AH, Ebrahim S. The prevalence of diagnoses, impairments, disabilities and handicaps in a population of elderly people living in a defined geographical area: the Gospel Oak project. *Age and Ageing* 1998; **27**(6): 707–14.

71. Staudinger UM, Freund A, Linden M, Maas I. Self, personality and life regulation: Facets of psychological resilience in old age. In: Baltes PB, Mayer KU (eds). *The Berlin Ageing Study: Ageing from 70 to 100*. New York: Cambridge University Press; 1999: 302–8.

72. Smith J, Baltes PB. Profiles of psychological functioning in the old and oldest old. *Psychology and Aging* 1997; **12**(3): 458–72.

73. Gunzelmann T, Schumacher J, Brahler E. Subjective body complaints in the elderly: Standardization of the Giessen subjective complaints list (GBB-24). *Zeitschrift fur Gerontologie und Geriatrie* 1996; **29**(2): 110–18.

74. Feder A, Olfson M, Gameroff M, Fuentes M, Shea S, Lantigua RA *et al.* Medically unexplained symptoms in an urban general medicine practice. *Psychosomatics* 2001; **42**(3): 261–8.

75. Rennemark M, Hagberg B. What makes old people perceive symptoms of illness? The impact of psychological and social factors. *Aging and Mental Health* 1999; **3**(1): 79–87.

76. Mora PA, Robitaille C, Leventhal H, Swigar M, Leventhal EA. Trait negative affect relates to prior-week symptoms, but not to reports of illness episodes, illness symptoms, and care seeking among older persons. *Psychosomatic Medicine* 2002; **64**(3): 436–49.

77. Schneider G, Driesch G, Kruse A, Wachter M, Nehen HG, Heuft G. Ageing styles: subjective well-being and somatic complaints in inpatients aged ≥60 years. *Psychotherapy and Psychosomatics* 2003; **72**(6): 324–32.

78. Schneider G, Driesch G, Kruse A, Wachter M, Nehen HG, Heuft G. What influences self-perception of health in the elderly? The role of objective health condition, subjective well-being and sense of coherence. *Archives of Gerontology and Geriatrics* 2004; **39**(3): 227–37.

79. Schneider G, Driesch G, Kruse A, Nehen HG, Heuft G. What influences subjective health in the eiderly? The roll of objective health factors, subjective wellbeing and the feeling of coherence. *Psychotherapie Psychosomatik Medizinische Psychologie* 2004; **54**(2): 111–12.

80. Schneider G, Wachter M, Driesch G, Kruse A, Nehen HG, Heuft G. Subjective body complaints as an indicator of somatization in elderly patients. *Psychosomatics* 2003; **44**(2): 91–9.

81. Schneider G, Driesch G, Kruse A, Nehen HG, Heuft G. Old and ill and still feeling well? Determinants of subjective well-being in ≥60 year olds: The role of the sense of coherence. *American Journal of Geriatric Psychiatry* 2006; **14**(10): 850–9.

82. Huibers MJ, Beurskens AJ, Bleijenberg G, van Schayck CP. The effectiveness of psychosocial interventions delivered by general practitioners. *Cochrane Database of Systematic Reviews* 2003; **2**: CD003494.

83. Kroenke K, Swindle R. Cognitive-behavioral therapy for somatization and symptom syndromes: a critical review of

controlled clinical trials. *Psychotherapy and Psychosomatics* 2000; **69**(4): 205–15.

84. Arnold IA, Speckens AEM, van Hemert AM. Medically unexplained physical symptoms: The feasibility of group cognitive-behavioural therapy in primary care. *Journal of Psychosomatic Research* 2004; **57**(6): 517–20.

85. Kirmayer LJ, Young A. Culture and somatization: Clinical, epidemiological, and ethnographic perspectives. *Psychosomatic Medicine* 1998; **60**(4): 420–30.

86. American Psychiatric Association. *Diagnostic and Statistical Manual of Mental Disorders – DSM-IV*, 4th edn. Washington: American Psychiatric Association; 1994.

87. Sumathipala A, Siribaddana SH, Bhugra D. Culture-bound syndromes: the story of dhat syndrome. *British Journal of Psychiatry* 2004; **184**: 200–9.

88. Guinness EA. Profile and prevalence of the brain fag syndrome: psychiatric morbidity in school populations in Africa. *British Journal of Psychiatry* 1992; **160**(Suppl 16): 53–64.

89. Morakinyo O, Peltzer K. 'Brain fag' symptoms in apprentices in Nigeria. *Psychopathology* 2002; **35**(6): 362–6.

90. Lin KM. Hwa-byung – a Korean culture-bound syndrome. *American Journal of Psychiatry* 1983; **140**(1): 105–7.

91. Sumathipala A, Siribaddana S, Hewege S, Sumathipala K, Prince M, Mann A. Understanding the explanatory model of the patient on their medically unexplained symptoms and its implication on treatment development research: a Sri Lanka Study. *BMC Psychiatry* 2008; **8**: 47.

92. Lee S, Kleinman A. Are somatoform disorders changing with time? The case of neurasthenia in China. *Psychosomatic Medicine* 2007; **69**(9): 846–9.

93. Lee S. Socio-cultural and global health perspectives for the development of future psychiatric diagnostic systems. *Psychopathology* 2002; **35**(2–3): 152–7.

94. Murphy HBM. Transcultural-psychiatry should begin at home. *Psychological Medicine* 1977; **7**(3): 369–71.

95. Leone SS, Wessely S, Huibers MJ, Knottnerus JA, Kant I. Two sides of the same coin? On the history and phenomenology of chronic fatigue and burnout. *Psychology and Health* 2010; **29**: 1–16.

96. Wessely S. Old wine in new bottles – neurasthenia and me. *Psychological Medicine* 1990; **20**(1): 35–53.

97. Cho HJ, Menezes PR, Bhugra D, Wessely S. The awareness of chronic fatigue syndrome: a comparative study in Brazil and the United Kingdom. *Journal of Psychosomatic Research* 2008; **64**(4): 351–5.

98. Cho HJ, Bhugra D, Wessely S. 'Physical or psychological?' – a comparative study of causal attribution for chronic fatigue in Brazilian and British primary care patients. *Acta Psychiatrica Scandinavica* 2008; **118**(1): 34–41.

99. Wessely S, Hotopf M, Sharpe M. *Chronic Fatigue and its Syndromes*. Oxford: Oxford University Press; 1998.

100. Patel V, Mann A. Etic and emic criteria for non psychotic mental disorder: a study of the CISR and care provider assessment in Harare. *Social Psychiatry and Psychiatric Epidemiology* 1997; **32**(2): 84–9.

101. Lee S, Yu H, Wing Y, Chan C, Lee AM, Lee DTS *et al.* Psychiatric morbidity and illness experience of primary care patients with chronic fatigue in Hong Kong. *American Journal of Psychiatry* 2000; **157**(3): 380–4.

102. Kirmayer LJ, Groleau D, Looper KJ, Dao MD. Explaining medically unexplained symptoms. *Canadian Journal of Psychiatry* 2004; **49**: 663–72.

103. Robbins L N, Regier D. *Psychiatric Disorders in America: The Epidemiologic Catchment Area Study*. New York: Free Press; 1991.

104. Canino IA, Rubiostipec M, Canino G, Escobar JI. Functional somatic symptoms – a cross-ethnic comparison. *American Journal of Orthopsychiatry* 1992; **62**(4): 605–12.

105. Escobar JI, Cooke B, Chen CN, Gara MA, Alegria M, Interian A *et al.* Whether

medically unexplained or not, three or more concurrent somatic symptoms predict psychopathology and service use in community populations. *Journal of Psychosomatic Research* 2010; **69**(1): 1–8.

106. Carstairs GM, Kapur RL. *The Great University of Kota. Stress, Change and Mental Disorder in an Indian Village.* London: Hogarth Press; 1976.

107. Kirmayer LJ, Robbins JM. Patients who somatize in primary care: a longitudinal study of cognitive and social characteristics. *Psychological Medicine* 1996; **26**(5): 937–51.

108. Bridges KW, Goldberg DP. Somatic presentation of DSM III psychiatric disorders in primary care. *Journal of Psychosomatic Research* 1985; **29**(6): 563–9.

109. Üstün TB, Sartorius N (eds). *Mental Illness in General Health Care. An International Study.* Chichester: John Wiley & Sons ; 1995.

110. Simon GE, VonKorff M, Piccinelli M, Fullerton C, Ormel J. An international study of the relation between somatic symptoms and depression. *New England Journal of Medicine* 1999; **341**(18): 1329–35.

111. Mak WWS, Zane NWS. The phenomenon of somatization among community Chinese Americans. *Social Psychiatry and Psychiatric Epidemiology* 2004; **39**(12): 967–74.

112. Kroenke K, Price RK. Symptoms in the community – prevalence, classification, and psychiatric comorbidity. *Archives of Internal Medicine* 1993; **153**(21): 2474–80.

113. Hiller W, Rief W, Brahler E, Hiller W, Rief W, Brahler E. Somatization in the population: from mild bodily misperceptions to disabling symptoms. *Social Psychiatry and Psychiatric Epidemiology* 2006; **41**(9): 704–12.

114. Gwee KA. Irritable bowel syndrome in developing countries – a disorder of civilization or colonization? *Neurogastroenterology and Motility* 2005; **17**(3): 317–24.

115. Kang JY. Systematic review: the influence of geography and ethnicity in irritable bowel syndrome. *Alimentary Pharmacology and Therapeutics* 2005; **21**(6): 663–76.

116. Gwee KA, Wee S, Wong ML, Png DJ. The prevalence, symptom characteristics, and impact of irritable bowel syndrome in an asian urban community. *American Journal of Gastroenterology* 2004; **99**(5): 924–31.

117. Husain N, Chaudhry IB, Jafri F, Niaz SK, Tomenson B, Creed F. A population-based study of irritable bowel syndrome in a non-Western population. *Neurogastroenterology and Motility* 2008; **20**(9): 1022–9.

118. Xiong LS, Chen MH, Chen HX, Xu AG, Wang WA, Hu PJ et al. A population-based epidemiologic study of irritable bowel syndrome in South China: stratified randomized study by cluster sampling. *Alimentary Pharmacology and Therapeutics* 2004; **19**(11): 1217–24.

119. Lee S, Wu J, Ma YL, Tsang A, Guo WJ, Sung J. Irritable bowel syndrome is strongly associated with generalized anxiety disorder: a community study. *Alimentary Pharmacology and Therapeutics* 2009; **30**(6): 643–51.

120. Farooq S, Gahir MS, Okyere E, Sheikh AJ, Oyebode F. Somatization – a transcultural study. *Journal of Psychosomatic Research* 1995; **39**(7): 883–8.

121. Gater R, Tomenson B, Percival C, Chaudhry N, Waheed W, Dunn G et al. Persistent depressive disorders and social stress in people of Pakistani origin and white Europeans in UK. *Social Psychiatry and Psychiatric Epidemiology* 2009; **44**(3): 198–207.

122. Mallinson S, Popay J. Describing depression: ethnicity and the use of somatic imagery in accounts of mental distress. *Sociology of Health and Illness* 2007; **29**: 857–71.

123. Weiss B, Tram JA, Weisz JR, Rescorla L, Achenbach TM. Differential symptom expression and somatization in Thai versus US children. *Journal of Consulting and Clinical Psychology* 2009; **77**(5): 987–92.

124. Kung WW, Lu PC. How symptom manifestations affect help seeking for mental health problems among Chinese Americans. *Journal of Nervous and Mental Disease* 2008; **196**(1): 46–54.

125. Husain N, Chaudhry I, Afsar S, Creed F. Psychological distress among patients attending a general medical outpatient clinic in Pakistan. *General Hospital Psychiatry* 2004; **26**(4): 277–81.

126. Sumathipala A, Hewege S, Hanwella R, Mann AH. Randomized controlled trial of cognitive behaviour therapy for repeated consultations for medically unexplained complaints: a feasibility study in Sri Lanka. *Psychological Medicine* 2000; **30**(4): 747–57.

127. Sumathipala A, Siribaddana S, Abeysingha MR, De Silva P, Dewey M, Prince M *et al.* Cognitive-behavioural therapy v. structured care for medically unexplained symptoms: randomised controlled trial. *British Journal of Psychiatry* 2008; **193**(1): 51–9.

128. Kleinman A, Benson P. Anthropology in the clinic: the problem of cultural competency and how to fix it. *PloS Medicine* 2006; **3**: 1673–6.

129. Yeung A, Shyu I, Fisher L, Wu S, Yang H, Fava M. Culturally sensitive collaborative treatment for depressed in primary care. *American Journal of Public Health* 2010; **100**(12): 2397–402.

130. Gater R, Waheed W, Husain N, Tomenson B, Aseem S, Creed F. Social intervention for British Pakistani women with depression: randomised controlled trial. *British Journal of Psychiatry* 2010; **197**(3): 227–33.

131. Yeiung A, Kam R. Ethical and cultural considerations in delivering psychiatric diagnosis: reconciling the gap using MDD diagnosis delivery in less-acculturated Chinese patients. *Transcultural Psychiatry* 2008; **45**(4): 531–52.

Chapter

7

Medically unexplained symptoms in children and adolescents

Emma Weisblatt, Peter Hindley and Charlotte Ulrikka Rask

Introduction

Medically unexplained or functional somatic symptoms, i.e. physical complaints with no known medical cause or clear physical pathology, are a common presentation in children and adolescents, with reported estimates of prevalence of recurrent symptoms varying from 2% to 30% [1;2;3;4;5]. These problems will, by definition, not usually present to child and adolescent psychiatrists or other mental health professionals, but in primary care or a paediatric medical setting. Understanding and expertise in assessing and managing these problems can thus vary considerably. Psychiatric paediatric liaison teams working in paediatric settings provide specific expertise and support to other staff when addressing medically unexplained symptoms, although provision of such teams is not universal. The aetiology and maintenance of medically unexplained symptoms are however complex and their assessment and treatment, particularly the engagement of families in the process, can still be problematic. The success of this process depends in large part on the family developing at least some degree of shared understanding of the links between emotional processes and physical symptoms, and a willingness to attempt to work on these (however ambivalently). However, medically unexplained symptoms in children often do not fit comfortably into International Classification of Diseases (ICD) or *Diagnostic and Statistical Manual of Mental Disorders* (DSM) diagnostic categories used in adults [6;7]. There is an extensive literature but most of it addresses single disorders, such as recurrent abdominal pain or chronic fatigue. Relatively little has so far been written about the area as a whole: Rutter and Taylor's *Child and Adolescent Psychiatry Textbook* devotes just over a page (of over 1500) specifically to medically unexplained symptoms [8]. Two recent reviews, however, do address the entire field, which does not lend itself to easy categorisation in children any more than in adults, and this account draws partly on these reviews [3;5].

Both the clinical presentation and the study of medically unexplained symptoms in children differ significantly from those in adults. Firstly, family influences are at their greatest, and are currently operating, in childhood (covered in more detail below): the interpretation, experience, and outcome of physical symptoms, as well as help-seeking behaviour and self-management, are all determined to a considerable extent by parents and other family members. This makes identification, engagement and management of medically unexplained symptoms in children profoundly different from that in adults, over and above issues of capacity and consent to treatment in children and adolescents. Secondly, children's physiology, neuro-endocrinology and cognitive abilities change profoundly during development, so that

Medically Unexplained Symptoms, Somatisation and Bodily Distress, ed. Francis Creed, Peter Henningsen and Per Fink. Published by Cambridge University Press. © Cambridge University Press 2011.

both their physical experiences and their descriptions of them are specific to the context of their developmental stage. Thirdly, as Eminson points out, participation in research is decided by parents for children under 16 years of age, and influenced by parents to some extent for older adolescents [3]. In addition, research instruments must be specifically designed and validated to be appropriate to the cognitive, verbal and emotional abilities of the age group being studied.

This chapter summarises current understanding and practice, emphasising particularly the role of the family and of the paediatric and child and adolescent mental health service multidisciplinary teams.

Classifications, definitions and current diagnostic categories

As in adult practice, the terminology used to describe medically unexplained symptoms is highly inconsistent and varies between countries, between specialties and disciplines, over time and between individuals. This reflects varying concepts of aetiology, physiology and appropriate management, and sometimes also appears to reflect the fear of paediatricians that any potentially 'mental health' label will frighten away the child and family for good. As mentioned in the introduction, the diagnostic options in ICD-10 are relatively limited and there are none specific to children and adolescents. In clinical practice, they are rarely used by either child and adolescent mental health service professionals or paediatricians.

Within paediatrics, a variety of terms are used to describe medically unexplained symptoms, including different functional somatic syndromes, single symptom diagnoses, and other clinical labels. Some of these overlap with those used in adults for somatic symptoms, for example: recurrent abdominal pain, non-epileptic seizures, psychogenic pain/vomiting/sensory loss or other symptom, fibromyalgia, irritable bowel syndrome, chronic pain, chronic fatigue, stress-related symptoms. Previously used terms such as 'hysteria' and 'supratentorial symptoms' are not regularly seen currently, although do still appear in referral letters occasionally. Child psychiatrists and other child and adolescent mental health service practitioners use many of the same terms, although they rarely go along with the more clearly 'medicalising' terminology such as 'fibromyalgia' on a long-term basis. The psychiatric terms available from ICD-10 are shown in Table 7.1.

Somatisation, in children as in adults, describes the presence of a range of physical symptoms not accounted for by physical pathology, which have an emotional or communicative function, but are attributed by child, family or both, to undiagnosed physical illness nonetheless. It could be argued that some version of this process underlies all presentations with medically unexplained symptoms. Older textbooks of child psychiatry include asthma and migraine, among others, in 'psychosomatic disorders'. This reflects the prominence of psychological factors in determining both the response to illness and the severity of symptoms. However, currently this would be considered as separate from 'medically unexplained' symptoms per se, and rather as an interaction between the child, the family and chronic illness.

Neurasthenia is more conventionally termed chronic fatigue syndrome, and its inclusion in ICD-10 (although not in DSM-IV) reflects the assumption that psychological factors are important in precipitating and/or maintaining the symptoms. Its nosological status remains controversial given the physiological findings associated, and the frequent viral illnesses at onset – but in the importance of emotional, family and behavioural factors in its continuation and severity, it fits with the other 'somatising' syndromes and is included here.

Table 7.1 Psychiatric terms available from ICD-10 [6]

ICD-10 category code	Category name	Diagnoses in category
F44	Dissociative disorders	• Motor
		• Convulsion
		• Sensory loss
		• Transient dissociative disorder of childhood
F45	Somatoform disorders	• Somatisation disorder
		• Undifferentiated somatoform disorder
		• Hypochondriacal disorder
		• Somatoform autonomic dysfunction
		• Persistent somatoform pain disorder
F48.0	Neurasthenia	

Three clinical presentations related to, but not identical to, medically unexplained symptoms are of significance in children and adolescents but are not themselves within the remit of this chapter, although they may co-exist and overlap with medically unexplained symptoms:

- *Abnormal response to illness, or apparently excessive symptoms in the setting of chronic illness*: this includes for example: problematic pain or nausea in oncology patients despite what would usually be adequate doses of medication; frequent presentations with shortness of breath in a child with documented asthma; perceived excessive pain in sickle cell disease. The borderline between these and entirely 'functional' symptoms is often not clear: pain may appear to some staff to be 'excessive' or 'psychogenic', while other staff feel the pain is explicable by the patient's illness. Sometimes the pain becomes manageable with specialist input from a palliative care team or a pain management team, or with explanation and reassurance. In other cases it remains intractable and can show clear features of medically unexplained symptoms. It is thus problematic to operationalise these presentations, which are common issues in paediatric liaison practice. Eminson describes the complexities of presentation of symptoms in some children as 'a mixture of explained, unexplained and uncertain physical symptoms', which neatly summarises the situation in children with a known serious medical illness [3]. Some of these symptoms can thus be seen as part of the medically unexplained symptoms spectrum but as yet have not been studied as such.
- *Factitious illness, particularly that evoked by a parent or carer (sometimes known as Munchausen's syndrome by proxy)*: this can present as, for example, recurrent abdominal pain, vomiting, or bleeding per vagina or per rectum. The illness may also be evoked by the child or adolescent themselves, with or without parental encouragement, example or collusion [9].
- *'Pervasive refusal syndrome'*: this is increasingly discussed by families and professionals, although the nosology is not yet established. A child or adolescent completely refuses

to eat, drink, walk, and often to speak or move at all. Attempts to carry out passive mobilisation or any other intervention can cause extreme pain and distress as well as active resistance. This clinical picture is familiar to paediatric liaison psychiatrists, and can cause severe and permanent damage, such as pressure sores and contractures, and potentially death from infection, dehydration or other complications. The assumption is generally made that this is an extreme manifestation of somatoform disorder, or possibly eating disorder [3;5], though it presents more with refusal to carry out activity and with intractable pain on activity rather than with more 'conventional' somatic complaints. In the authors' experience there are similar family issues to those seen in patients with 'medically unexplained' symptoms, but engagement and intervention are even more challenging, particularly in light of the serious medical situation often requiring extended periods of care in a medical setting.

Perhaps because of the (largely unhelpful) debates about whether somatic symptoms are 'physical' or 'mental', classification of somatic symptoms without known medical cause has long been contentious. The classifications are in the process of reassessment and change, and are discussed in detail elsewhere in this volume. The diagnostic categories available to child psychiatrists will therefore be somewhat different in years to come. The new category of complex somatic symptom disorder has been recently reviewed in relation to children and adolescents, and found to be more appropriate than the older classification [10]. The authors of this study recommend that parental concern should be included in the diagnostic criteria, an area of great importance in child and adolescent practice, and this is discussed below.

Normal development and age-appropriate coping mechanisms

As with all disorders of childhood, psychiatric or otherwise, developmental considerations are absolutely central, and all symptoms must be assessed in the developmental context of the child, with a sound understanding of normal developmental stages. Abdominal pain or headache are so common in children between the ages of 3 and 11 years as to be seen as normal by most parents and clinicians. For example, a prevalence study in a Spanish sample of over 800 children between the ages of 3 and 5 years found that 56% of the children displayed at least one somatic symptom in the preceding two weeks, and 20% of the children had frequent reports of somatic symptoms [11]. Only if presented as a problem by school, parents or medical staff, do such symptoms become clinically significant and are given a label such as 'recurrent abdominal pain'. Families have their own understandings and ways of dealing with physical symptoms, ranging from seeing them as evidence of minor illness – 'upset tummy' – through seeing them as expressions of distress such as not wanting to go to school on a particular day, to seeing them as evidence of serious illness that needs the sick role to be taken on. In this last case, the symptoms may become severe and impairing, and the worse the symptoms the more certain the family may become that a serious illness is being missed. This can lead to more and more investigation, and extremely strong resistance to consideration of emotional or psychiatric factors. Physical symptoms that can be seen as part of normal development can therefore nonetheless become a serious and impairing illness, if family and other factors, such as school or the health system, come into play. It can thus be seen that family beliefs, responses and behaviours are of primary importance in medically unexplained symptoms in children, and this will be returned to.

Epidemiology

Counting cases is an important first step toward measuring the social burden caused by a specific health problem; population-based studies are therefore needed to measure the extent of need and unmet need for prevention or treatment. A major task facing the area of medically unexplained symptoms in children is to develop assessment measures that accurately identify true cases, i.e. children with clinically significant symptoms. Two reviews in the 1990s agreed that significant medically unexplained physical symptoms were present in up to 1 in 10 children in the general population, more common in girls (particularly older girls), and most often recurrent abdominal pain and headache [12;13]. Interestingly, headache is common as a presentation in adults, recurrent abdominal pain much less so (an example of change in symptoms with development). Limb pains were also noted to be common. However, somatoform disorders as such, as in adults, were uncommon. A large population study in the USA found headaches in 10% of children, stomach pains in 2.8% and musculoskeletal pains in 2.2%, all at the lower end of the rates found in such studies [14]. The Illness Attitudes Scales developed for adults [15] have been adapted for use in children: higher scores on these scales were associated with higher somatic symptom scores, with more distress about illness and with more experience of medical treatment [16].

Formal epidemiological studies using validated questionnaire measures designed specifically for somatic symptoms in children and adolescents are increasingly being used to give reliable information about the epidemiology of medically unexplained symptoms and associated impairment. A recent study in the UK [17] using the Children's Somatization Inventory [18] confirmed that multiple physical symptoms were common at around 10% of children, commoner in girls, and were associated with impairment in everyday life and with emotional symptoms. Interestingly, a quarter of participants did feel that their symptoms were made worse by 'stress', showing some understanding of the link between emotional state and physical symptoms. A parental interview measure has recently been designed and validated specifically to assess functional somatic symptoms in children, the Soma Assessment Interview [4;19]. This has found impairing symptoms in 4% of 5- to 7-year-olds in a general population, confirming once again that significant and problematic medically unexplained symptoms are very common. This scale is designed for use in both clinical and research settings.

As described above, the more severe disorders as seen in adults are thought to be very uncommon in children, and this has recently been formally confirmed in an Australian study that found conversion disorder occurred in only 2–4 per 10 000 children (0.02–0.04%) [20].

Systemic considerations (family)

There are extensive effects of family factors on expression of emotional distress, illness behaviour, attribution of symptoms and consultation behaviour for children and adolescents of all ages [3]. Parents with mood disorders and/or physical symptoms (including somatisation and medically unexplained symptoms) consult more frequently for their children as well as themselves, and parental beliefs and attitudes strongly affect the amount of time children have off school both for medically unexplained symptoms and after surgery or documented medical illness. Two principal groups of family style have been reported, one being chaotic with multiple physical and psychiatric complaints in multiple family members, and the other being high-functioning, outwardly stable families that may have difficulty putting emotional issues into words and strenuously deny any emotional issues. These latter families may bear a striking resemblance to the families of children with anorexia nervosa.

As parents are usually firmly in control of the consulting behaviour of their children, and family belief systems have a powerful influence on the beliefs and behaviours of children, these factors take on primary importance in children and young people in both the genesis and maintenance of physical symptoms as an expression of emotional distress. In addition, parents frequently give all or most of the history even for adolescents, which will also be influenced by their own beliefs and interpretations of physical symptoms. A further area of significance in the family is of course that of parental mental health (affecting both the child's genetic inheritance and their environment). For example, parental somatisation is associated with somatic symptoms and school absence in children [21]. This demonstrates intergenerational transmission, although it does not elucidate the gene–environment relationships. Parental anxiety and depression are both associated with recurrent abdominal pain in children [22], while parental anxiety (as well as child temperament) during the first year of a child's life predicts recurrent abdominal pain in later childhood [23]. A clear demonstration of the impact of parental beliefs directly on somatic symptoms in the child is the finding that distraction behaviours by parents reduce the symptoms of recurrent abdominal pain (particularly in girls), while attention increases them [24]. Of particular note in this study is the finding that while children reported decreasing symptoms with distraction, parents felt that distraction made their child worse – this difference of opinion has therapeutic implications. Relationship problems and family illness are frequently reported in children with conversion disorders [25]. Children with recurrent abdominal pain report excess daily stressors at home and at school, with strong associations between stressful events and pain symptoms [26]. The association was stronger in those children who also reported negative affect traits, possibly marking a vulnerability to emotional disorders, as well as negative cognitive appraisals of events.

This finding does not distinguish between 'objective' excess of life events, and 'subjective' appraisal of events as excessively 'stressful'. However, if it is the appraisal of events, that is to say 'perceived stress', that is important in the genesis of recurrent abdominal pain in a vulnerable child, perhaps this distinction is unnecessary. This was explored by a further study, which assessed (perceived) stressful events, appraisal of the events and coping with pain in children with recurrent abdominal pain [27]. The children with pain reported decreased confidence in their ability to change or adapt to stress and were less likely to describe using coping strategies that involved accommodating to the stressful events. Such traits may thus not be specific to medically unexplained symptoms, but be vulnerability factors shared between children with medically unexplained symptoms (who often but not always have emotional disorders) and children with emotional disorders without prominent somatic symptoms.

Little is yet known about the relationship of other disorders such as factitious disorder with childhood medically unexplained symptoms, though it is suggested that the two may be associated on clinical and theoretical grounds [28]. Similarly, it can be hypothesised that family bereavements, and abuse, particularly sexual, within a family, may be associated with medically unexplained symptoms in some children, either as non-specific stressors, or *perhaps* as specific associations. In fact there is often an assumption that medically unexplained symptoms very frequently arise from abuse, to the point where abuse may be thought by some clinicians to be present in most children with medically unexplained symptoms. This is certainly not the case, and it should not be assumed that a child (or adult) with medically unexplained symptoms is likely to have experienced abuse. The association of childhood abuse with *adult* medically unexplained symptoms may in fact be more relevant. The recent development of quantitative scales for medically unexplained symptoms in children will facilitate research in this area from now on.

Genetics and biological factors

As well as 'environmental' family factors in the broadest sense, involving behavioural and emotional modelling and family 'narratives' of illness, the importance of inherited factors, while largely unknown in the genesis of medically unexplained symptoms, is likely to be significant. Almost all quantitative behavioural and physiological traits studied to date have shown significant heritability, ranging from as low as 20% to over 80%. Some of these are of obvious relevance to 'personality' traits relevant to medically unexplained symptoms or emotional disorders, such as the 'novelty-seeking' trait associated with the dopamine D4 receptor, behavioural inhibition traits, or traits related to perfectionism, obsessionality or anxiety. Other relevant traits that show significant heritability include startle response (associated with glutamate receptor loci) and markers of autonomic nervous system function such as galvanic skin response and heart rate variability. Detailed review of this field is beyond the scope of this chapter; see, for example, Plomin *et al.* for further coverage of heritability in behavioural traits [29].

While twin and adoption studies can demonstrate heritability, most children are brought up by their genetic parents, with whom they share both genes and environment, the interaction of both thus being central to the development of any clinical problem, and perhaps particularly to one where interpretation of symptoms is central, as with medically unexplained symptoms. For example, a physiological diathesis, caused initially by inherited physiological factors affecting the gastrointestinal tract, might cause discomfort in a child placed in an anxiety-provoking situation (gene–environment interaction). A child with this diathesis might only display symptoms in certain circumstances. The response and narrative of the family will, however, play a crucial role in the response of child, family and professionals to this discomfort (gene–environment correlation). It has been proposed that serotonergic dysregulation might play a part in both gastrointestinal distress and emotional symptoms, on the grounds that serotonin is an important neurotransmitter in both the gastrointestinal tract and brain, and it is known to influence symptoms of nausea and gut motility [30]. While an engaging idea, and all the more so given the gastrointestinal as well as emotional manifestations of carcinoid syndrome, this theory so far awaits formal testing. If gastrointestinal sensations in response to serotonergic activity are indeed found to be associated with emotional disorder, the genesis of problematic medically unexplained symptoms would still involve the interpretation of the symptoms as medically caused and potentially serious, by the child and family. In general, this area has not yet been well studied in humans, although it is a very active area of research. For example, child temperament in the first year of life (as measured by feeding and sleeping behaviours) is associated with recurrent abdominal pain later in childhood [23]. It should be borne in mind, however, that the heritability of such early behaviours has not been shown to be extremely high, and factors such as maternal mental health, particularly depression and anxiety, are also likely to be important (and independently associated with recurrent abdominal pain).

Psychiatric comorbidity

In a study of children with recurrent abdominal pain attending primary care services, over 75% had an anxiety disorder, and about half had a depressive disorder [31]. These are of course strikingly high rates of comorbidity (or perhaps primary disorder) and these should be treated in their own right. More than 50% of children admitted to hospital with conversion disorders have a psychiatric disorder [25] and about 75% of young people with chronic fatigue syndrome have a psychiatric disorder (mainly emotional disorder) documented in the year prior to interview [32]. Some of these disorders, though almost certainly not all, can be seen as response to loss of independence, friends or other life experiences, but there is increasing evidence that anxiety disorders may precede the onset of, and persist after recovery from, somatoform disorders [5].

Wider systemic considerations

The beliefs and behaviours of other health professionals, particularly paediatricians, as well as the structure of paediatric liaison services, are also of great importance. Most children with medically unexplained symptoms will present in primary care and may be managed in that setting alone. A proportion will be referred to paediatricians for further assessment and medical investigations. Paediatricians are thus the primary determinant of referral to or joint work with liaison services (in the UK many liaison services will not take referrals directly from primary care services). Paediatricians vary widely in their attitudes to medically unexplained symptoms and their referral rates to liaison services. There is some consensus among paediatric liaison psychiatrists that joint working, co-located in the paediatric setting, is highly desirable, rather than a model of referring on to child and adolescent mental health services once all medical avenues are exhausted. Clinical experience suggests that families are much more likely to engage with a collaborative, 'curious' approach with paediatric and mental health services working together, where conversations and terminology can be tailored to the beliefs and understanding of the family, and gradual agreement can be reached on a helpful approach to the child's symptoms. Families are almost always seeking the best for their children, and this must be respected and built on by all professionals with the family as part of the team, experts on their own children. The wider system is also critical, including primary care professionals, school teachers, nurses and other mental health professionals, and the community child and adolescent mental health team local to the child.

Summary and formulation

Medically unexplained symptoms in children can be seen to occur as a result of multiple factors, biological, familial and historical. This section describes a working model based on current knowledge in the area. Although there is no single formulation that can describe the various complex situations of children with medically unexplained symptoms, some themes, based on empirical evidence as well as clinical experience, can be drawn together. Some characteristics are shared by children with conversion disorder, chronic fatigue syndrome and other medically unexplained symptoms presentations (and similarities can also be seen in some cases with anorexia nervosa patients). Families may not easily express emotions verbally, and may attempt not to express negative emotions such as anger at all. Psychological explanations for bodily sensations or symptoms are discouraged, and some of the children may be high achievers, and extremely compliant and well behaved. If a child then finds that they are not performing as expected by the family, or they are experiencing negative emotions such as

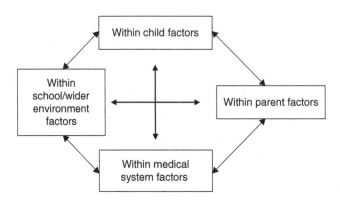

Figure 7.1 An interactive approach to medically unexplained symptoms in children (after Eminson [3])

anger or anxiety, bodily symptoms may allow 'escape' from a situation which will otherwise be intolerable, particularly to the parents. The symptoms will elicit care and sympathy from the family (which might not be forthcoming for angry outbursts or emotional symptoms), and will legitimise retreat from stressful situations such as school. This will occur in the context of a child who may have unusually severe reactions to stressful situations, either physiologically or emotionally. This formulation may apply most clearly to children with (rare) conversion syndromes [33], but can be seen in many other contexts in clinical practice.

Assessment and management of medically unexplained symptoms in children and young people

Children and young people present with medically unexplained symptoms as a result of an interaction between child factors, family factors, factors within the wider social system (e.g. school) and the medical care system (Figure 7.1) [3]. The factors shown in this model may all include both pathogenic and protective factors, interacting to produce the outcome in the child.

In many children who present with medically unexplained symptoms there are familial factors contributing to the development or maintenance of symptoms in either well-organised or disorganised families [3]. Assessment and engagement of the family as well as the child are thus of primary and central importance.

Initial engagement and assessment

The majority of children and young people with medically unexplained symptoms will be managed in primary care. The key intervention will be the primary care physician listening carefully to the presenting symptoms and history, medically examining the child and using a limited range of investigations. In doing so they will be able to exclude underlying organic pathology and reassure the family and young person. If the child lies within the first group of children described by Eminson [3], in an organised family structure, and a clear precipitating factor can be identified, the primary care physician can explain psychosomatic mechanisms and reassure the parents that they are able effectively to support the child to recover from his or her symptoms [3]. This can be termed psychoeducation and may be seen as empowering the parents or the whole family. If the child comes from a family with a more chaotic style of functioning, the doctor's main aim is to limit investigations and encourage the family to engage with appropriate services such as social care. It seems likely that the majority of children and young people presenting with medically unexplained symptoms, in primary and secondary care, will respond to these simple strategies, and they form the basis of current management of these children in primary care and paediatric practice. However, there is as yet no research evidence to support this approach.

Additional strategies, such as psychological therapies and/or drug therapies (for example specific serotonin reuptake inhibitors), are needed when children present with persistent symptoms or symptoms which are associated with high levels of impairment, as well as comorbid psychiatric disorders such as emotional disorders. This can be seen as a stepped-care approach analogous to that common in adult practice. Some examples of psychological therapies are given below. However, all of these strategies are dependent on meaningful engagement with the young person and their families or carers. It is suggested that reassuring and containing parental fears about possible undiscovered organic pathology is a central component to this engagement [34]. Campo and Fritz have summarised the key elements of initial assessment and management [35]:

- acknowledge patient suffering and family concerns
- investigate patient and family fears provoked by the symptoms
- remain alert to the possibility of physical disease and communicate an unwillingness to prejudge the aetiology of the symptoms
- avoid unnecessary tests and procedures
- avoid diagnosis by exclusion
- explore symptom timing, context and characteristics
- state the diagnostic impression clearly, frankly and directly
- build a foundation for intervention.

Many children and families can be helped by consultation and liaison with paediatrics: some children are managed by discussion with paediatric and nursing colleagues without direct input. In any case, the liaison team has a role in discouraging further investigations and supporting the paediatric team to stick to this decision in the face of pressure from the family for 'just one more opinion'. Sharing of the uncertainty with the family, admitting the limitations of knowledge and avoiding a 'diagnosis by exclusion' model are all agreed to be important.

If a decision is taken to involve mental health professionals directly, there is then the challenge for the paediatrician or other referrer of how best to engage mental health professionals. Some families have no concerns but some may see this as implying that the child's symptoms are 'all in their mind'. Using the principles outlined by Campo and Fritz should facilitate this process, as should having mental heath professionals present on the paediatric ward, in ward rounds and with ready availability in outpatient clinics as a well-integrated and 'routine' part of the clinical team. However, it is also important to bear in mind that, as described above, psychiatric disorders such as anxiety disorders and depression are common comorbid conditions in children with medically unexplained symptoms, and that their detection and management form a crucial component of effective intervention [31]. The factors affecting the emergence of somatic (physical) symptoms can be usefully summarised in a visual biopsychosocial formulation (Figure 7.2).

This approach can be supported by an 'informing conference' involving the paediatrician and family, with or without the paediatric liaison psychiatrist present [36]. In this meeting, the paediatrician conveys the biopsychosocial formulation and outlines the suggested treatment programme. The authors suggest that if families have a sense that the paediatrician

Factor	Predisposing	Precipitating	Maintaining	Protective
Biological				
Psychological				
Social				
Medical				

Figure 7.2 A biopsychosocial formulation of the factors affecting the emergence of somatic symptoms.

understands and empathises with the distress that somatic symptoms is causing, the family is more likely to engage in ongoing management [36]. If the family refuses child mental health intervention, the paediatric liaison psychiatrist can provide ongoing consultation to the paediatric team as they manage the child.

Management and treatment models

The majority of paediatricians and child mental health practitioners advocate a rehabilitation model for the management of medically unexplained symptoms [35]. This entails a shift away from curing symptoms towards a return to as normal function as possible. Patients and families become active partners in recovery and parents are encouraged to regard their children as capable, strong and competent, rather than passive, helpless and fragile [36]. Realistic, collaborative goal setting is an essential component of this process. This approach can be seen to have much in common with solution-focused approaches (see below).

This approach to management involves a close collaboration between physiotherapy and occupational therapy to promote physical functioning, supported by cognitive, behavioural and motivational approaches. Most children can be managed as outpatients but children with severe presentations may need inpatient assessment on a paediatric or psychiatric ward, and those with very severe presentations may need admission to services specialising in working with children with medically unexplained symptoms, where these are available. Admission can also give an insight into the role that families may be playing in maintaining symptoms and so aid outpatient management. Some paediatric or adolescent medicine units have well-resourced liaison teams and admit young people with very severe medically unexplained symptoms, for example, chronic pain, pervasive refusal to eat or unexplained weight loss without clear evidence of anorexia nervosa. In other services, these children are admitted to psychiatric inpatient units with paediatric input available. Some clinicians are critical of this approach, seeing the involvement of physiotherapy and occupational therapy as reinforcing abnormal illness beliefs. They suggest that this can, potentially, unnecessarily prolong somatic symptoms and that the key interventions should be paediatric, psychiatric and psychological [37].

Specific psychosocial interventions

The evidence as to which interventions are most appropriate for which conditions is limited and variable in quality. For specific syndromes there is greatest research evidence for the effectiveness of cognitive behavioural therapy in syndromes in which pain is the predominant characteristic (see below), and this is therefore discussed in some detail. Biofeedback has been found to be effective for medically unexplained symptoms in adults and there is growing evidence for its effectiveness in children and adolescents. There is also a growing body of evidence for intervention in chronic fatigue syndrome in children and young people [32]. There is less research-based evidence for dynamic psychotherapy and systems-based therapies. However, there are case series and expert evidence to support these approaches. There is emerging evidence to support a limited role for pharmacotherapy [36]. The rehabilitation approach is often particularly acceptable to families with a child who has chronic fatigue syndrome, although this can be a mixed blessing as it can perpetuate adherence to a medical model.

Cognitive behavioural therapy and pain syndromes

There are four studies which support the use of cognitive behavioural therapy in recurrent abdominal pain: a small, retrospective case study [38]; a small case-controlled series [39]; a moderately sized, randomised controlled trial [40]; and a larger randomised controlled trial using intention-to-treat analysis [42]. All of these studies used recognised outcome measures, and manualised cognitive behavioural therapy with both children and parents. Two studies (40 and 41) compared standard medical care (SMC only) with a combination of standard medical care and cognitive behavioural therapy (CBT+SMC). The study by Sanders et al. included 44 children [40]. Children and parents were assessed pre- and post-treatment, at six months' and at 12 months' a combination of follow-up. The proportion of children who were pain-free was significantly greater in the CBT+SMC group immediately post-treatment and at 12 months but not at six months. Children and parents' ratings of pain intensity and parents' ratings of pain behaviour were significantly reduced. Using regression analysis, the authors identified the following active treatment components: child positive self-talk and parental strategies which promoted adaptive coping (acknowledging the pain, distracting the child, encouraging independence and ignoring pain complaints). Parental expectations of treatment outcomes did not predict outcome, but parents in the CBT+SMC group had higher satisfaction ratings than parents in the SMC-only group.

Robins et al. enrolled in their study 86/108 children [41]. They were assessed pre-treatment, three months into treatment, immediately post-treatment, and six and 12 months after treatment had ended. The children in the CBT group received five two-weekly sessions, three of which were with their parents. The aims of the sessions were to: develop a greater understanding of the child's pain; increase the child's repertoire of pain management techniques; increase the child and parents' understanding of the link between pain and stress; encourage the child to take control of pain; increase the child's awareness of the impact of positive and negative self-talk on pain; and increase the partnership between children and parents. Parent and child pain scores were reduced immediately post-treatment and at follow-up (effect reduction 3.4–5.4); the number needed to treat was 1/3. However, differences between the treatment and control groups in somatisation scores and functional impairment were not statistically significant. There was no significant difference in the number of visits to physicians at 12 months post-treatment, but there were significantly fewer school absences in the group receiving cognitive behavioural therapy (t = 2.04, df (67); p = 0.047) and the mean number of days lost was less (9 versus 14.5 for the SMC group). Robins et al. concluded that CBT+SMC is a useful intervention in the management of recurrent abdominal pain.

Degotardi *et al.* developed a manual for the psychological management of juvenile fibromyalgia [42]. Unfortunately they did not use a randomised controlled trial design to assess its effectiveness. Using a moderate-sized case series (n = 67, age 8–20 years), they administered pre- and post-treatment measures but did not carry out any follow-up assessments. The cognitive behavioural therapy intervention consisted of eight weeks of cognitive behavioural therapy plus family therapy and interpersonal therapy, weekly parent meetings, psychoeducation, sleep improvement, pain management and activities of daily living. Children and young people reported significant improvements in pain and sleep (p<0.006), with 24% becoming pain-free. They also reported improvements in fatigue (p<0.05) and psychological symptoms improved (p<0.006). Unfortunately, because of the study design, the effect size, a more conventional approach to reporting the effectiveness of interventions, could not be used.

Lee *et al.* conducted a randomised controlled trial of standard physiotherapy combined with cognitive behavioural therapy compared with more intensive physiotherapy combined with cognitive behavioural therapy in the management of complex regional pain syndrome [43]. The cognitive behavioural therapy consisted of psychoeducation, pain management, relaxation, breathing exercises, biofeedback, guided imagery, problem solving and coping. All subjects received six sessions of cognitive behavioural therapy and were assessed pre- and post-treatment and at 6–12 months' follow-up. The two groups differed only in the number of physiotherapy sessions offered. A total of 56 children and young people enrolled in the study; 22/28 children attended 80% of physiotherapy sessions and 23/28 attended 80% of cognitive behavioural therapy sessions. There was a significant improvement in all complex regional pain syndrome symptoms in both groups: pain; allodynia (pain to light touch or other neutral stimuli); stair climbing; and gait (p<0.001), at the end of treatment. These changes were sustained at follow-up with further improvements in pain and stair climbing. None of the subjects were using physical mobility devices. However, 10 patients had recurrence of severe pain which did not respond to physiotherapy and required lumbar sympathetic and epidural infusions of local anaesthesia. This study did not however assess the effect of cognitive behavioural therapy alone.

In summary, these studies suggest that cognitive behavioural therapy can play a significant part in the management of children with medically unexplained symptoms in which pain is a significant feature. The studies suggest that cognitive behavioural therapy should involve both children and their parents.

Headaches, biofeedback and relaxation

Headaches are common among children and adolescents. Biofeedback has been found to be particularly effective for migraines in children with an average effect size of 2.2 [44]. Nanke and Rief suggest that biofeedback may be even more effective in children than in adults [45]. Many of the psychological interventions, both cognitive behavioural therapy and biofeedback, use relaxation as a principal component. Shaw and DeMaso provide a useful summary of relaxation techniques, using either breathing or progressive muscular relaxation [36]. For children who cannot use either of these techniques, 'safe place' guided imagery can be very effective.

Dynamic psychotherapy and systemic psychotherapies

Both psychodynamic psychotherapy and the systemic psychotherapies can play a vital role in understanding the intrapsychic and systemic functions of somatic symptoms [46;47]. Kozlowska has used a large case series and service description to propose that a systemic, family-based approach can be effective in the management of chronic pain [48]. The central feature of this approach is including somatic, psychological and social systems in the therapy to make sense of the child's subjective experience of pain. Kaplan *et al.* suggest that the dynamic psychotherapies are not only effective in the management of medically unexplained symptoms but also lead to lowered overall healthcare expenditure [46]. Lask and Fosson provide a useful approach to the assessment and management of medically unexplained symptoms within a systemic framework, with a particular emphasis on the role that somatic symptoms play in communication within families (analogous to the concept of 'talking with the body' in eating disorders) [47]. Sometimes, in clinical practice where child psychotherapy is available (not always the case, particularly in hospital practice), the child engages with a child psychotherapist and other team members work with the mother or other family members, to identify and address underlying emotional issues or family tensions. The authors have seen this approach produce spectacular results in some otherwise difficult-to-engage families, notably where there is unacknowledged anger or suspected but never proven (non-life-threatening) factitious illness. However, the effectiveness of these treatment methods has not yet been assessed using clinical trials methodology.

Solution-focused approach

Usually led by clinical psychologists, this approach does not directly explore underlying emotional conflicts, but supports the child and family to identify factors that improve the symptoms and build on them (not dissimilar to the approach often taken in individual psychotherapy, but using different language). This is generally felt to be more effective if it includes the whole family, although the evidence base in medically unexplained symptoms is as yet lacking. It may be part of a wider multidisciplinary and systemic approach integrated into paediatric settings [49], where it is likely to be most effective, as discussed earlier. There is as yet no evidence for efficacy of this intervention, although results in clinical practice are encouraging.

Relationship to adult disorders

There is limited literature on the outcomes of children with severe medically unexplained symptoms, although retrospective studies of adults with severe medically unexplained symptoms report onset in childhood or adolescence in most patients. However, a recent prospective study found that the larger the number of unexplained symptoms in childhood, the more likely they were to persist into adulthood [50]. Recurrent abdominal pain in childhood is associated with later anxiety and/or depression and also increased medical consultations. Given the association of parental psychiatric disorder, including medically unexplained symptoms, with medically unexplained symptoms in children, there is likely to be a 'cycle of medically unexplained symptoms' analogous to the cycle of abuse (although there are also likely to be genetic influences).

Medically unexplained symptoms in children thus present in many ways similarly to those in adults, but family influences on both symptomatology and consulting behaviour are of primary importance in children and adolescents, and much of the intervention is negotiated with and aimed at other family members, usually parents. Medically unexplained symptoms in children can be severe and can disrupt critical developmental stages, particularly schooling and interaction with peers, which can have lifelong consequences. This makes it all the more important that these symptoms are identified and effectively treated.

Improving treatment

As there are an increasing number of randomised controlled trials now attesting to the efficacy of psychological therapies (see above), medically unexplained symptoms in children need to be identified, assessed and managed appropriately to improve both short- and long-term outcomes. Close and collaborative working between primary care, hospital paediatrics and mental health services, both hospital and community, is needed to achieve this. We propose four developments, building on the areas reviewed above, which are likely to lead to an improvement in the management of medically unexplained symptoms in children and adolescents. Firstly, improved recognition in primary care, for example, by increased awareness among professionals and use of screening instruments. Secondly, early psychoeducation of parents and children (starting in primary care) is likely to reduce or prevent the entrenchment of emerging medically unexplained symptoms. Thirdly, closer cooperation between paediatricians, primary care and mental health workers (psychiatrists, psychotherapist, clinical psychologists and others) so that care is genuinely integrated from the first presentation. This is likely to lead to better engagement in psychological interventions and lower drop-out rates when children and families are referred for management in paediatric liaison services. Critical to this is integrated working among the different mental health disciplines. Fourthly, greater use of evidence-based therapies, such as cognitive behavioural and family behavioural interventions: the evidence base is rapidly increasing and is likely to include more psychodynamic and systemic interventions in the future.

References

1. Aro H. Life stress and psychosomatic symptoms among 14–16 year old Finnish adolescents. *Psychological Medicine* 1987; **17**: 191–201.

2. Goodman JE, McGrath, PJ . The epidemiology of pain in children and adolescents: a review. *Pain* 1991; **46**: 247–64.

3. Eminson DM. Medically unexplained symptoms in children and adolescents. *Clinical Psychology Review* 2007; **27**: 855–71.

4. Rask CU, Olsen EM, Elberling H, Christensen MF, Ørnbøl E, Fink P, Thomsen PH, Skovgaard AM. Functional somatic symptoms and associated impairment in 5–7-year-old children: the Copenhagen Child Cohort 2000. *European Journal of Epidemiology* 2009; **24**: 625–34.

5. Garralda ME. Unexplained physical complaints. *Child and Adolescent Psychiatric Clinics of North America* 2010; **19**: 199–209.

6. World Health Organization. *International Statistical Classification of Diseases and Related Health Problems. 10th Revision*

(ICD-10). Geneva: World Health Organization; 1992.

7. American Psychiatric Association. *Diagnostic and Statistical Manual of Mental Disorders*, 4th edn. Washington: American Psychiatric Association, 1994.

8. Mrazek MD. Psychiatric aspects of somatic disease and disorders. In: Rutter M, Taylor E, eds. *Child and Adolescent Psychiatry*, 4th edn. Oxford: Blackwell; 2002: 817–18.

9. Libow JA. Child and adolescent illness falsification. *Pediatrics* 2000; **105**: 336–42.

10. Schulte IE, Petermann F. Somatoform disorders: 30 years of debate about criteria. What about children and adolescents? *Journal of Psychosomatic Research* 2011; **70**: 218–28.

11. Domenech-Llaberia E, Jane C, Canals J, Ballespi S, Esparo G, Garralda E. Parental reports of somatic symptoms in preschool children: Prevalence and associations in Spanish sample. *Journal of the American Academy of Child and Adolescent Psychiatry* 2004; **43**: 598–604.

12. Garralda ME. A selective review of child psychiatric syndromes with a somatic

presentation. *British Journal of Psychiatry* 1992; **161**: 759–73.

13. Campo JV, Fritsch SL. Somatization in children and adolescents. *Journal of the American Academy of Child and Adolescent Psychiatry* 1994; **33**(9): 1223–35.

14. Egger HL, Costello EJ, Erkanli A, Angold AC. Somatic complaints and psychopathology in children and adolescents: stomach aches, muscular-skeletal pains and headaches. *Journal of the American Academy of Child and Adolescent Psychiatry* 1999; **38**(7): 852–60.

15. Kellner R. *Abridged Manual of the Illness Attitude Scales*. Albuquerque, NM: Department of Psychiatry: 1987.

16. Eminson DM, Benjamin S, Shortall A, Woods T, Faragher B. Physical symptoms and illness attitudes in adolescents: an epidemiological study. *Journal of Child Psychology and Psychiatry* 1996; **37**: 519–27.

17. Vila M, Kramer T, Hickey N. Assessment of somatic symptoms in British secondary school children using the Children's Somatization Inventory (CSI). *Journal of Pediatric Psychology* 2009; **34**: 989–98.

18. Garber J, Walker L, Zeman J. Somatization symptoms in a community sample of children and adolescents: further validation of the Children's Somatization Inventory. *Psychological Assessment* 1991; **3**: 588–95.

19. Rask CU, Christiansen MF, Borg C. The SOMA assessment interview: new parent interview on functional somatic symptoms in children. *Journal of Psychosomatic Research* 2009; **6**(5): 456–64.

20. Kozlowska K, Nunn KP, Rose D. Conversion disorder in Australian pediatric practice. *Journal of the American Academy of Child and Adolescent Psychiatry* 2007; **46**(1): 68–75.

21. Craig TK, Cox AD, Klein K. Intergenerational transmission of somatization behaviour: a study of chronic somatizers and their children. *Psychological Medicine* 2002; **32**: 805–16.

22. Campo JV, Bridge J, Lucas A, Savorelli S, Walker L, Di Lorenzo C *et al*. Physical and emotional health of mothers of youth with functional abdominal pain. *Archives of Pediatric and Adolescent Medicine* 2007; **161**: 131–7.

23. Ramchandani PG, Stein A, Hotopf, M. Early parental and child predictors of recurrent abdominal pain at school age: results of a large population-based study. *Journal of the American Academy of Child and Adolescent Psychiatry* 2006; **45**(6): 729–36.

24. Walker LS, Williams SE, Smith CA, Garber J, Van Slyke DA, Lipani TA. Parent attention versus distraction: impact on symptom complaints by children with and without chronic functional abdominal pain. *Pain* 2006; **122**(1–2): 43–52.

25. Pehlivanturk B, Unal F. Conversion disorder in children and adolescents: clinical features and comorbidity with depressive and anxiety disorders. *Turkish Journal of Pediatrics* 2000; **42**: 132–7.

26. Walker LS, Garber J, Smith CA, van Slyke DA, Claar RL. The relation of daily stressors to somatic and emotional symptoms in children with and without recurrent abdominal pain. *Journal of Consulting and Clinical Psychology* 2001; **69**(1): 85–91.

27. Walker LS, Smith CA, Garber J, Claar RL. Appraisal and coping witn daily stressors by pediatric patients with chronic abdominal pain. *Journal of Pediatric Psychology* 2007; **32**(2); 206–216.

28. Glaser D. Personal communication 2010.

29. Plomin R, Defries JC, Craig IW, McGuffin P (eds). *Behavioral Genetics in the Postgenomic Era*. Washington: American Psychiatric Association; 2002.

30. Campo JV, Dahl RE, Williamson DE. Gastrointestinal distresss to serotonergic challenge: a risk marker for emotional disorder? *Journal of the American Academy of Child and Adolescent Psychiatry* 2003; **42**(10): 1121–6.

31. Campo JV, Perel JM, Lucas A, Bridge J, Ehmann M, Kalas C *et al*. Citalopram treatment of pediatric recurrent abdominal pain and comorbid internalizing disorders: an exploratory study. *Journal of the American Academy of Child and Adolescent Psychiatry* 2004; **43**(10): 1234–42.

32. Garralda ME, Chalder T. Practitioner review: chronic fatigue syndrome in childhood. *Journal of Child Psychology and Psychiatry* 2005; **46**(11): 1143–51.

33. Kozlowska K. Good children presenting with conversion disorder. *Clinical Child Psychology and Psychiatry* 2001; **6**(4): 575–91.

34. Hardwick JP. Engaging families who hold strong medical beliefs in a psychosomatic approach. *Clinical Child Psychology and Psychiatry* 2005; **19**: 601–16.

35. Campo JV, Fritz G. A management model for pediatric somatization. *Psychosomatics* 2001; **42**: 467–76.

36. Shaw RJ, DeMaso DR. *Clinical Manual of Pediatric Psychosomatic Medicine: Mental Health Consultation with Physically Ill Children and Adolescents.* Washington: American Psychiatric Association: 2006.

37. Hedderly T. Personal communication, 2010.

38. Youssef NN, Rosh JR, Loughran M, Schuckalo SG, Cotter AN, Verga BG et al. Treatment of functional abdominal pain in childhood with cognitive behavioural strategies. *Journal of Pediatric Gastroenterology and Nutrition* 2004; **39**: 192–6.

39. Sanders MR, Rebgetz M, Morrison M, Bor W, Gordon A, Dadds M et al. Cognitive-behavioural treatment of recurrent abdominal pain in children: an analysis of generalization, maintenance and side-effects. *Journal of Consulting and Clinical Psychology* 1989; **57**: 294–300.

40. Sanders, MR, Shepherd RW, Gleghorn G, Woolford H. The treatment of recurrent abdominal pain in children: a controlled comparison of cognitive-behavioural family intervention and standard medical care. *Journal of Consulting and Clinical Psychology* 1994; **62**: 306–14.

41. Robins PM, Smith SM, Glutting JJ, Bishop CT. A randomized controlled trial of a cognitive-behavioural family intervention for paediatric recurrent abdominal pain. *Journal of Pediatric Psychology* 2005; **30**: 397–408.

42. Degotardi PJ, Klass ES, Rosenberg BS, Fox DG, Gallelli KA, Gottlieb BS. Development and evaluation of a cognitive behavioural intervention for juvenile fibromyalgia. *Journal of Pediatric Psychology* 2006; **31**: 714–23.

43. Lee BH, Scharff L, Sethna NF, McCarthy CF, Scott-Sutherland J, Shea A et al. Physical therapy and cognitive-behavioural therapy for complex regional pain syndromes. *Journal of Pediatrics* 2002; **141**: 135–40.

44. Hermann C, Blanchard EB. Biofeedback and the treatment of headache and other childhood pain. *Applied Psychophysiology and Biofeedback* 2002; **27**: 143–62.

45. Nanke A, Rief W. Biofeedback in somatoform disorders and related syndromes. *Current Opinion in Psychiatry* 2004; **17**; 133–8.

46. Kaplan HI, Sadock BJ, Grebb JA. Somatoform Disorders. In: Kaplan HI, Sadock BJ (eds). *Kaplan and Sadock's Synopsis of Psychiatry: Behavioural Sciences/Clinical Psychiatry.* Baltimore, MA: Williams and Wilkins; 1994.

47. Lask B, Fosson A. *Childhood illness: the psychosomatic approach.* Chichester: Wiley; 1989.

48. Kozlowska K, Rose D, Khan R, Kram S, Lane L, Collins J. A conceptual model and practice framework for managing chronic pain in children and adolescents. *Harvard Review of Psychiatry* 2008; **16**(2): 136–50.

49. Griffin A, Christie D. Taking the psycho out of psychosomatic: using systemic approaches in a paediatric setting for the treatment of adolescents with unexplained physical symptoms. *Clinical Child Psychology and Psychiatry* 2008; **13**(4): 531–42.

50. Steinhausen H-C, Winkler-Metzke C. Continuity of functional-somatic symptoms from late childhood to young adulthood in a community sample. *Journal of Child Psychology and Psychiatry* 2007; **48**: 508–13.

Chapter

8

Identification, assessment and treatment of individual patients

Francis Creed, Christina van der Feltz-Cornelis,
Else Guthrie, Peter Henningsen, Winfried Rief,
Andreas Schröder and Peter White

Introduction

This chapter provides an overview of the assessment and treatment of individual patients with bodily distress syndromes. It includes contributions from different clinicians who have experience of treating such patients and describes a range of techniques that are used for patients with these disorders. Efficacy of these treatments is described in Chapter 3.

It is important to appreciate that techniques may vary greatly across the range of severity of patients with this type of disorder. For example, patients in primary care who present with bodily distress may be quite open from the outset to a psychological approach to their symptoms, whereas patients with more severe and persistent disorders may be initially very resistant to this approach. Thus recommendations for management of mild or transient disorders may be inappropriate for patients with severe disorders and vice versa.

While the concept of somatisation disorder arose in specialist clinics in the USA, much has been written in the past concerning the management of patients with severe and disabling bodily distress syndromes. Some of these patients have marked difficulties in their relationships with doctors and the healthcare system. Such descriptions are not necessarily relevant to the large number of patients seen every day in primary and secondary care with less severe forms of bodily distress. In order to match the intensity of treatments to the severity of the disorder, the first part of this chapter concerns assessment of the patient. The extent of the assessment will vary according to the situation and the severity of the disorder. Where necessary, the assessment is aimed at enhancing the patient's motivation for further therapy. The second part of the chapter is concerned with further clinical management in primary and secondary care, including specialised treatment. It is not possible to provide in a single chapter all the details of treatment for this large group of patients, so the text refers throughout to more detailed descriptions of the different management techniques.

Assessment
Aims of the assessment

The first aim of the assessment is to establish whether the patient has a diagnosis of a bodily distress disorder, either alone or in conjunction with concurrent physical or psychiatric disorders. The second step is to establish the level of severity of such a disorder. While performing the assessment, the health professional should also attempt to be supportive of the

Medically Unexplained Symptoms, Somatisation and Bodily Distress, ed. Francis Creed, Peter Henningsen and Per Fink. Published by Cambridge University Press. © Cambridge University Press 2011.

patient, acknowledge the reality of the symptoms and understand the patient's views regarding their cause. The health professional should be prepared to provide a tangible explanation for the symptoms by the end of the assessment and outline the next steps of management, providing clear reasons why some form of psychological treatment would be helpful if this is appropriate. The assessment may be completed at a single interview or further investigations may be required before it can be completed.

Identification of patients with bodily distress

There is no single way to identify those patients with bodily distress syndromes who require treatment. In clinical practice, a clinician must make a judgement according to the number and severity of symptoms, their chronicity, the level of impairment and healthcare use. Unfortunately, the *Diagnostic and Statistical Manual of Mental Disorders* (DSM)-IV definitions are not very helpful as the threshold for diagnosis of somatisation disorder is too high and excludes many people who require treatment. On the other hand, undifferentiated somatisation disorder has a low threshold and some patients with this disorder would not require specific treatment.

Often in research studies, in preference to the DSM-IV definitions, a cut-off point on a self-administered questionnaire has been used, as these correlate well with impairment of function and increased healthcare use. For example, scores on the Patient Health Questionnaire (PHQ)-15 questionnaire in the highest 10% or 20% correlate with considerable disability and increased healthcare costs [1;2;3]. The same is true for people who score high on the Whiteley Index of health anxiety. These two measures, number of somatic symptoms and level of health anxiety, appear to be the most important dimensions determining clinically important bodily distress. These questionnaires alone are inadequate to define people who need treatment, but they are very useful as screening questionnaires [4]. Additional psychological dimensions, such as excessive concern or rumination about illness, catastrophising about the consequences of symptoms and avoidance behaviours are additional factors that may require specific attention during treatment.

There are clear definitions of the functional somatic syndromes but, nevertheless, clinicians generally use their own judgement about these diagnoses and the need for treatment [5;6;7]. In addition to the bodily distress disorder itself, it is necessary at the first assessment to identify whether the patient has an anxiety or depressive disorder. This is best done clinically, but questionnaires such as the Hospital Anxiety and Depression Scale (HADS) or PHQ-9 for depression and PHQ-7 for anxiety, can be helpful aids, especially in general medical settings.

Stratification according to levels of severity

A disease management approach to assessment

A disease management approach for bodily distress syndromes can be helpful as a comprehensive treatment plan should recognise the risk of these symptoms becoming chronic, disabling and leading to frequent healthcare use. Because of the wide range of severity of bodily distress syndromes, it is important to try to identify, at an early stage in treatment, the risk level and to define the treatment plan accordingly. In this way one can match the intensity, type and setting for the treatment with the level of risk, an approach described in the Dutch Multidisciplinary Guideline for medically unexplained symptoms and somatoform disorders [8]. The Dutch model uses a biopsychosocial assessment of patients in all risk levels (see below).

As well as risk of becoming chronic and disabling, bodily distress syndromes are also heterogeneous in terms of complexity. This complexity has several aspects. One aspect concerns comorbidity – with both physical and psychiatric disorders. Comorbidity with medical illness is seen in the common situations where chronic widespread pain (fibromyalgia) co-occurs with rheumatoid arthritis, non-cardiac chest pain with heart disease and irritable bowel syndrome with inflammatory bowel disease. Comorbidity with psychiatric disorders includes the very common concurrent anxiety and depressive disorders.

Another level of complexity is the association of these disorders with stress. During the assessment phase stress levels are explored to identify biological stressors, such as painful physical illness that leads to lack of sleep, psychosocial stressors such as external life events and cognitive aspects including negative thinking. The biopsychosocial model of Engel is a useful means to chart this complexity and to identify cues for treatment [9].

The third level of complexity is the illness behaviour of the patient. In mild or transient bodily distress, this is not an issue. In more serious bodily distress syndromes, patients may be visiting many doctors and a chaotic pattern of health services use can occur, without adequate communication between those treating the patient. Such complexity is best handled by systematic case management, and one of the aims of assessment for treatment is to identify the most suitable case manager and the most appropriate healthcare setting for the case management to be successful.

In terms of risk, three levels can be discerned.

Low risk

This is the least complex level of bodily distress syndrome with the most favourable prognosis. In this group, patients tend to experience somatic symptoms for short periods of time, especially in stressful circumstances. As well as presenting somatic symptoms, such patients are usually quite ready to discuss psychosocial factors, provided they are invited to do so by the physician. These symptoms are not so severe that they lead to serious impairment of function. If the patient is on sick leave, this is for a period not longer than 3–6 weeks and resumption of work should be anticipated [10].

Intermediate risk

This group includes patients with some degree of complexity in terms of comorbidity, either concurrent medical illness or psychiatric disorder. This comorbidity can complicate the choice of treatment for both doctor and patient as the focus tends to be on the distinct medical and/or psychiatric disorder rather than on the factors which lead to multiple somatic symptoms and high health anxiety. Such comorbidity has a negative influence on treatment outcome if no attention is paid to it at this level of complexity [1;3;11;12;13;14;15;16]. If this comorbidity is recognised and addressed, however, the prognosis should be good.

High risk

This group includes patients with persistent bodily distress that is markedly disabling. These patients may have serious problems in their relationships with doctors, so requests for second opinions and numerous transfers between clinics are evident. Extensive diagnostic procedures, admissions and even surgery may occur. Patients may be entrenched in legislation procedures for disability pensions or other claims, which often predict a poor outcome. Case management is the preferred format for management.

Complicated or uncomplicated functional somatic syndromes

Functional somatic syndromes, such as chronic fatigue syndrome, irritable bowel syndrome and fibromyalgia, which are so common in many medical clinics, may be categorised as complicated or uncomplicated. In the latter group, patients only have the symptoms which characterise the functional somatic syndrome itself. In contrast, in complicated functional somatic syndromes the patient also has numerous somatic symptoms outside of the relevant bodily system of the functional syndrome. For example, patients with irritable bowel syndrome who have numerous 'extraintestinal' symptoms or patients with fibromyalgia who also have numerous other somatic symptoms outside the musculoskeletal system would be regarded as complicated.

A questionnaire that screens for somatic symptoms is useful in this context. Prior to the use of such a questionnaire the attention of both patient and doctor is usually focused on the presenting symptoms of the functional somatic syndrome and investigations for possible organic disease are also focused on this complaint. The questionnaire may highlight the fact that the presenting symptom is only one of several somatic symptoms throughout the body and this may alert the doctor to the fact that the presenting symptom is part of a complicated functional somatic syndrome.

For example, when a patient presents with chest pain, the main concern of patient and doctor is to exclude heart disease. This is quite proper if the pain sounds like angina. If the investigations for cardiac disease are negative, however, the search can quickly lead to investigations for possible gastrointestinal disorders that might cause chest pain. At this point it is helpful if the doctor ask about headaches, fatigue, pains in the limbs and joints, dizziness, etc., which would indicate that the chest pain may be part of a wider bodily distress syndrome. A questionnaire that elucidates all of these somatic symptoms helps to broaden the search for the cause of the chest pain. This broadening of the search for a cause may not occur if the anxieties about heart, chest or gastrointestinal disease are high, and the doctor and patient get locked into a series of investigations aimed at identifying one of the many possible organic diseases that can cause chest pain.

Enhancing patient motivation for further therapy

An important aspect of the assessment should be to motivate the patient for further therapy if this is going to be necessary. This can usually be achieved if the assessment:

- is seen to cover both physical and psychological aspects of the patient's complaints
- includes understanding the patient's views regarding the cause and the seriousness of the symptoms
- is carried out by a health professional who is viewed as supportive, rather than rejecting or dismissive, of the patient's symptoms
- includes an explanation for the symptoms in a tangible way that promotes self-management [17].

Assessment in primary and secondary medical care settings

The extent of the assessment will depend on the situation. A brief assessment is usual in primary care as so many symptoms resolve spontaneously [18]. For patients with a more persistent disorder, this may be followed by longer interviews which allow more detailed assessment. For the patient who has been investigated in one or more medical departments in the general hospital, a much more detailed assessment by a mental health professional is usually required. An outline of a detailed assessment is provided in this chapter as many health professionals in both general medical and mental health practice have not had adequate training in this area of practice. References to more detailed descriptions are provided to which the reader can refer. A useful brief assessment for primary care is provided by Hatcher and Arroll [19]. More detailed descriptions are provided by Fink and others [20;21;22;23].

The following description of detailed assessment is derived in part from the widely used reattribution model and The Extended Reattribution and Management (TERM) model, as these have been developed in primary care and encapsulate widely held views about the assessment of patients presenting with bodily distress syndromes in that setting [20;24]. More details are provided, which will be applicable to the assessment of complicated cases of bodily distress that are usually seen in secondary or tertiary care.

Sources of information

Although much of the assessment can be completed during the interview with the patient, in severe or prolonged bodily distress further information from a relative or close friend can be helpful and a thorough examination of previous notes is essential to elicit details of all previous symptoms and treatments. This examination of the notes aims to elucidate whether there have been previous episodes of bodily distress . It is also necessary to become fully aware of all the previous investigations for possible organic disease that have been performed, together with all the details of any coexisting or previous physical illnesses and their treatment.

In primary care, multiple, rather than single bodily distress symptoms, persistence or disability are indicators of a worse outcome [18]. Therefore the assessment should indicate whether the disorder is sufficiently serious to merit intensive treatment. This requires careful assessment of several dimensions, most notably, the number of somatic symptoms and degree of health anxiety, possibly using formal measures (Table 8.1).

1) *The doctor takes the history of:*
   - presenting physical symptom(s)
   - other associated physical symptoms
   - emotional problems and psychosocial factors, including direct enquiry about symptoms of anxiety and depression
   - any recent stressful life events, or other external factors (work-related, family and broader social life)
   - any previous similar symptoms or episodes
   - the person's beliefs about the cause of their symptom(s)
   - the degree of illness worry associated with the symptom and whether family members share these fears
   - the person's current functional level (physical, social, and family)
   - the person's expectations of treatment and examinations.

2) *The doctor's immediate actions:*
   - include a brief, focused physical examination and, if clinically indicated, arrange necessary laboratory investigations. Warn the patient that the results may be negative if this seems likely. Avoid redundant investigations only 'to calm' the patient.
   - provide feedback on the results of the physical examination and any investigations (including no or minor abnormalities) and state whether these are, or are not, related to the present symptoms.
   - acknowledge the reality of the symptoms and the concern they raise, even if the physical examinations are negative.

Table 8.1 Dimensions and instruments of assessment in patients with bodily distress syndromes

	Dimension	Measure
Presenting and other somatic symptoms	Number of somatic symptoms	PHQ-15 [2], SSI [26]
Symptoms of distress	Anxiety and depression	HADS [27], PHQ-9 and PHQ-7 [28;29]
Degree of illness worry	Health anxiety	Whiteley Index of hypochondriasis [30], HAQ [31]
Level of functioning	Health status	SF-36 [32]
Patient's view of cause	Attribution	Open questions or illness attribution questionnaire (IPQ-R [33;34])
Patient's expectation of treatment		Open questions
Recent stress or difficulties	Life events	Brief list of threatening events [25]
Medical help-seeking	Number of consultations and number of doctors: (a) in last year; (b) in lifetime	Medical notes

PHQ, Personal Health Questionnaire; SSI, Somatic Symptom Inventory; HADS, Hospital Anxiety and Depression Scale; PHQ-9 and -7, HAQ, Health Anxiety Questionnaire; SF-36, Short Form 36 (health status); IPQ-R, Illness Perception Questionnaire – revised.

The detailed assessment of patients referred to a specialist mental health professional

This section outlines the assessments to be used when patients are referred to a specialist mental health professional for treatment of more severe bodily distress disorder. For a full description of this assessment see House in Mayor *et al.* [23]. It is important to discuss at the outset the patient's attitude to the referral to a mental health professional. Sometimes this interview can be dominated by the patient's resentment at the referral to a psychiatrist or psychologist. People with such an aversion to seeing a psychiatrist usually do not attend an outpatient appointment, but if the patient is an inpatient in a medical ward it is hard for them to avoid a consultation when this has been requested by the patient's usual physician. Thus, in this setting, the mental health professional may have to deal with resentment, hostility or frank bewilderment about the referral.

If the patient is undergoing a series of investigations for possible organic disorders, they may feel that the main aim of the hospital admission is to find which of these will produce positive results. Therefore, they may be unwilling to discuss psychological causes for the symptoms [25]. If this occurs, it is appropriate to offer the patient the opportunity for discussion at a later occasion when the investigations are complete.

Specific points of the history and examination

Assess the presenting symptom

Taking a thorough history is often the most important part of the diagnostic process in patients with bodily distress. First, the doctor can assess each symptom and:

- consider carefully whether it is typical of an organic disease or not (e.g. whether chest pain occurs primarily with exertion and whether it is relieved by drinking milk or taking antacids)
- identify whether the presenting symptom occurs alone or with other somatic or psychological symptoms (e.g. whether headaches occur alone, with visual disturbance or with other symptoms, such as sweating, tachycardia and musculoskeletal pains, suggestive of tension)
- identify the exact time course of the symptom, paying particular attention to the circumstances of its onset and whether it has fluctuated in severity subsequently or even disappeared intermittently
- whether there have been previous episodes that have resolved spontaneously or in response to particular treatments.

Second, a detailed assessment of all the patient's symptoms, both physical and psychological, is not only helpful in order to arrive at the correct diagnosis, but may also help to establish the doctor–patient relationship. It should assure the patient that their somatic symptoms are being taken very seriously and the doctor is interested in all aspects of the patient's problem. The doctor can show equal interest in the patient's somatic and psychological symptoms, thereby re-establishing a balance that may have been lost when previous medical interviews and investigation concentrated only on the former. Patients sometimes comment that their symptoms have not been assessed as thoroughly previously, reflecting the rapid use of investigative techniques in modern medicine.

A problem occurs if the patient has many symptoms. If time is limited, the doctor may find it useful to note that the patient has many symptoms, but then ask the patient to name the most worrying two or three symptoms and deal with those in great detail at the first consultation. The fact that there are numerous somatic symptoms is an important finding in itself, as there are few organic diseases which lead to multiple symptoms, and concurrent anxiety and depression is often the reason for multiple somatic symptoms [36].

It is important to assess the degree of disability that accompanies the symptoms and any important maintaining factors. These may include being off sick from work – is the patient motivated to return to work or are there problems at the workplace? Is there any claim for compensation in progress? Sometimes the symptoms play an important part in the person's close relationships, such as avoidance of a sexual relationship or the shift to another of responsibility for child care. The person may hope that the symptom could lead to early retirement from a job that they find stressful.

Personal, developmental and past history of illness and mental state, including abuse and prior severe life events

A full psychiatric history must be taken. It is important to take a personal history in such a way that the previous illness episodes can be fitted in to the patient's life history. It is often best to document all previous illness episodes and identify when these occurred, and then work out at which point in the patient's biography each one occurred. In this way it should become clear whether or not somatic symptoms develop at times of stress in the person's life. The assessment will also indicate the person's attitude to illness and doctors, and family history should also assess whether the person has grown up in a family where illness and medical help-seeking were common or not.

It is important to assess childhood experiences. This includes exposure to illness either in themselves or close relatives. It also includes specific questioning about childhood adversity, including possible abuse, and this can only be done satisfactorily once good rapport has been developed between the patient and the mental health professional.

A number of features increase the probability that psychological factors are important in the development of somatic symptoms [37;38]:

- the presenting bodily symptom is accompanied by psychological symptoms or other somatic symptoms typical of anxiety or depression
- the presenting bodily symptom is not typical of organic disease
- there have been previous episodes of the bodily distress
- the symptom may have been precipitated by stress and alleviated by the alleviation of stress
- there is a family or past personal history of psychiatric disorder
- the symptom responds to psychological treatment, when there has been no previous response to medical treatments.

Special features of the mental state examination [37]:

- Observe any evidence of abnormal illness behaviour, such as constantly returning to the symptoms during conversation and interrupting the flow of conversation in order to emphasise their severity.
- It should also be noted whether certain topics of conversation, such as discussion of recent stressful life events, leads to the accentuation of such behaviours. Are there repeated demonstrations or complaints of severe pain even when the patient appears to be sitting comfortably most of the time?
- Assess the level of denial, usually denial of psychological aspects of the illness. A patient may deny depression even when he or she appears close to tears. Does the patient deny depression claiming that they have nothing to be depressed about, even while stating that the illness and lack of successful treatment is ruining their life?
- Assess whether the patient believes strongly that their physical symptoms must have a physical cause. Does he or she repeat that this is the case even when extensive investigations have failed to show any organic illness that might cause the symptoms? Some patients claim that the investigations are inadequate. There may be overvalued ideas concerning their cause, and occasionally bizarre hypochondriacal beliefs, which, if challenged, may lead to hostility.
- Does the patient openly state that they feel psychiatric referral is totally inappropriate as the cause is physical?
- Does the patient have catastrophic thoughts that their life is going to be ruined by a symptom, which does not, objectively, seem so severe?
- Is there obsessional rumination about the symptoms and their effect on the patient's life?
- Is there any abnormal hostility expressed towards doctors who have previously treated the patient? Are doctors and their treatments blamed for making the symptoms worse?
- Does the patient appear to be in great discomfort? Does the patient repeatedly touch or check a particular part of the body? Is there evidence that the patient is emphasising severe pain or more disability when observed but not at other times? Does the patient tense up markedly or shy away when the doctor carries out a physical examination?

Clinical assessment at the Research Clinic for Functional Disorders, Denmark

An example of a detailed assessment is provided by the biopsychosocial assessment model used at the Research Clinic for Functional Disorders and Psychosomatics, Aarhus University Hospital, Denmark. This unit treats currently patients with severe and disabling bodily distress of at least two years' duration. This threshold has been used to ensure that the unit is concerned primarily with severe disorders and is not swamped with milder disorders that should be managed in primary and secondary medical care. The Danish team uses a biopsychosocial assessment of patients with marked bodily distress. The assessment aims to:

- ensure a patient's symptoms are not due to an undiagnosed medical or psychiatric condition
- provide the patient with a positive and evidence-based understanding of their illness
- enhance acceptability of psychosocial interventions for a patient's bodily complaints.

The assessment includes:

- a review of clinical records
- the World Health Organization (WHO)-endorsed, semi-structured psychiatric interview Schedule for Clinical Assessment in Neuropsychiatry (SCAN), which includes an extensive section about physical symptoms [39]
- a physical and neurological examination
- a laboratory screening battery.

The SCAN interview asks about 76 somatic symptoms and the interviewer tries to decide whether each is due to a medical condition or side effect of medication, or whether it is 'functional'. The interview establishes whether the patient has a formal anxiety, depressive or other psychiatric disorder, including a somatoform disorder.

All patients are given individualised information about the nature, course and treatment options for their somatic symptoms. Moreover, each patient's primary care doctor and referring hospital ward are informed of the patients' diagnosis (see below) with a summary of their illness history and previous examinations. If an undiagnosed medical condition is suspected, patients are referred to the relevant department. If comorbid anxiety and depression is present, written individualised advice on treatment is given to the patient's primary care physician, in the expectation that they will treat this psychiatric disorder.

Impact of the diagnostic label

The way multiple bodily complaints are labelled is important [40]. A diagnosis shapes a patient's beliefs about what is wrong with them, and it claims authority and legitimises medical procedures and litigation [41;42]. A diagnostic strategy based on pathological findings and the exclusion of serious organic disease, rather than on patients' impairment and suffering is not helpful to most patients. On the one hand, many people have been told that investigations for organic disease have shown that 'nothing is wrong' with them, and they often feel that the doctor implies there is no need for healthcare intervention. Such reassurance often fails [43;44;45]. On the other hand, diagnostic labels that indicate serious, chronic conditions may act as self-fulfilling prophecies. It has been shown, for instance, that the term myalgic encephalopathy (ME) is associated with poorer outcome than a more neutral term, chronic fatigue [40;46;47]. Yet providing psychological explanations in a way that rejects the patient's experience of disabling and painful physical symptoms does not solve the problem

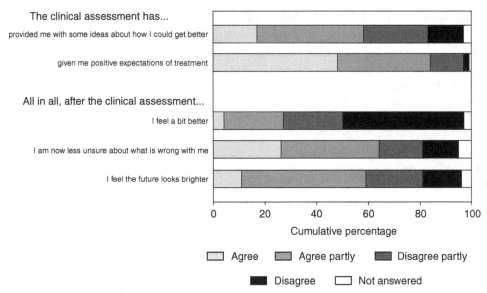

Figure 8.1 Effect of a thorough clinical assessment, as perceived by patients (N = 118 [51]).

either. In this difficult area of medicine, doctors are often not able to give alternative explanations for bodily symptoms in a way that is acceptable to patients [48;49].

In Aarhus, over recent years the diagnosis of bodily distress syndrome has been used [50;51]. This diagnosis has been introduced as an empirically based diagnostic category that encompasses the functional somatic syndromes and the somatoform disorders without making assumptions about physical or psychological aetiology. For patients with severe, multi-organ bodily distress, a thorough biopsychosocial assessment based on the concept of bodily distress syndrome may have favourable effects on their perceived bodily distress, anxiety and depression, and illness worry (Figure 8.2). The thorough clinical assessment is, however, not intended as part of the intervention for this patient group; it aims to provide an alternative illness model and motivate patients to engage in treatments that are based on active patient involvement, such as exercise or cognitive behavioural therapy (CBT). An extract of the information given to patients at the Aarhus research unit is given in Appendix 8.1.

Acceptability of the biopsychosocial assessment used in Aarhus

Patients' perceptions of the clinical assessment at the Research Clinic for Functional Disorders have been collected, and they show that the majority of these patients had positive treatment expectations after the clinical assessment, and many had developed some ideas about how they could get better (Figure 8.1) However, most patients did not feel any better immediately after the assessment, which was in contrast with the finding of a moderate symptom relief in the weeks after the clinical assessment (Figure 8.2).

Interpretation and communicative aspects of diagnostic tests

Much is written about the need to avoid investigations for organic disease; this is one of the tenets of the Smith model, described above. In clinical practice, however, there may be a clinical indication to do another such investigation because a particular organic

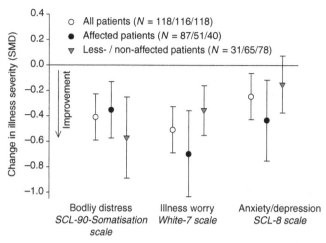

Figure 8.2 Effect of a thorough clinical assessment, expressed as reduction in illness severity from before to median seven weeks after the clinical assessment [51]. Change (standardised mean difference, SMD) of illness severity scores, from a few days before the clinical assessment to approximately six weeks after the assessment. Besides the overall effect on all patients, SMD is shown for affected and less-affected patients separately. 'Affected' refers to the following subgroups: for the SCL-90 somatisation scale, to severely impaired patients according to the clinician; for the Whitely-7 scale, to patients with comorbid health anxiety; and for the SCL-8 scale, to patients with a DSM-IV- diagnosis of comorbid major depression, anxiety disorder or dysthymia. N states number of analysed change scores in the different groups for bodily distress, illness worry, and anxiety/depression, respectively. Error bars indicate 95% confidence intervals.

disease has not been ruled out. When it is necessary to do such a test, the doctor may feel that the result is likely to be negative because the overall picture is typical of a bodily distress disorder. In this case, before ordering the investigation, the doctor should spend some time explaining to the patient that s/he expects a normal result in view of the overall clinical picture. The doctor can describe possible reasons for the symptom(s) other than the organic disease under investigation and state clearly that when the normal test result comes back, the patient can embark on the agreed course of treatment with greater confidence.

When a patient has had numerous investigations for organic disease, the notion that this is the likely cause of the symptom tends to be reinforced. Many patients agree, however, that having raised expectations prior to each test, only to be followed by disappointment, is a demoralising experience. In this case, the doctor can point out that there is an alternative strategy and suggest that the main investigations that might yield positive results have usually not been performed. These are investigations to assess the extent of anxiety, depression, health anxiety etc. As an illustration of this phenomenon, a report from London concerning 22 patients with functional abdominal pain revealed that, between them, these patients had seen 76 consultants, undergone numerous investigations and 38 abdominal operations [52]. The only investigation which provided abnormal results was the Hamilton Rating Scale for Depression: 14 had moderate or severe depression and four had mild depression.

As can be seen from the above, it is necessary to assess the patient on a number of dimensions. For each of these, there is an appropriate questionnaire and some examples are given below. The first two of these should be considered in most cases.

(1) *Number of somatic symptoms.* This is a crucially important dimension and is an important predictor of health status (see Chapter 1). If the patient has numerous somatic symptoms which they find bothersome, this is suggestive of accompanying anxiety or depression but is also an independent predictor of poor outcome. There are numerous instruments; the most common are PHQ-15 [2], Somatic Symptoms Inventory [26;53] and the Symptom Checklist (SCL)-90 somatisation scale [54]. A high score may occur in the presence physical illness or depression/anxiety, which commonly accompany bodily distress syndromes.

(2) *Health anxiety.* It is necessary to assess the degree to which a person is anxious about their symptoms. The most common instrument is the Whiteley Index [30].

(3) *Anxiety and depression.* HADS is widely used in Europe [26]. The PHQ-9 (depression) and PHQ-7 (anxiety) are also widely used [27;28].

Further clinical management in primary and secondary care

Aims of management

The aim of management depends on the severity of the condition. In mild to moderate bodily distress, the aim is to reduce the symptom and promote full functioning, but with very severe bodily distress the aims may be to improve functioning/health status and reduce healthcare use even if the primary symptom changes little. A thorough assessment, as described in the previous section, should enable the health professional to identify the aim of management. It should also have led the patient to recognise the nature of his or her disorder and the types of treatment that are available.

An immediate aspect of management is to commence treatment for concurrent psychiatric disorder if necessary and optimise treatment for any concurrent physical disorder. It is important to remember that medically unexplained and explained symptoms can coexist and the pattern may change with time. The doctor should be prepared to review the whole disorder if new symptoms occur, but at the same time should try to avoid unnecessary tests and procedures. The doctor should not perform repetitive investigations only to calm the patient or him or herself and be prepared to state to the patient his or her diagnostic impression clearly, frankly and directly.

Two examples of the stepped-care approach to treatment are presented here. They are similar in content, but vary in style and other details. The first is described in the Dutch Multidisciplinary Guideline for MUS [medically unexplained symptoms] and Somatoform Disorder [8].

Stepped-care approach to treatment

Based on risk management as used in the Dutch Multidisciplinary Guideline for MUS and Somatoform Disorder [8]

All patients being treated for bodily distress need a clear treatment plan and this should be established, as far as possible, in accord with the preference and agreement of the patient. This should be developed after a thorough diagnostic examination, including clarification of symptoms, assessment of the attribution of the symptoms by the patient, and assessment of psychosocial stressors. The clinician should provide a full explanation of the likely reasons for the person's symptoms and recommend non-specific interventions which are applicable at all risk levels. These include attention to good sleep, hygiene, regular moderate physical exercise and stress management.

First step

In a case of low risk, a two-track disease management approach is recommended in which the doctor follows up the patient in relation to both somatic as well as psychiatric diagnostic procedures, and assesses the adherence to and outcome of the recommendations for a healthy lifestyle. Usually, this treatment is provided in the primary-care setting by the general practitioner (GP), who can refer the patients to the primary-care psychologist for a short course of CBT, if the symptom does not subside spontaneously.

Second step

In a case of moderate risk, attention should be paid to any concurrent medical or psychiatric conditions, and these should be treated optimally. This may be straightforward if adjustment of the dose of a drug is required. Common symptoms are pain and fatigue, and such symptoms are ambiguous – they can be attributed to either a medical or psychological disorder or both.

When such symptoms are prominent, the clinician should try to decide whether these symptoms are principally associated with a concomitant medical illness or psychological disorder in order to direct treatment. It is helpful to try to understand whether the pain or fatigue fluctuates according to the patient's general medical condition or whether it fluctuates according to stress or anxiety and depression. In the latter case, close attention to optimal treatment of anxiety or depression is necessary. In either case, however, antidepressants, particularly tricyclics, even at low doses, may be very helpful in relieving the pain. If depression is evident, the dose should be increased to that which is appropriate to treat depression. Once the depression is treated satisfactorily, pain and fatigue may be reassessed to see whether they have also improved. If not, adjustment of the therapy for a concurrent medical condition may be tried. In a complex situation like this, it is preferable to make one change at a time so the effect of each change in medication can be assessed before proceeding to the next.

In addition, any relief of pain or fatigue should be accompanied by an appropriate increase in activity to minimise the impairment associated with the patient's illness. It is worth exploring with the patient the extent to which his or her general functioning can be improved in spite of any restrictions imposed by the concurrent medical illness. Many patients in this situation underestimate their capacity for exercise because of fears of worsening their condition, so a very cautious but persistent approach is required. A specific programme of exercise can be helpful for pain, fatigue and depression, and careful monitoring of these dimensions can be helpful. If a relative or carer is involved in this monitoring a somewhat more objective view is possible.

Sometimes this aim of optimal treatment of both physical and psychiatric disorders requires shared care between the mental health professional and the medical doctor. If the treatment setting is primary care, the GP may need psychiatric expertise. The most consistent evidence in terms of the benefit of psychiatric consultation, exists in the form of a consultation by the psychiatrist resulting in a consultation letter for the GP. If the treatment setting is the general hospital because of comorbid medical illness, the psychiatric treatments may be provided to the medical specialist by the psychiatric consultation-liaison service.

Third step

In the third step, there is considerable risk that the patient will undergo numerous diagnostic procedures with consequent high healthcare costs and no specific treatment for their symptoms and associated disability. Outside the healthcare system, there is the potential for unemployment and deteriorating social relationships. For such complex cases, some form of case management is the method of choice to decrease health service use and to diminish the patient's suffering and disability. If the case manager is the GP, she or he would be helped by psychiatric consultation. The principles guiding such care have been developed by Smith [55]. These are:

- Provide brief, regularly scheduled visits so that the patient need not develop new symptoms in order to see the physician.
- Establish a strong patient physician relationship in which only one physician is providing the majority of the care.
- Perform a physical examination of the relevant part of the body when new symptoms arise.
- Search for signs of disease instead of relying on symptoms.
- Understand the somatic symptoms as an emotional communication rather than necessarily being a harbinger of new disease.
- Avoid diagnostic tests and laboratory or surgical procedures unless clearly indicated by signs of disease.
- Gradually encourage the patient to view their symptoms in such a way that he or she is prepared to receive care from a mental health professional.

However, it may be necessary to treat the patient in the setting of a multidisciplinary team, possibly in a specialised ward, if such a facility is available.

Improving adaptation should be the main focus of a comprehensive treatment approach, rather than attempting to remove symptoms. The approach should aim to improve the patient's awareness of his or her current situation, which is usually dominated by sickness and disability, and motivate him or her to change this so that functioning improves. The treatment plan should be focused specifically on improving the coping skills of each particular patient with a view to improved functioning. It is necessary to develop the doctor–patient or therapist–patient relationship by emphasising a joint approach towards helping the patient to improve their health-related quality of life.

If legislation for a disability pension is ongoing, it may be preferable to refrain from treatment until the legal procedure has come to an end. This may take a long time, however, so efforts at rehabilitation should be attempted if the patient is willing. If it becomes clear that a relative or carer reinforces sickness behaviour, by doing most daily tasks for the patient and protecting him or her from any demands, the relative must be involved in the treatment plan, starting with motivation for change.

Vignette

In order to show how the use of the biopsychosocial assessment model leads on to a treatment approach, the case history of a patient with bodily distress in the primary care setting is presented, where a psychiatric consultation and a consultation letter to the GP as well as the patient were provided, in a consultation model that was developed and found to be effective in the Dutch primary care setting [13;56;57].

A 48-year-old, married woman with two children, aged 16 and 13 years, visited the GP frequently with bodily distress. She was insisting on referral to the cardiologist because of dizziness and cardiac chest pain that frightened her. Previous referrals to the cardiologist for similar complaints had not shown any evidence of cardiac pathology and previous referrals to a neurologist for headaches had also not yielded any evidence of serious disease. Therefore, the GP did not consider the present complaints adequate reason for a referral. The GP found the ongoing requests of the patient for referrals difficult to handle. It made her feel incompetent.

During a joint consultation with the GP and a consultant psychiatrist, who visited the practice, the patient's pattern of asking for referral for bodily distress was discussed together with its consequent impact on the GP and the patient. It turned out that the patient was content if the referral did not yield evidence of disease. It reassured her. For the GP as well as the patient, it was a relief to discuss this during the consultation. A situation ensued that made it possible to negotiate the amount of reassurance that was required by the patient. In the end, the patient was willing to accept an examination by the GP with exercises to improve her condition, instead of referral to the cardiologist. The GP came to realise that a lack of positive findings during her physical examination would suffice to reassure the patient.

In addition, it transpired during the consultation that the patient felt stressed by tantrums of her eldest son, who had entered puberty with vigour. The GP, the psychiatrist and the patient discussed several strategies that she might use to avoid becoming so stressed and to set proper limits to her son's behaviour. The psychiatrist provided a consultation letter to the GP and the patient (Box 8.1). After six weeks, the psychiatrist contacted the GP for follow-up and it was clear that the doctor–patient interactional problem had been solved and no further referrals had been necessary.

Consultation letter

After the consultation, the psychiatrist provided the GP and the patient with a consultation letter with recommendations regarding their interaction (Box 8.1). The details of this case vignette can best be displayed using the biopsychosocial scheme [57]. Table 8.2 summarises the biological, psychological and social aspects of the history, consultation findings, diagnosis and treatment recommendations.

In this case, the patient had problems in her interactions with her son. She had trouble setting limits to his behaviour in the context of his pubertal mood swings. She did not turn

---

Box 8.1 Recommendations in connection with consultation on account of non-cardiac chest pain and dizziness

During the conversation, you explained that from time to time you feel the need to be reassured about the nature of your bodily symptoms. You do think this has to do with your personality and your upbringing. You need certainty. As you felt dizzy and experienced some chest pain, you wanted to be sure that they were not due to a cardiac problem, although you visited the cardiologist for these complaints recently and he did not find any evidence of a cardiac problem in a rigorous check-up. You told us that your eldest son had started puberty tantrums and you find it hard to cope with them. This made you nervous. If people have to endure stress daily, they can suffer from chest pain which results from the reactions of the nervous system to stress. It is important to keep in mind that you need reassurance, especially if you experience stress in your daily life. This reassurance can only be partial with regard to the exclusion of an imminent heart attack. You will have to discuss with your GP whether a referral to a cardiologist is needed or not. You can start exercising to improve your condition, as this will lower your stress levels. Also, you will find that talking about your questions on how to cope with your son's behaviour, i.e. with your spouse or with your GP, will give relief, mentally as well as physically.

Table 8.2 Biopsychosocial scheme for the case of non-cardiac chest pain [56]

	History	Consultation findings	Diagnosis (ICD)	Treatment
Biological	Female, 48 years	Non-cardiac chest pain and dizziness Stress-related	Non-cardiac chest pain	Exercise
Psychological	Obsessive compulsive traits	Health anxiety. Needs reassurance	Somatoform autonomous dysfunction, cardiac system Obsessive compulsive personality traits	Explain link between stress and medically unexplained symptoms
Health services	Multiple referrals; no findings by cardiologist	Referrals give security	Patient–GP interaction insecure	Discuss security needs Avoid referrals
Social system	No history in family	Eldest son has tantrums	Difficulty setting limits to son in puberty	Improve coping with son by strengthening bond with spouse or by providing suggestions

to her husband for help, but experienced stress-related non-cardiac chest pain for which she requested a referral to a cardiologist. The GP felt inadequate because the patient had been referred recently and there was no evidence of cardiac pathology, yet the patient continued to visit the GP frequently and request further referrals.

In fact, the patient's problem of difficult interaction with her son could be partly resolved by explicit discussion during the consultation, exploration of the background and recommendations mentioned in the consultation letter about managing the son's demands and the patient's specialist referral requests. This led to a situation with more treatment possibilities aimed at the underlying problem, namely physical activity to reduce stress and health anxiety, and efforts aimed at better coping with the son's behaviour.

This vignette provides an example of the use of a biopsychosocial model and consultation letter in the situation of a psychiatric consultation in the primary-care setting. However, this model can be used in every treatment setting to assess the problems and symptoms of the patient at every relevant level. In this case there was a low risk level and the treatment strategy was in line with that and had good results. In a later trial, this consultation model proved effective in patients with medically unexplained symptoms in primary care [13].

Complicated or uncomplicated functional somatic syndromes – review by Henningsen and colleagues [58]

In routine medical care, the workup and diagnosis of functional somatic syndromes is usually reasonably straightforward and often leads on to one or more medical treatments for the presenting symptom(s): pain, fatigue etc. The importance of a stepped-care model for such patients is the early consideration as to whether the functional somatic syndrome is complicated or uncomplicated [58;59]. The management strategy should be based on the decision as to which of these is the case.

Step 1

(a) In *uncomplicated* functional somatic syndromes, the following actions should be taken:
- Reassure the patient about the fact that no organic disease has been found and that the doctor is confident about the diagnosis of the particular functional somatic syndrome. This should be accompanied by a clear and positive explanation of how stress, anxiety, depression or other psychological factors can lead to the development or perpetuation of pain or fatigue. The diagnosis should be presented in this positive way and not couched in terms of negative investigation results.
- Provide symptomatic treatments such as pain relief.
- Advise the patient to adopt a healthy lifestyle. This may require dietary change for patients with irritable bowel syndrome, or graded activation leading to regular exercise in the case of fatigue.

(b) With *complicated* functional somatic syndromes, the following actions should be taken:
- Reassure the patient with positive explanation of the symptoms as described below. Consider antidepressant medication either at a low dose as an analgesic or, if appropriate, at a full dose to treat depressive disorder. In the latter case, the dose would need to be increased slowly as patients with bodily distress may tolerate these drugs poorly.
- Identify and provide advice on any dysfunctional attributions and illness behaviour and encourage reframing of symptoms within a biopsychosocial framework (i.e. incorporate both the patient's beliefs about the organic nature of their symptoms and how these can be affected by a range of psychological and contextual factors).
- If appropriate, make appointments at regular intervals rather than letting them be patient-initiated.

Step 2

If either step 1a or step 1b prove insufficient:
- prepare referral to psychotherapist or mental-health specialist with reappointment
- ensure that traumatic stressors and maintaining context factors, such as litigation, are assessed
- continue with appointments at regular intervals rather than their being patient-initiated
- liaise with psychotherapist or mental-health specialist on further treatment planning and difficulties.

Step 3

If step 2 proves insufficient and if appropriate in your country, initiate multidisciplinary treatment including symptomatic measures, activating physiotherapy, and psychotherapy.

Explanation, reassurance, broadening the explanatory model

Two initial key factors of management are a clear positive explanation to the patient as to the likely causes of the symptoms and an agreed management plan that gives some responsibility to them for managing their symptoms. These are described in more detail now.

- Summarise the problem – somatic and psychological symptoms, the results of examination and any investigations. Acknowledge (again) the reality of symptoms and the patient's distress.
- Express degree of certainty in doctor's mind. Explain that the doctor will keep an open mind and that new or changed symptoms will lead to reconsideration of the whole problem.
- Provide a positive explanation of the likely causes of problem – which symptoms can be attributed to known physical health problems (if any), which can be attributed to known psychological disorders (if relevant) and those whose cause remains unclear. Try to relate fluctuation of symptoms to fluctuation in any of the following: physical illness, mood, stress or lifestyle. Mention the fact that these symptoms are sometimes regarded as being 'all in the mind', but that modern research shows that mind and body interact continuously and such 'dualism' is outdated.
- Develop with the patient a preliminary management plan. This should take into account the patient's expectations (elicited above), the doctor's view of the likely cause of the problem and the appropriate treatment. This should mention the possibility of further appointments and the doctor's willingness to reassess symptoms fully if they change. If any further investigations are needed, these should be mentioned here to make clear that these could be investigations for psychological problems and not only to detect organic disease.
- Negotiate any specific requests from the patient for investigations to discover organic disease. It is usual to balance such investigations with those for psychological problems (see Table 8.1). There should be a discussion of the likelihood of negative investigations and the implications for further management.
- Outline the main avenues of treatment. These may include: symptomatic treatment, either 'peripheral' or 'central' acting drugs (see below); specific treatment of concurrent physical illness; specific treatment for depression, anxiety or other psychiatric disorder (e.g. obsessive-compulsive or eating disorder); self-management strategies; or no specific treatment but 'watchful waiting' to see if the symptoms resolve spontaneously.
- Some forms of therapy strongly emphasise a model which provides a physical explanation for the symptoms. The TERM model stresses a biological basis for somatisation [20]; a Spanish model explains the somatic symptoms as an hormonal response to stress [60]. It is not known whether such explanations are helpful therapeutically, but a positive explanation is considered to be important [61].

Four important tasks

- *Explanation of how somatic symptoms can develop in the absence of underlying physical illness.* This may include: how symptoms get worse at times of stress, e.g. symptom(s) worsen at work, or at weekends, or in situations of conflict or tension; recognise the symptoms of autonomic arousal, e.g. while waiting to go into the dentist or doing an exam; pain resulting from holding a heavy book on an outstretched arm; onset or worsening of symptoms when one hears bad news of illness or death affecting others; and how depression lowers the pain threshold.

- *Specific actions that the patient can take to manage the symptoms themselves.* This includes: keeping a symptom diary; taking regular exercise; practising relaxation or some other form of stress management; attending to lifestyle, including a healthy diet, reduction of alcohol intake and smoking cessation if necessary.
- *Self-treatment.* Many patients take analgesics, dietary supplements and other 'over-the-counter' remedies, and some use complementary medicine, which may not be helpful and may be expensive. It is worth discussing these with the patient to see which are helpful and which are not, and whether it is worth pursuing them. Make it clear you have an open mind about such treatments and be prepared to discuss which might have proven efficacy.
- *Reassure the patient that you will continue to try to help them in a collaborative way with a view to attaining better coping and less impairment.* This requires a collaborative effort with the patient taking an active role in treatment and not a passive one. Usually there is no pill to cure the problem.
- In view of the complexity of these explanations, consider giving the patient written material to reinforce these discussions.

The reattribution model has been widely recommended in primary care but it is not of proven efficacy. The main limitation of this model is that it focuses on only one of several psychological processes that are important in this group of patients. The important dimensions associated with disability and high healthcare use are: numerous somatic symptoms, depression, presence of concurrent medical illnesses, avoidance of physical activities, catastrophising, body-focused attention, somatic illness beliefs and a tendency to seek medical care rapidly for bodily symptoms [3;62;63].

Activation

Activation is an important component of the treatment of most bodily distress disorders, because inactivity, subjective fatigue, is a regular feature, not only where it appears in the diagnostic label as in chronic fatigue, but also where the lead symptom(s) comprise pain and other functional complaints, as in fibromyalgia, chronic low back pain, chronic dizziness etc. Activation means to support the patient in increased self-generated bodily activity, i.e. increased walking, exercising etc.

Despite the more general relevance of this sort of treatment, the specific and most prominent example of chronic fatigue will be used to illustrate points about it.

Activation treatments for chronic fatigue syndrome

The two effective forms of treatment for chronic fatigue syndrome are CBT and graded exercise therapy (GET). The former is described in the next section, the latter is described here [64;65]. See also the National Institute for Health and Clinical Excellence (NICE) guidance (guidance.nice.org.uk/CG53). CBT is often accompanied by some form of graded increase in activity as the exercise may provoke the unhelpful cognitions (e.g. the catastrophic interpretation of symptoms following a transient increase in activity) which need to be tackled in CBT.

Graded exercise therapy (GET) focuses on stabilising and then gradually increasing physical activity, particularly exercise (defined as any physical activity that demands exertion). This initially occurs at a low level of intensity, but later the aerobic intensity is gradually increased. So, GET starts as a behavioural graded exposure therapy and then moves into a physiological training programme. This therapy is usually given on a one-to-one basis by a physiotherapist, but can be organised in groups which usually combine education, CBT and GET techniques. While there is good evidence for the effectiveness of individual programmes, there is less good evidence for group approaches [66].

Graded exercise therapy should be delivered by a suitably qualified therapist (usually a physiotherapist) who has been trained to give GET for chronic fatigue syndrome. Appropriate clinical supervision is essential. As with CBT, audio-recorded sessions, with a patient's consent, can be invaluable. Fears of physical activity are openly discussed and the reasons for providing GET are explored. A daily activity diary can help to establish whether a patient is pervasively inactive or in the boom-and-bust cycle. Therapeutic goals are agreed. A baseline of physical activity is determined empirically, incorporating a low intensity exercise that is sustainable even on a 'bad' day. The commonest exercise chosen is walking, but swimming and cycling are sometimes chosen, or a mixture. Most importantly the exercise needs to be at a light level, with no significant aerobic or metabolic load. Stretches before and after exercise can be helpful. Once the baseline is established, the duration of exercise is increased by 20% weekly or fortnightly increments. For example, increasing exercise duration from 10 minutes a day to 12 minutes. So long as the patient is not more symptomatic, then the duration can be increased a week or two later. If symptoms increase, then a further period for the same duration should be applied until symptoms abate. Interval exercise, such as breaking up the periods of exercising to more than one a day can be helpful. When exercise duration has reached 30 minutes a day in total on five days a week, exercise intensity may be increased, sometimes using set heart rate maximums, assessed by ambulatory heart rate monitors. Pedometers offer an alternative way of doing this. Again the increase in intensity depends on symptomatic response. After completing the GET programme, strategies to maintain exercise and incorporate it within a normal day are put in place, along with a set-back plan. Ongoing review sessions at longer intervals support recovery.

A *pragmatic rehabilitation programme*, provided by nurses and incorporating education with elements of CBT and GET, has recently been shown to be more effective than supportive listening and usual medical care, when provided in primary care [67]. Although the differences in efficacy were statistically significant, the effects were mild to moderate. This may be related to the dose (only 10 sessions), the delivery (half over the telephone) or the non-specialised staff employed (general nurses).

Pacing is an energy management approach, which is often a self-help approach, but is sometimes guided by healthcare professionals, to plan and restrict daily physical activity so as not to exacerbate symptoms. The model of therapy is based on the envelope theory of energy [68], which suggests that available energy is fixed and finite and exceeding it produces symptoms. The key to pacing is to stay within these fixed limits of energy by restricting activity or balancing it with rest or different activities. This avoids boom-and-bust cycles, hence minimising setbacks and relapses. There is little empirical evidence to support the use of pacing, although surveys of patient charities support its popularity [64, for recent evidence see Chapter 3].

Specialised treatment
Aims of specialised treatment

The main types of specialised psychological therapy for bodily distress disorders are CBT and psychodynamic interpersonal therapy. These therapies may appear to be very different but they probably have many similarities in terms of non-specific ingredients, including developing a close relationship with the patient and cooperative work to understand and overcome symptoms [69]. CBT aims to identify triggers in daily life that are associated with bodily distress and break the vicious circles of cognitions and behaviours that maintain symptoms and the person's concern about them. Psychodynamic interpersonal therapy, on the other hand, is based on the assumption that bodily distress symptoms reflect underlying emotional difficulties that continue to bother the person but which are not shared or discussed. This kind of psychotherapy aims to increase patients' insight into their emotional and interpersonal conflicts in the hope that their interpersonal difficulties can be faced and then improve. It is hoped that their somatic symptoms will then lessen or resolve.

In both of these rather different approaches to treatment, the therapist aims to be understanding and sympathetic to the patient and to take their symptoms seriously. Some patients comment that this attitude contrasts with that they have experienced previously from doctors who appeared to become frustrated by the patient's continued anxiety about somatic symptoms even after negative investigations. Both types of treatment aim to put some responsibility on patients to become active partners in treatment and may include use of symptom diaries as a means of trying to help the patient to understand the link between psychosocial difficulties and symptom exacerbation.

Although both types of therapy are usually found in secondary medical care settings, including departments of psychiatry or psychology, they may also be found in primary care. The modified reattribution model of Blankenstein and colleagues employed several techniques of CBT modified for the primary-care setting [70]. The modified model developed in Spain used psychodynamic interpersonal ingredients in its communication techniques and it is also employed in primary care [60]. The details of treatment of the individual functional somatic syndromes is beyond the scope of this book. The reader is referred to the relevant publications: references 64, 71, 72, 73, 74, 75, 76 and 77].

Outpatient psychotherapy
Cognitive behavioural therapy

Cognitive behavioural treatments have been shown to be effective in patients with multiple somatic symptoms/somatoform disorders (Chapter 3). For other subgroups of patients with disorders such as hypochondriasis, the reported effect sizes for CBT are substantially higher than those reported for CBT in somatisation disorder [78;79].

Getting CBT treatment started

Many patients with somatoform disorders have a history of disappointing treatment attempts, and they are reluctant to participate in psychological interventions. Therefore engaging patients with CBT is the first and sometimes most crucial task of the therapist. Expressing sympathy for patients' attempts to cope with the symptoms, empathy for seeking different treatments and the associated personal disappointments after these treatment attempts have failed are just a few techniques that should be used during the first sessions.

One additional task at the start of treatment is emphasising that the patient will be an active partner in the therapy, as this may be different from the patient's expectations and previous experience. Another important aspect is the development of a positive explanation for the symptoms. This will contrast with the rather negative statements that the patient would have heard repeatedly, that 'there is no organic disease responsible for the symptoms'.

Symptom diaries help to analyse the relationship between daily stressful events and symptom perception/symptom annoyance. These can temporarily lead to deterioration in symptoms because of increased body-focused attention, but this can be used to advantage as it establishes the link between body focusing and symptom experience. During the diagnostic period, the therapist should identify the key aspects that are relevant for treatment planning. These commonly include selective attention to bodily processes, attribution of bodily symptoms to physical illness, illness worrying and catastrophising, emotional reactions including comorbid depressive episodes, physical avoidance and help-seeking behaviour, social and communication aspects.

The process of change

In contrast to former formulations of CBT, the major task of the therapist is not a 'reattribution' of illness explanations, but an expansion of the explanations for physical symptoms. Patients should be encouraged during the whole process of therapy to detect further influences and determinants of symptom perception. Specific intervention tools of CBT are:

- *Relaxation, stress reduction.* The results of the symptom diary can be used to demonstrate the association between stressful events, feelings of distress and depressed mood, and symptom annoyance. Additionally, biofeedback techniques can be used to highlight this association and to demonstrate to the patient the close link between psychological well-being and physiological reactions [80]. After demonstrating the close link between stressful life events and bodily symptoms, relaxation techniques and techniques to reduce stress should be applied. Progressive relaxation is one potential strategy, but if more powerful stress reduction techniques are necessary, programmes such as the one described by Meichenaum and Deffenbacher should be used [81].
- *Modifying selective attention.* Many patients with multiple somatic symptoms focus their attention on bodily processes; this fact is the core of Barsky's model of somatosensory amplification [82]. Before trying to modify selective attention in CBT programmes, their negative role has to be demonstrated, e.g. by using *behavioural experiments* [83]. These behavioural experiments should demonstrate to the patient that focusing attention on bodily symptoms is a process relevant to symptom persistence. In this way patients are encouraged to change the focus of their attention from internal perceptions to the perception of external events. Modern approaches of CBT combine this period of treatment with acceptance and commitment techniques, and/or mindfulness techniques [84;85;86].
- *Changing functional beliefs and cognitions.* Symptom appraisal is necessary and general health beliefs which are not helpful in overcoming the bodily problems have to be identified. Many patients with bodily distress report an over-inclusive concept of 'being healthy' (i.e. not having any somatic symptoms at all). Other cognitions are highly specific (e.g. a headache is a typical sign of a brain tumour), but broader cognitive concepts are also relevant (e.g. a life with these symptoms is worthless). Typical cognitive techniques have been developed to reattribute these cognitions. One of them is the conversation technique of the 'Socratic dialogue' or guided detection. The major goal of these cognitive techniques is not to falsify the specific cognition of the patient,

but rather to encourage him or her to use multiple explanations for symptoms, to broaden the perspective and to reduce absolutism.

- *Increased physical activity, reducing avoidance behaviour.* Avoidance behaviour in bodily distress syndromes can be manifold. However a crucial aspect is the avoidance of physical activity, which has been shown to be a major predictor of symptom persistence [63;87]. In pain research, the avoidance of physical activity is considered as one of the 'yellow flags' indicating an unfavourable course of pain. Before trying to change the avoidance, behaviour therapists have to establish the motivational basis for it. This is usually done by demonstrating the difference between short- and long-term effects of avoidance behaviour. The typical short-term effect of reducing physical activity in somatisation syndrome is positive; this is the reason why the patient developed this behaviour pattern. The long-term consequences, however, are negative and symptoms may become chronic or even deteriorate. This distinction between short- and long-term effects is also necessary to explain the rationale of changing avoidance behaviour: the short-term effects of changing avoidance behaviour will be more negative (increasing aches and some pains), but the long-term effect can be considered to be positive (remission of symptoms). After establishing the motivational bases for change, a physical fitness programme can be planned and implemented. Patients with serious health anxiety show additional aspects of avoidance behaviour. 'Seeking reassurance' (e.g. from doctors and relatives) is very common in hypochondriasis. The more reassurance is provided from significant others, the less the patient is able to reassure himself or herself. Therefore, encouraging patients to reassure him or herself can be an additional major goal.

- *Additional tools.* As mentioned above, acceptance and commitment therapy and also mindfulness techniques can be implemented in CBT programmes. Modern approaches also emphasise the role of emotion regulation techniques, which include techniques to accept these emotions that have to be accepted, and developing abilities to modify those emotions that should be changed. Notably, in the highly successful programme of Allen and colleagues, additional emotion regulation techniques were implemented [88]. This programme also emphasised the role of significant others, and it suggested guidelines for helpful support from partners, instead of reinforcing less helpful illness behaviour [89;90]. Some authors also emphasise the need to improve communication skills in patients with somatisation syndrome [91]. After suffering long periods of somatic complaints, many people have changed their communication techniques, and use symptom complaining to regulate communication and to express personal needs. In these cases, it is necessary to re-establish adequate communication strategies. Finally, it has also been emphasised that many patients with multiple somatic symptoms need further support to detect the enjoyable parts of life [90]. Again this can be combined with mindfulness techniques.

General comments

CBT programmes have been developed both in individual settings and group format, and have been shown to be effective not only in developed countries but also in developing countries [92]. It should be borne in mind, however, that the effect sizes for the improvement of symptoms are typically in the medium range and do not reach the high effect sizes for CBT in anxiety disorders or depression. While some methodological aspects might partly contributes to this fact (e.g. the sensitivity of outcome measures), the medium effect sizes also indicate that there is still a need to improve the efficiency of psychological interventions in somatoform disorders. Further details of CBT in somatoform disorders can be found in several review articles [90;93;94].

An example of manualised CBT for severe bodily distress syndrome

This section describes Specialised Treatment for Severe Bodily Distress Syndromes (STreSS), a complex intervention based on a cognitive behavioural approach developed at The Research Clinic for Functional Disorders and Psychosomatics at Aarhus University Hospital in Denmark. It aims to provide an evidence-based guide to improved functioning and enhanced quality of life for patients with severe bodily distress. STreSS was designed to be delivered as a group treatment at a general hospital and targets patients with severe functional somatic syndromes (combined under the unifying diagnosis 'bodily distress syndrome, multiorgan type' – see Chapter 2).

Does the use of cognitive and behavioural strategies, as they are used in the STreSS intervention, indicate that bodily distress syndromes are mental disorders? Patients frequently ask this question, and the answer depends on the understanding of the term 'mental disorder'. It is important to explain to patients that bodily distress syndromes are *not* mental disorders in the sense that the bodily symptoms are 'all in the mind', 'not real' or 'the result of psychological problems' (see Appendix 8.1). Current knowledge suggests that bodily distress syndromes are diseases with a complex multifactorial aetiology. Nonetheless, patients with chronic bodily distress are often trapped in a vicious circle in which dysfunctional cognitions and behaviours worsen their symptoms and contribute to the maintenance of disability. Moreover, patients' health beliefs or illness perceptions are very strongly related to outcome. More importantly, however, cognitive and behavioural treatments have proven effective in various functional somatic syndromes (see Chapter 3). In other words, the techniques used in STreSS are based on firm evidence.

STreSS is not a self-help guide, and should only be provided by experienced psychiatrists with comprehensive knowledge and skills in the field of functional somatic syndromes and training in CBT, or by other skilled therapists in close collaboration with patients' primary care physicians.

Assessment

A thorough clinical assessment, aimed at excluding relevant physical diseases, initiating treatment for possible comorbid psychiatric disorders and enhancing patients' motivation to engage in a cognitive behavioural group treatment, is a basic prerequisite of STreSS (the clinical assessment is described in detail on pp. 183–185). STreSS may initially trigger or aggravate depression or anxiety, and all efforts should be made to prevent premature, patient-initiated termination of treatment. At the clinic, patients who get worse or who are at high risk for dropping out are offered individual consultations with their contact psychiatrist.

Intervention

The STreSS intervention consists of several elements, some of which are aimed at the patient's doctors and may indirectly influence patient care. At the outset, a letter is sent to patient's primary care physician with recommendations for management of the bodily distress syndrome. In addition, there is a telephone consultancy service for primary care physicians or specialists involved in the care of patients in the programme. We also have close cooperation with social authorities and patients' employers, when needed.

The treatment itself consists of nine modules, each lasting 3.5 hours as a group activity, with the group consisting of nine patients and two psychiatrists who have at least two years of training in CBT, experience with group treatment and expertise in the field of functional somatic syndromes. Each patient also receives two supplementary individual consultations with their contact psychiatrist in case new important physical symptoms or psychiatric problems occur. The psychiatrist does not prescribe drug treatment or make referrals to other specialists themselves, but can give advice to the patient's primary care doctor.

The treatment manual given to the patients includes educational material, a symptom diary, worksheets and homework assignment for the nine treatment modules [94]. Patients are given the relevant chapters at the beginning of each module. This is sent by post if patients do not attend the module. The details of the nine modules have been published in Danish (www.functionaldisorders.dk) and are available in English [94]. The introduction includes enhancing motivation to deal with painful and disabling bodily symptoms, and an introduction to CBT. Subsequent modules cover:

- the interpretation of bodily symptoms and challenging inflexible symptom attributions
- biopsychosocial factors involved in the development and maintenance of bodily distress and the impact of illness perceptions
- the connection between bodily symptoms and emotions, thoughts and behaviours; individual identification of perpetuating factors
- identification of cognitive distortions and enhancing emotional awareness
- recognising further the connection between life events and bodily stress, but aiming towards boosting pleasurable activities
- restoring normal sleep pattern, balanced diet and appropriate physical exercise;
- evaluating one's own social network and interpersonal relationships
- adapting lifestyle to improved functioning, developing problem-solving skills and an individual treatment plan for possible relapse.

Effect of the STreSS intervention

The efficacy of STreSS has been tested in a randomised controlled trial, and the results showed an immediate, clinically relevant effect on patients' self-reported physical health, bodily distress and illness worry [95]. This effect was sustained one year after the treatment was completed. However, before recommending STreSS to be implemented in routine clinical care, large multicentre trials are needed to explore the (cost-)effectiveness of STreSS or similar complex interventions.

Modifications of CBT for hypochondriasis (health anxiety)

In the largest trial of CBT for hypochondriasis, the CBT was administered individually in six 90-minute sessions at weekly intervals [78]. Each session was tightly scripted and a manual is available from the authors. The therapy covered the factors that cause patients to amplify somatic symptoms and misattribute them to serious disease: (i) attention focused on bodily symptoms – hypervigilance; (ii) beliefs about symptom aetiology; (iii) circumstances and context; (iv) illness and sick role behaviours; and (v) mood. Each session consisted of presentation of educational information about the symptom amplifiers, an illustrative exercise and a discussion to personalise the material presented.

In addition, it was considered necessary to coordinate patients' ongoing medical management with the CBT so a consultation letter is sent to each patient's primary care physician. A copy of this letter is also available from the authors [78]. It included five suggestions for medical management to augment the individual therapy: (i) aim medical management towards improved coping with somatic symptoms rather than trying to 'cure' the symptoms; (ii) schedule regular appointments with the physician rather than arranging appointments only when the patient is troubled by their complaints; (iii) provide only limited reassurance (see below); (iv) use a model of symptom amplification to explain the patient's symptoms; and (v) try to limit investigations and medical treatments within the bounds of appropriate medical practice.

Health anxiety: the need to change the doctor's response to patient worries

Doctors frequently reassure patients who express concern about their symptoms and their health. Patients who are anxious about their health keep asking for reassurance, but if this is always dealt with by reassurance from the doctor, they come to rely on this source of reassurance and seek it each time they become worried – hence frequent attendance at primary care clinics and increased likelihood of more investigations. This tends to leave the patient without skills to reassure themselves [70]. In the CBT model, it is necessary to try to break vicious cycles of cognitions leading to maladaptive behavioural responses (in this case: I am worried by a symptom therefore I must seek reassurance from the GP). It is difficult for doctors to change this behaviour but in the Dutch modified reattribution model it is recommended that GPs reassuring patients being treated for multiple somatic symptoms should shift to an alternative approach [70]. The suggested approaches are:

- The GP can challenge the patient to consider the most alarming thought or outcome about the symptom and then to consider how likely it is that this will come about. The patient should then be asked to come up with alternative, less alarming explanations for the symptom.
- If the patient persists in mentioning as a possible cause for the symptom a particular disease, for which there is a well-recognised diagnostic test, it is reasonable to negotiate with the patient that such a test be ordered, but make it clear that this is solely with the aim of enabling the patient to stop worrying. The doctor will predict that the result will be negative.
- If the patient avoids situations that might provoke illness/worry then gradual exposure to threatening thoughts may be used to diminish such worry. This is a well-recognised procedure used to treat other anxieties.

Symptom diary

Many of the treatments mentioned in this chapter include use of a symptom diary. This is a useful way of ensuring active participation of the patient in their treatment and, eventually, some degree of mastery of their symptoms. After the detailed assessment of the patient's complaints (see above), he or she is asked to keep a symptom diary. This usually has three columns to record: (i) severity of symptoms; (ii) activities; and (iii) thoughts, worries and feelings regarding the symptoms. The diary is discussed with the patient at each appointment.

The symptom diary enables the patient to realise firstly that symptoms vary considerably and most are not present much of the time. This in itself may be reassuring, as it is not the typical pattern of serious organic disease. Secondly, the patient becomes aware, gradually, of the situations or activities that are associated with symptoms getting worse or improving. Third, the cognitions that either precede or follow the symptoms can be identified. The former (e.g. thought of an ill relative or reminder of a stressful situation) can be regarded as triggers to symptom exacerbation. Cognitions which follow the symptoms (e.g. there is that pain again, it must be something serious) can be seen as unhelpful cognitive responses. Lastly, the symptom diary may enable the patient to realise the importance of psychosocial precipitants of the symptom experience, rather than always believing symptoms are caused by medical illness.

Psychodynamic interpersonal therapy

This section describes psychodynamic interpersonal therapy as it has been used in severe irritable bowel syndrome because the model has been fully developed in relation to this condition. The therapy can be used for other bodily distress syndromes and has recently been tested in somatoform disorders.

The therapy developed by Hobson has been adapted to treat patients who present with numerous somatic symptoms [96;97;98]. Key features of the model include: (i) the assumption that the patient's problems arise from, or are exacerbated by disturbances of significant personal relationships; (ii) a tentative, encouraging, supportive approach on behalf of the therapist, who seeks to develop deeper understanding with the patient through negotiation, exploration of feelings and metaphor; (iii) the linkage of the patient's distress to specific interpersonal problems; and (iv) the use of the therapeutic and transference relationship to address problems and test out solutions in the 'here and now'.

The therapy was developed in the context of a randomised controlled trial in which the cost-effectiveness of psychotherapy and antidepressant treatment for severe irritable bowel syndrome was demonstrated [99]. Patients entered the study if they had severe irritable bowel syndrome which had not responded to usual treatment and for which the gastroenterologists could offer no further specific treatment. Thus the patients had sought help with a medical problem; they were not seeking psychotherapy. None had been assessed for their suitability for psychotherapy. The therapy had, therefore, to be accessible to a broad range of patients. In the study, the therapy consisted of one long initial session and seven further sessions over a 12-week period. The long first session lasted approximately three hours and focused on the patient's symptoms, the physical sensations involved, their impact on the patient's life and the context in which they occurred. In developing the conversation, the therapist tried to obtain a detailed picture of the patient's suffering, taking note of the words, phrases and expressions used by the patient to describe his/her symptoms.

Key aspects of the model helped to facilitate this process. These included a particular regard for cue-based responses, development of physical body metaphors and a negotiating, tentative style. The intention was to move seamlessly from a focus on physical problems to a conversation that included an emotional or interpersonal/dynamic dimension. A full interpersonal history was also taken during this session, and patients were invited to reflect on illnesses and medical interventions in the course of their life, and the lives of those close to them. Towards the end of this long first session, the therapist tentatively presented a verbal formulation, reflecting on the key emotional events in the patient's life, the possible emotional significance of the patient's symptoms, and the connection between symptoms and problems in interpersonal relationships. The aim was to develop a shared understanding, so that one or two specific problem areas in the patient's life could be addressed over the course of the therapy.

The remaining seven sessions, each of 45 minutes' duration, focused on the issues raised in the first long first session. Towards the end of therapy, usually in the fifth session, the therapist, in referring to the forthcoming end of therapy, told each patient that she would be writing them a personal farewell letter that would aim to tell the story of their therapy. She explained that this would be something for them to keep when therapy was over, to draw the work of the therapy together, to remind them of what had happened as therapy started to recede into the past, and to help them carry forward the work that was begun together in therapy. The sixth session focused specifically on the important goodbyes the person had experienced in their life. These were linked to his or her feelings about the end of therapy, with an emphasis on the importance of not denying the emotional impact that loss entails, while at the same time looking at what the person would be able to hold onto and take away with them from the therapy.

The farewell letter referred to the patient's symptoms as he or she had described them in the initial session. It then gave a summary of the history of emotional events in the patient's life, highlighting the way in which the situation at the time had dictated how the patient dealt with painful emotions, and how this pattern had continued in subsequent relationships and situations. The formulation discussed at the end of the first session, which included the link between emotional functioning and bowel symptoms was restated in writing. The progress that the patient had made in changing these patterns was then set out, with some indication of what the patient would need to continue working on after therapy had ended. The draft letter was read aloud to the patient and discussed in detail so the patient felt they had ownership of the content of the letter.

The rationale for using a farewell letter in psychodynamic interpersonal therapy with patients with bodily distress disorder is based on three assumptions. First, the therapy is more active than traditional interpretative models in that patients are encouraged from the beginning to collaborate fully in the work. This includes completing bowel questionnaires and diaries, actively testing out new solutions to interpersonal difficulties, and making practical changes to their lives. Second, a key part of the therapeutic process is the exploration of the patient's physical symptoms, with a view to discovering connections with important emotional and interpersonal issues. This is reiterated and reinforced in the farewell letter. Third, the therapy is very brief, and not all work can be completed within the allotted time. A farewell letter may help the patient to continue working on their problems after the therapy has finished.

A case vignette illustrates the therapy with one patient.

Vignette

A 36-year-old female patient had irritable bowel syndrome. She suffered abdominal pain, nausea, diarrhoea and constipation, bloating and constant tiredness, none of which were helped by antispasmodics or other medication for irritable bowel syndrome. Her symptoms had started at the age of 11 when her father began to sexually abuse her. She described a harsh and loveless childhood, during which she had been afraid to tell anyone of the abuse, not even her grandmother, with whom she had a good relationship. After a brief first marriage, in which she was again abused, she met her present husband, eight years before starting therapy. There were sexual difficulties in the marriage, for which the patient blamed herself.

Around that time, fearing for the safety of the young children in the family, she reported the incest, and her father was imprisoned. The patient was ostracised by the rest of the family, and when her grandmother died soon afterwards, she was devastated, feeling that her disclosure had contributed to her grandmother's death. At the end of the first session, the therapist offered the formulation that her bowel symptoms, starting at the time of the abuse, may be a physical expression of all the pain she had been unable to express; the pain of the abuse, of feeling worthless and unvalued, of the self-blame, of the loss of her grandmother. Through it all she had tried to be strong and carry on coping. The therapist suggested that her symptoms were an expression of the vulnerable hurt self inside, which she could not escape from, no matter how hard she tried.

During the early part of therapy the patient was flooded with terrifying and painful memories of the abuse and humiliation she had suffered from both parents. She wrote down her thoughts and brought them for the therapist to read. The therapist's continued acceptance of her, after reading and discussing the incidents about which she felt so ashamed, was a key factor in her own self-acceptance and a belief that others could accept her. In this way, the only good relationship in her childhood (with her grandmother) was re-enacted in the therapeutic relationship. Initially her symptoms got worse, as her fear of being rejected by the therapist intensified. As she faced and overcame these anxieties, however, her symptoms started to improve, and by the end of therapy had all but disappeared. She became more confident, assertive and detached from her parents. She was able to express her feelings of loss and anxiety about the end of therapy, while being determined to take forward the issues she was tackling. The farewell letter restated the formulation, acknowledged the courage the patient had shown in dealing with painful memories and commented on how she had moved forward emotionally. It encouraged her to prioritise her own needs appropriately and to communicate more fully with her husband.

Psychopharmacotherapy

A wide variety of drugs are used for patients with bodily distress, principally in patients who have a functional somatic syndrome. For example, pharmacological management of fibromyalgia includes tramadol and other analgesics, antidepressants (such as amitriptyline, fluoxetine, duloxetine, milnacipran, moclobemide) and other drugs including pirlindole, tropisetron, pramipexole, pregabalin and cyclobenzaprine [73;100]. The pharmacological treatments for irritable bowel syndrome include antispasmodics, laxatives, antimotility and antidepressant drugs. Only antidepressants will be discussed in this section. Further information, including the use of other drugs, can be found in the relevant publications concerning fibromyalgia [73;100;101], irritable bowel syndrome [71;77;102;103], somatisation [100;104] and chronic pain [105;106]. For an algorithm for the pharmacological treatment of bodily distress disorder, see Lydiard [100].

The role of drugs in bodily distress disorders has not been fully evaluated and has, therefore, not been discussed widely in the relevant texts [107]. Although there is reasonable evidence of their efficacy in the short term [108;109;110;111], bodily distress disorders are often chronic and respond best to active treatment methods [58;112]. There is very little information about the long-term use of antidepressants for bodily distress disorders. Furthermore, the mode of action of antidepressants in these disorders is not clear. The systematic reviews described in Chapter 3 generally concluded that the beneficial effects of these drugs was independent of change in level of psychological distress. In addition to the well recognised analgesic effect, serotonin selective reuptake inhibitors (SSRIs) may have beneficial, possibly cognitive, effects and it has been suggested that antidepressants have an anti-stress action through their effect on corticotrophin-releasing factor [100;113]. On the other hand, an advantage of antidepressants over psychological treatment is that they can be prescribed in a medical clinic without referral to a mental-health professional.

A further complication of antidepressants is the fact that patients with bodily distress disorders tend to react strongly to side effects and often stop the drug at the first sign of one. Since patients with bodily distress experience worrying somatic symptoms, additional somatic symptoms as side effects of drugs inevitably make them worry about the additional new symptoms. This can cause difficulties in the patient–doctor relationship as some patients can be resentful that they were persuaded to take drugs that went on to produce new somatic symptoms. Therefore, antidepressants should only be used when there is a clear indication and there are specified potential benefits that can be monitored.

There are several reasons for considering antidepressants drugs in patients with bodily distress disorders. These include their use as:

- an analgesic
- an antidepressant for concurrent depressive or related disorder
- a non-specific agent to reduce somatic symptoms
- an aid to commencing exercise or other active treatment.

The drug may be used alone, and low-dose antidepressants are often used in this way for chronic painful conditions. In bodily distress disorders, however, it is preferable to use antidepressants as only part of a treatment programme. If the antidepressant allows the patient to feel better and this leads to better compliance with an exercise programme, for example, it may be possible to reduce or stop the antidepressant once the beneficial effects of the exercise programme are evident. Antidepressants appear to have greater effect on pain than exercise programmes do, but the reverse is true for fatigue, so initial treatment with an antidepressant may be useful to enable a patient to commence an exercise programme.

One of the key features of using antidepressants for patients with bodily distress disorders is a full and open discussion with the patient about why the drug is being prescribed, the expected benefits and the importance of continuing the drug, provided side effects are not intolerable. If the doctor does not explain that the drug is an antidepressant, if the patient discovers later that this is the case, they may be annoyed that the doctor has not been fully open and honest. If the drug is being prescribed as a short-term analgesic, this should be made clear. If the intention is to increase the dose to an effective one for depressive disorder, the reasons for this course of action should be explained fully. Crucially, however, it is necessary to understand the patient's attitude towards taking medication prior to prescription. If the patient is not at all keen to take an antidepressant, this view should be respected; and it paves the way for early commencement of psychological treatment, which might be the preferred treatment in the longer run. Harris and Roberts found that, although many people with functional somatic syndromes dislike the idea of taking drugs in the long term, most people with irritable bowel syndrome said they will accept tablets if recommended by the doctor [114].

Where possible, it is preferable to assess the severity of pain, other somatic symptoms and depression before and during treatment to assess progress [115]. Depression, for example, can be assessed using HADS, which does not include somatic symptoms [27;100;116]. A high score is useful in explaining to the patient that they have depressive symptoms and repeated administration of this questionnaire will be a good way of monitoring this aspect of treatment. Similarly, repeated assessment of the number of somatic symptoms (e.g. using PHQ-15) is helpful; it appears that during treatment of depressed patients with somatic symptoms, an immediate improvement in somatic symptoms precedes improvement in depression but the former reaches a plateau after one month whereas depression continues to improve over nine months [117]. Assessment of pain severity and coping with pain (e.g. using the Coping Strategies Questionnaire, which includes a measure of pain catastrophising) is very helpful in monitoring progress of treatment [118;119]. A complete series of assessments would also include a measure of health status (e.g. Medical Outcome Survey Short Form 36 (SF-36)), as improvement of somatic symptoms may be accompanied by improvement in the dimensions of physical function, whereas improved depression is accompanied by improvement in social functioning [99;117]. An assessment battery of this nature has not been common in many psychological therapies but it is important because a patient's global impression cannot reflect accurately all of these different dimensions, each of which may be important within the treatment plan. The choice of assessment(s) should be made according to the patient's particular needs and symptom profile.

The treatment of pain in somatoform disorders is very important [106]. A recent review has suggested the following stepped-care approach to the treatment of pain [105]:

(1) simple analgesics (acetaminophen or nonsteroidal anti-inflammatory drugs (NSAIDs))
(2) tricyclic antidepressants (if neuropathic, back or fibromyalgia pain) or tramadol
(3) gabapentin, duloxetine or pregabalin if neuropathic pain
(4) cyclobenzaprine, pregabalin, duloxetine, or milnacipran for fibromyalgia
(5) topical analgesics (capsaicin, lidocaine, salicylates) if localised neuropathic or arthritic pain
(6) opioids.

The analgesic properties of the tricyclic antidepressants are well recognised as can be seen from the fact that they are recommended as first-line drugs in neuropathic pain [120]. The serotonin–norepinephrine reuptake inhibitors (SNRIs) duloxetine and venlafaxine are also recommended for this condition. In view of the risk of side effects, low starting doses are recommended [100;120]. Interaction with other drugs for concurrent medical conditions and adverse effects on the heart and other organs needs to be considered carefully in those patients who have such conditions [107]. There is some evidence of short-term benefit in bodily listress syndromes with St John's wort or opipramol, but this evidence relates only to patients who do not have concurrent psychiatric disorders including depression [121;122].

Venlafaxine was not superior to placebo in patients with depression and multisomatoform disorder, although it did help relieve pain [123]. Antidepressants have generally been found to be effective in reducing back pain severity, but not in improving functional status; CBT may achieve better results [108]. Tricyclic antidepressants are effective for headache, but SSRIs are not effective for migraine headaches and not as effective as tricyclic antidepressants for tension headaches [124]. Since CBT, relaxation therapy and biofeedback are beneficial for migraine and tension headaches, these are preferred [125].

Antidepressant treatment of hypochondriasis and body dysmorphic disorder

The SSRI antidepressants paroxetine and fluoxetine at a dose of 40–50 mg daily are moderately effective treatments for hypochondriasis over three to four months [126;127]. One of these trials suggested that paroxetine is virtually as effective as CBT and appears to be tolerated just as well [127]. Patients need to be warned about the side effects of sexual dysfunction, fatigue and perspiration with paroxetine. At least part of the improvement is independent of reduction of anxiety or depressive symptoms so, if these symptoms remain, it is appropriate to try increasing the dose if this is tolerated. One of the few long-term trials showed that the improvement gained over the initial treatment period can be expected to persist up to 18 months, though this requires continuation of the antidepressant or additional psychological treatment [128]. There is some evidence that fluoxetine and clomipramine are beneficial for body dysmorphic disorder, but the evidence base is limited [129].

Functional somatic syndromes

In a recent systematic review of antidepressants in fibromyalgia, the results of which are likely to be relevant for other bodily distress disorders, pain reduction was most successfully treated with tricyclic antidepressants followed by monoamine oxidase inhibitors, and least successfully with SSRIs and SNRIs [101]. Since depression and pain so often occur together, the treatment of depression is important [115]. Tricyclics at full dose can lead to troublesome side effects in this population, therefore one of the other antidepressant drugs may be preferable. Duloxetine has been shown to be superior to milnacipran and pregabalin in improving depressed mood in fibromyalgia; however, patients should be warned that headache, nausea and diarrhoea are side effects of duloxetine [130]. There is only weak evidence that depressed patients with somatic symptoms who have not responded to an SSRI may improve when switched to duloxetine [131].

Psychopharmacotherapy is considered as an alternative to CBT for moderate irritable bowel syndrome [102;103]. A low dose of antidepressant (tricyclic, SSRI or SNRI) can be tried for four to six weeks and the dose increased if necessary. The advantage of pharmacotherapy over psychological treatment is that it can be administered in the gastroenterology clinic without referral to a mental-health professional. It is possible to increase the dose of the antidepressant, provided side effects do not interfere with treatment. If there is no response, the patient should be referred to a mental-health professional, either for a psychological treatment alone or, if necessary, psychological treatment in combination with an antidepressant. Further details are provided in the relevant publications [102;103]. In severe irritable bowel syndrome, treatment with paroxetine is as effective as psychodynamic interpersonal therapy, both in the short and long term, in terms of health status [99]. This beneficial effect of the paroxetine cannot be explained in terms of reduction of depression or pain.

Current guidelines indicate that antidepressants are used as a second line of treatment in irritable bowel syndrome if laxatives, loperamide and antispasmodics have not been helpful [71;77]. CBT administered in primary care together with mebeverine helps the symptoms in the short term, and helps work and social adjustments in the long term [132].

In fibromyalgia, tricyclic antidepressants are one of the recommended first-line treatments; the others are aerobic exercise, CBT and multicomponent treatment [133]. There is some doubt about the efficacy of antidepressants in fibromyalgia beyond 12 weeks [73].

There is no convincing research evidence to suggest that pharmacological interventions are useful in directly helping chronic fatigue syndrome [64]. Low dose tricyclic and related antidepressants, may be useful for both pain and insomnia [64]. SSRIs may help comorbid anxiety or depression. Duloxetine and pregabalin are efficacious central pain modulators in patients with associated fibromyalgia [74;134].

Multicomponent treatment

Since there is evidence that psychological treatments and antidepressants can benefit patients independent of reduction of psychological distress, it is logical to use combined treatment for people with bodily distress syndromes that do not respond to either alone. This policy has been recommended for severe irritable bowel syndrome, but the evidence base for this is extremely limited [102]. More intensive treatment may be required for the very severe bodily distress syndromes which may be accompanied by personality disorders and/or a history of childhood abuse. Specialist psychiatric treatment is usually required for these conditions; the refractory somatic symptoms may be only part of a wider set of psychiatric symptoms.

In Germany, the term 'multimodal treatment' refers to the different forms of therapy received by patients in inpatient units. CBT or psychodynamic interpersonal psychotherapy is accompanied by stress management, biofeedback, graded activation, physiotherapy, body psychotherapy and usual somatic diagnostics and therapy, where indicated. This integration of body-oriented therapies makes it easier for patients to accept psychotherapeutic elements; it is particularly suited to the subgroup of patients with severe disabilities. The therapy has been described and evaluated in the German literature but there are very few randomised controlled trials [135;136;137;138].

Conclusion

This chapter has provided an overview of the assessment and treatment of individual patients with bodily distress syndromes. The first important message concerns matching intensity of treatment with severity of the bodily distress syndrome. This is important as bodily distress syndromes are so numerous; it is pointless providing treatment for a condition which will spontaneously resolve. On the other hand, inadequate treatment will not be helpful if more intense treatment is required. There is evidence that this is often the case. The second message concerns the availability of more intensive, specialist treatment. In many centres this is simply not available. The individual treatments described briefly in this chapter should be used more widely by doctors of all specialties. Prior to such treatments, the assessment of the overall clinical picture and the explanation to the patient is paramount. This requires skills that need to be learned by all doctors.

Appendix 8.1

Part of the document text given to patients about bodily distress syndrome at the Research Clinic for Functional Disorders, Aarhus, Denmark.

About bodily distress syndrome

Bodily distress syndrome is a new diagnosis used for research purposes, so you probably have not heard about the illness before. Individuals with bodily distress syndrome (hereafter BDS) experience daily bothersome physical symptoms. Typical symptoms are headache, pains in the back, muscles or joints, stomach trouble, breathlessness, excessive fatigue and many more. In some individuals, the distressing symptoms are so pronounced that they cannot go to work. Even normal daily chores such as shopping, doing the dishes or vacuuming can become impossible because of the symptoms.

Many patients with BDS have gone through numerous examinations by their GPs, by specialists, or at hospitals without the doctors finding a good explanation for their symptoms. Unfortunately, some patients feel that they have been misunderstood and that some doctors become less sympathetic when they notice that no signs of well-known disease have been found. Some patients report having been told that they are not 'genuinely' ill, that the symptoms are imaginary, or that it is a 'mental' problem. Most patients find this extremely distressing. Some patients with BDS have received diagnoses such as fibromyalgia, whiplash-associated disorder, irritable bowel syndrome, chronic pain disorder or others. Today, we regard these all as subtypes of BDS.

We emphasise that BDS is a genuine disorder and that the symptoms are not imaginary.

How is BDS diagnosed?

Based on an interview and your medical records, a doctor at our department assesses your symptoms. The doctor decides the severity of the symptoms and whether your symptoms could be due to other disease, for instance if pains in the joints are better explained by arthritis or if breathlessness can be explained by asthma. If the symptoms are better explained by another disease, it is not considered part of BDS. The diagnosis is thus only made on the basis of the symptoms, their severity and duration. Presently, no examinations such as blood tests or a scan can determine if an individual has BDS.

What are the causes of BDS?

Unfortunately, our knowledge about BDS is limited, and it will probably take some time before we fully understand the disorder. We know that the cause of the disorder is very complex and that several factors are involved in the onset of BDS. There are five known factors that influence BDS: (i) the brain; (ii) heredity; (iii) other disease/injury; (iv) illness worries; and (v) longstanding stress or strain.

The brain

We know that part of the explanation can be found in the brain – and thus not in the body, although that is where the symptoms are felt. Research has shown that other parts of the brain for registering pain are involved in patients with BDS compared with healthy individuals. Also, there are demonstrable biological changes in the brain.

Long-standing stress and strain

We know that exposure to long-standing stress and strain increases the risk of getting BDS. This is particularly true of stresses in childhood, but also strains in adulthood. Many people with BDS have for years exceeded the limits of what they are capable of. If you exceed your limits over a long period of time, you can react with stress, which can trigger BDS.

How do we treat BDS?

BDS is treatable. It is possible to rehabilitate the body, to learn to be less worried about your symptoms, and learn strategies to cope with stress and strain. At the same time, medical treatment can change the symptom experience in the brain so that the symptoms are less bothersome. Some of our patients get completely well, others experience that their symptoms are relieved and that they get more energy. You can discuss with your doctor which kind of treatment is the best for you.

References

1. Barsky AJ, Orav EJ, Bates DW. Somatization increases medical utilization and costs independent of psychiatric and medical comorbidity. *Archives of General Psychiatry* 2005; **62**(8): 903–10.

2. Kroenke K, Spitzer RL, Williams JB. The PHQ-15: validity of a new measure for evaluating the severity of somatic symptoms. *Psychosomatic Medicine* 2002; **64**(2): 258–66.

3. Harris AM, Orav EJ, Bates DW, Barsky AJ. Somatization increases disability independent of comorbidity. *Journal of General Internal Medicine* 2009; **24**(2): 155–61.

4. Toft T, Rosendal M, Ornbol E, Olesen F, Frostholm L, Fink P. Training general practitioners in the treatment of functional somatic symptoms: Effects on patient health in a cluster-randomised controlled trial (the functional illness in primary care study). *Psychotherapy and Psychosomatics* 2010; **79**(4): 227–37.

5. Drossman DA. *Rome III The Functional Gastrointestinal Disorders*, 3rd edn. McLean, VA: Degnon Associates; 2006.

6. Fukuda K, Straus SE, Hickie I, Sharpe MC, Dobbins JG, Komaroff A *et al.* The chronic fatigue syndrome – a comprehensive approach to its definition and study. *Annals of Internal Medicine* 1994; **121**(12): 953–9.

7. Wolfe F, Smythe HA, Yunus MB, Bennett RM, Bombardier C, Goldenberg DL *et al.* The American College of Rheumatology 1990 criteria for the classification of fibromyalgia. Report of the multicenter criteria committee. *Arthritis and Rheumatism* 1990; **33**(2): 160–72.

8. Multidisciplinary Guideline Working Group. Multidisciplinairy Guideline for MUS and Somatoform Disorder. Netherlands: CBO/Trimbos Instituut; 2011.

9. Engel GL. The clinical application of the biopsychosocial model. *American Journal of Psychiatry* 1980; **137**: 535–44.

10. van der Feltz-Cornelis CM, Hoedeman R, de Jong FJ, Meeuwissen JA, Drewes HW, van der Laan NC *et al.* Faster return to work after psychiatric consultation for sicklisted employees with common mental disorders compared to care as usual. A randomized clinical trial. *Journal of Neuropsychiatric Disease and Treatment* 2010; **6**: 375–85.

11. Huijbregts KML, van der Feltz-Cornelis C, van Marwijk HWJ, de Jong FJ, van der Windt DAWM, Beekman ATF. Negative association of concomitant physical symptoms with the course of major depressive disorder: a systematic review. *Journal of Psychosomatic Research* 2010; **68**(6): 511–19.

12. Huijbregts KML, van Marwijk HWJ, de Jong FJ, Schreuders B, Beekman ATF, van der Feltz-Cornelis CM. Adverse effects of multiple physical symptoms on the course of depressive and anxiety symptoms in primary care. *Psychotherapy and Psychosomatics* 2010; **79**(6): 389–91.

13. van der Feltz-Cornelis CM, van Oppen P, Adèr HJ, van Dyck R. Randomised controlled trial of a collaborative care model with psychiatric consultation for persistent medically unexplained symptoms in general practice. *Psychotherapy and Psychosomatics* 2006; **75**(5): 282–9.

14. van der Feltz-Cornelis CM. [Unexplained or undiagnosed? To a DSM-V for somatoform disorder. Comment on van Dieren & Vingerhoets.] (article in Dutch) *Tijdschrift voor Psychiatrie* 1997; **49**(11): 839–43.

15. Sha MC, Callahan CM, Counsell SR, Westmoreland GR, Stump TE, Kroenke K. Physical symptoms as a predictor of health care use and mortality among older adults. *American Journal of Medicine* 2005; **118**(3): 301–6.

16. Kroenke K, Zhong X, Theobald D, Wu JW, Tu WZ, Carpenter JS. Somatic symptoms in patients with cancer experiencing pain or depression prevalence, disability, and health care use. *Archives of Internal Medicine* 2010; 170(18): 1686–94.

17. Salmon P, Peters S, Stanley I. Patients' perceptions of medical explanations for somatisation disorders: qualitative analysis. *British Medical Journal* 1999; 318(7180): 372–6.

18. Jackson JL, Passamonti M. The outcomes among patients presenting in primary care with a physical symptom at 5 years. *Journal of General Internal Medicine* 2005; 20(11): 1032–7.

19. Hatcher S, Arroll B. Assessment and management of medically unexplained symptoms. *British Medical Journal* 2008; 336(7653): 1124–8.

20. Fink P, Rosendal M, Toft T. Assessment and treatment of functional disorders in general practice: the extended reattribution and management model – an advanced educational program for nonpsychiatric doctors. *Psychosomatics* 2002; 43(2): 93–131.

21. Bass C, Murphy M. Somatisation, somatoform disorders and factitious illness. In: Guthrie E, Creed F (eds). *Seminars in Liaison Psychiatry*. London: Royal College of Psychiatrists; 1996: 103–56.

22. Bass C, Benjamin S. The management of chronic somatisation. *British Journal of Psychiatry* 1993; 162: 472–80.

23. House A. The patient with medically unexplained symptoms: making the initial psychiatric contact. In: Mayou R, Bass C, Sharpe M (eds). *The Treatment of Functional Somatic Symptoms*. Oxford: Oxford University Press; 1995: 89–102.

24. Morriss R, Dowrick C, Salmon P, Peters S, Rogers A, Dunn G et al. Turning theory into practice: rationale, feasibility and external validity of an exploratory randomized controlled trial of training family practitioners in reattribution to manage patients with medically unexplained symptoms (the MUST). *General Hospital Psychiatry* 2006; 28(4): 343–51.

25. Brugha T, Bebbington P, Tennant C, Hurry J. The list of threatening experiences: a subset of 12 life event categories with considerable long-term contextual threat. *Psychological Medicine* 1985; 15(1): 189–94.

26. Derogatis LR, Lipman RS, Rickels K, Uhlenhuth EH, Covi L. The Hopkins Symptom Checklist (HSCL): a self-report symptom inventory. *Behavioral Science* 1974; 19(1): 1–15.

27. Zigmond AS, Snaith RP. The hospital anxiety and depression scale. *Acta Psychiatrica Scandinavica* 1983; 67: 361–70.

28. Kroenke K, Spitzer RL, Williams JB. The PHQ-9: validity of a brief depression severity measure. *Journal of General Internal Medicine* 2001; 16(9): 606–13.

29. Spitzer RL, Kroenke K, Williams JBW, Lowe B. A brief measure for assessing generalized anxiety disorder – the GAD-7. *Archives of Internal Medicine* 2006; 166: 1092–7.

30. Fink P, Ewald H, Jensen J, Sørensen L, Engberg M, Holm M, Munk- Jørgensen P. Screening for somatization and hypochondriasis in primary care and neurological in-patients: a seven-item scale for hypochondriasis and somatization. *Journal of Psychosomatic Research* 1999; 46(3): 261–73.

31. Lucock MP, Morley S. The health anxiety questionnaire. *British Journal of Health Psychology* 1996; 1: 137–50.

32. Ware JE Jr, Sherbourne CD. The MOS 36-item short-form health survey (SF-36). I. Conceptual framework and item selection. *Medical Care* 1992; 30(6): 473–83.

33. Moss-Morris R, Weinman J, Petrie KJ, Horne R, Cameron LD, Buick D. The revised Illness Perception Questionnaire (IPQ-R). *Psychology and Health* 2002; 17(1): 1–16.

34. Broadbent E, Petrie KJ, Main J, Weinman J, Broadbent E, Petrie KJ et al. The brief illness perception questionnaire. *Journal of Psychosomatic Research* 2006; 60(6): 631–7.

35. Bridges KW, Goldberg DP. Psychiatric illness in inpatients with neurological disorders – patients views on discussion of emotional problems with

neurologists. *British Medical Journal* 1984; **289**(6446): 656–8.

36. Katon W, Lin EHB, Kroenke K. The association of depression and anxiety with medical symptom burden in patients with chronic medical illness. *General Hospital Psychiatry* 2007; **29**(2): 147–55.

37. Creed F, Guthrie E. Techniques for interviewing the somatising patient. *British Journal of Psychiatry* 1993; **162**: 467–71.

38. Guthrie E, Creed FH. Basic skills. In: Guthrie E, Creed FH (eds). *Seminars in Liaison Psychiatry*. London: Royal College of Psychiatrists; 1996: 21–52.

39. World Health Organization, Division of Mental Health. *Schedules for Clinical Assessment in Neuropsychiatry*. Geneva: World Health Organization; 1994.

40. Huibers MJ, Wessely S. The act of diagnosis: pros and cons of labelling chronic fatigue syndrome. *Psychological Medicine* 2006; **36**(7): 895–900.

41. Wolfe F. Fibromyalgia wars. *Journal of Rheumatology* 2009; **36**(4): 671–8.

42. Feinstein AR. The Blame-X syndrome: problems and lessons in nosology, spectrum, and etiology. *Journal of Clinical Epidemiology* 2001; **54**(5): 433–9.

43. Rief W, Heitmüller AM, Reisberg K, Rüddel H. Why reassurance fails in patients with unexplained symptoms – an experimental investigation of remembered probabilities. *PLoS Medicine* 2006; **3**(8): e269.

44. Jackson JL, Kroenke K. Managing somatization: medically unexplained should not mean medically ignored. *Journal of General Internal Medicine* 2006; **21**(7): 797–9.

45. Dowrick CF, Ring A, Humphris GM, Salmon P. Normalisation of unexplained symptoms by general practitioners: a functional typology. *British Journal of General Practice* 2004; **54**(500): 165–70.

46. Hamilton WT, Gallagher AM, Thomas JM, White PD. The prognosis of different fatigue diagnostic labels: a longitudinal survey. *Journal of Family Practice* 2005; **22**(4): 383–8.

47. Woodward RV, Broom DH, Legge DG. Diagnosis in chronic illness: disabling or enabling – the case of chronic fatigue syndrome. *Journal of the Royal Society of Medicine* 1995; **88**(6): 325–9.

48. Salmon P. Conflict, collusion or collaboration in consultations about medically unexplained symptoms: the need for a curriculum of medical explanation. *Patient Education and Counseling* 2007; **67**(3): 246–54.

49. Salmon P, Wissow L, Carroll J, Ring A, Humphris GM, Davies JC et al. Doctors' responses to patients with medically unexplained symptoms who seek emotional support: criticism or confrontation? *General Hospital Psychiatry* 2007; **29**(5): 454–60.

50. Fink P, Schröder A. One single diagnosis, bodily distress syndrome, succeeded to capture 10 diagnostic categories of functional somatic syndromes and somatoform disorders. *Journal of Psychosomatic Research* 2010; **68**(5): 415–26.

51. Fink P, Toft T, Hansen MS, Ornbol E, Olesen F. Symptoms and syndromes of bodily distress: an exploratory study of 978 internal medical, neurological, and primary care patients. *Psychosomatic Medicine* 2007; **69**(1): 30–9.

52. Kingham JGC, Dawson AM. Origin of chronic right upper quadrant pain. *Gut* 1985; **26**: 783–8.

53. Weinstein MC, Berwick DM, Goldman PA, Murphy JM, Barsky AJ. A comparison of three psychiatric screening tests using receiver operating characteristic (ROC) analysis. *Medical Care* 1989; **27**(6): 593–607.

54. Derogatis LR. *SCL-90-R: Administration, Scoring, and Procedures Manual II – For the R(evised) Version*, 1st edn. Towson: Clinical Psychometric Research; 1983.

55. Smith RG. Treatment of patients with multiple symptoms. In: Mayou R, Bass C, Sharpe M (eds). *Treatment of Functional Somatic Symptoms*. Oxford: Oxford University Press; 1995: 175–87.

56. Adler RH. Engel's biopsychosocial model is still relevant today. *Journal of Psychosomatic Research* 2009; **67**(6): 607–11.

57. van der Feltz-Cornelis CM, Wijkel D, Verhaak PFM, Collijn DH, Huyse FJ, van Dyck R. Psychiatric consultation for somatizing patients in the family practice setting: a feasibility study. *International Journal of Psychiatry in Medicine* 1996; **26**(2): 223–39.

58. Henningsen P, Zipfel S, Herzog W. Management of functional somatic syndromes. *The Lancet* 2007; **369**(9565): 946–55.

59. Creed FH. Somatisation and pain syndromes. In: Mayer EA, Bushnell MC (eds). *Functional Pain Syndromes: Presentation and Pathophysiology.* Seattle, WA: IASP; 2009: 227–44.

60. Aiarzaguena JM, Grandes G, Gaminde I, Salazar A, Sanchez A, Arino J. A randomized controlled clinical trial of a psychosocial and communication intervention carried out by GPs for patients with medically unexplained symptoms. *Psychological Medicine* 2007; **37**(2): 283–94.

61. Thomas KB. General-practice consultations – is there any point in being positive. *British Medical Journal* 1987; **294**(6581): 1200–2.

62. Barsky AJ, Ettner SL, Horsky J, Bates DW. Resource utilization of patients with hypochondriacal health anxiety and somatization. *Medical Care* 2001; **39**(7): 705–15.

63. Rief W, Mewes R, Martin A, Glaesmer H, Braehler E. Are psychological features useful in classifying patients with somatic symptoms? *Psychosomatic Medicine* 2010; **72**(7): 648–55.

64. National Institute for Health and Clinical Excellence. *Chronic fatigues syndrome/ Myalgic encephalomyelitis: diagnosis and management of CFS/ME in adults and children.* London: NICE; 2007.

65. Fulcher KY, White PD. Chronic fatigue syndrome: a description of graded exercise treatment. *Physiotherapy* 1998; **84**: 223–6.

66. Edmonds M, McGuire H, Price J. Exercise therapy for chronic fatigue syndrome. *Cochrane Database of Systematic Reviews* 2004; **3**: CD003200.

67. Wearden AJ, Dowrick C, Chew-Graham C, Bentall RP, Morriss RK, Peters S *et al.* Nurse-led, home-based self-help treatment for patients in primary care with chronic fatigue syndrome: randomised controlled trial. *British Medical Journal* 2010; **340**: c1777.

68. Pesek JR, Jason LA. An empirical investigation of the envelope theory. *Journal of Human Behavior in the Social Environment* 2000; **3**(59): 77.

69. Brown RJ. Introduction to the special issue on medically unexplained symptoms: background and future directions. *Clinical Psychology Review* 2007; **27**: 769–80.

70. Blankenstein AH, van der Horst HE, Schilte AF, de Vries D, Zaat JO, Andre KJ *et al.* Development and feasibility of a modified reattribution model for somatising patients, applied by their own general practitioners. *Patient Education and Counseling* 2002; **47**(3): 229–35.

71. Spiller R, Aziz Q, Creed F, Emmanuel A, Houghton L, Hungin P *et al.* Guidelines on the irritable bowel syndrome: mechanisms and practical management. *Gut* 2007; **56**(12): 1770–98.

72. Häuser W, Arnold B, Eich W, Felde E, Flügge C, Henningsen P. Management of fibromyalgia syndrome – an interdisciplinary evidence-based guideline. *German Medical Science* 2008; **6**: Doc 14.

73. Carville SF, Arendt-Nielsen S, Bliddal H, Blotman F, Branco JC, Buskila D *et al.* EULAR evidence-based recommendations for the management of fibromyalgia syndrome. *Annals of the Rheumatic Diseases* 2008; **67**(4): 536–41.

74. Arnold LM. Strategies for managing fibromyalgia. *American Journal of Medicine* 2009; **122**(Suppl 12): S31–S43.

75. American College of Gastroenterology Task Force on Irritable Bowel Syndrome, Brandt LJ, Chey WD, Foxx-Orenstein AE, Schiller LR, Schoenfeld PS *et al.* An evidence-based position statement on the management of irritable bowel syndrome. *American Journal of Gastroenterology* 2009; **104**(Suppl 1): S1–S35.

76. Brosseau L, Wells GA, Tugwell P, Egan M, Wilson KG, Dubouloz CJ *et al.* Ottawa Panel evidence-based clinical practice guidelines for aerobic fitness exercises in the management of fibromyalgia: Part 1. *Physical Therapy* 2008; **88**(7): 857–71.

77. National Institute for Health and Clinical Excellence. *Irritable Bowel Syndrome in Adults. Diagnosis and Management of Irritable Bowel Syndrome in Primary Care.* London: NICE; 2008.

78. Barsky AJ, Ahern DK. Cognitive behavior therapy for hypochondriasis: a randomized controlled trial. *Journal of the American Medical Association* 2004; **291**(12): 1464–70.

79. Clark DM, Salkovskis PM, Hackmann A, Wells A, Fennell M, Ludgate J *et al.* Two psychological treatments for hypochondriasis. A randomised controlled trial. *British Journal of Psychiatry* 1998; **173**: 218–25.

80. Nanke A, Rief W. Biofeedback-based interventions in somatoform disorders: a randomized controlled trial. *Acta Neuropsychiatrica* 2003; **15**(4): 249–56.

81. Meichenbaum DH, Deffenbacher JL. Stress inoculation training. *Counseling Psychologist* 1988; **16**(1): 69–90.

82. Barsky AJ. Amplification, somatization, and the somatoform disorders. *Psychosomatics* 1992; **33**(1): 28–34.

83. Salkovskis PM, Warwick HMC. Meaning, misinterpretations and medicine: a cognitive-behavioural approach to understanding health anxiety and hypochondriasis. In: Starcevic V, Lipsitt DR (eds). *Modern Perspectives on an Ancient Malady.* Oxford: University Press; 2002: 203–22.

84. Segal ZV, Williams JMG, Teasdale JD. *Mindfulness-Based Cognitive Therapy for Depression.* New York: Guildford Press; 2002.

85. Lau MA, Mcmain SF. Integrating mindfulness meditation with cognitive and behavioural therapies: the challenge of combining acceptance- and change-based strategies. *Canadian Journal of Psychiatry* 2005; **50**(13): 863–9.

86. Hayes SC, Luoma JB, Bond FW, Masuda A, Lillis J. Acceptance and commitment therapy: model, processes and outcomes. *Behaviour Research and Therapy* 2006; **44**(1): 1–25.

87. Chou R, Shekelle P. Will this patient develop persistent disabling low back pain? *Journal of the American Medical Association* 2010; **303**(13): 1295–302.

88. Allen LA, Woolfolk RL, Escobar JI, Gara MA, Hamer RM, Allen LA *et al.* Cognitive-behavioral therapy for somatization disorder: a randomized controlled trial. *Archives of Internal Medicine* 2006; **166**(14): 1512–18.

89. Thieme K, Gromnica-Ihle E, Flor H. Operant behavioral treatment of fibromyalgia: a controlled study. *Arthritis and Rheumatism* 2003; **49**(3): 314–20.

90. Woolfolk RL, Allen LA. *Treating Somatisation: A Cognitive Behavioural Approach.* New York: Guildford Press; 2006.

91. Rief W, Hiller W. The psychological treatment of somatoform disorders. In: Ono Y, Janca A, Asai M, Sartorius N (eds). *Somatoform Disorders: A Worldwide Perspective.* New York: Springer; 1999.

92. Sumathipala A, Hewege S, Hanwella R, Mann AH. Randomized controlled trial of cognitive behaviour therapy for repeated consultations for medically unexplained complaints: a feasibility study in Sri Lanka. *Psychological Medicine* 2000; **30**(4): 747–57.

93. Witthöft M, Hiller W. Psychological approaches to origins and treatments of somatoform disorders. *Annual Review of Clinical Psychology* 2010; **6**: 257–83.

94. Allen LA, Woolfolk RL. Cognitive behavioral therapy for somatoform disorders. *Psychiatric Clinics of North America* 2010; **33**(3): 579–93.

95. Schröder A. *Syndromes of bodily distress Assessment and treatment. PhD dissertation.* Faculty of Health Sciences. Aarhus University, Denmark, 2010.

96. Hobson RF. *Forms of Feeling.* London: Tavistock; 1985.

97. Guthrie E, Creed F, Dawson D, Tomenson B. A controlled trial of psychological

treatment for the irritable bowel syndrome. *Gastroenterology* 1991; **100**: 450–7.

98. Guthrie E. Brief psychotherapy with patients with refractory irritable bowel syndrome. *British Journal of Psychotherapy* 1991; **8**: 175–88.

99. Creed F, Fernandes L, Guthrie E, Palmer S, Ratcliffe J, Read N *et al.* The cost-effectiveness of psychotherapy and paroxetine for severe irritable bowel syndrome. *Gastroenterology* 2003; **124**(2): 303–17.

100. Lydiard RB. Pharmacotherapy for functional somatic conditions. In: Mayer EA, Bushnell MC (eds). *Functional Pain Syndromes: Presentation and Pathophysiology.* Seattle, WA: IASP Press; 2009: 465–89.

101. Hauser W, Klose P, Langhorst J, Moradi B, Steinbach M, Schiltenwolf M *et al.* Efficacy of different types of aerobic exercise in fibromyalgia syndrome: a systematic review and meta-analysis of randomised controlled trials. *Arthritis Research and Therapy* 2010; **12**(3): R79.

102. Creed FH, Levy R, Bradley L, Drossman DA, Francisconi C, Naliboff BD *et al.* Psychosocial aspects of functional gastrointestinal disorders. In: Drossman DA, Corazziari E, Delvaux M, Spiller RC, Talley NJ, Thompson WG *et al.*, eds. *Rome III. The Functional Gastrointestinal Disorders*, 3rd edn. McLean, VA: Degnon Associates; 2006: 295–368.

103. Levy RL, Olden KW, Naliboff BD, Bradley LA, Francisconi C, Drossman DA *et al.* Psychosocial aspects of the functional gastrointestinal disorders. *Gastroenterology* 2006; **130**(5): 1447–58.

104. Fallon BA. Pharmacotherapy of somatoform disorders. *Journal of Psychosomatic Research* 2004; **56**(4): 455–60.

105. Kroenke K, Krebs EE, Bair MJ. Pharmacotherapy of chronic pain: a synthesis of recommendations from systematic reviews. *General Hospital Psychiatry* 2009; **31**(3): 206–19.

106. Birket-Smith M. Somatization and chronic pain. *Acta Anaesthesiologica Scandinavica* 2001; **45**(9): 1114–20.

107. Malt UF, Lloyd G. Psychopharmacological treatment in liaison psychiatry. In: Lloyd GG, Guthrie E (eds). *Handbook of Liaison Psychiatry.* Cambridge: Cambridge University Press; 2007: 763–94.

108. Jackson JL, O'Malley PG, Kroenke K. Antidepressants and cognitive-behavioral therapy for symptom syndromes. *CNS Spectrums* 2006; **11**(3): 212–22.

109. O'Malley PG, Jackson JL, Santoro J, Tomkins G, Balden E, Kroenke K. Antidepressant therapy for unexplained symptoms and symptom syndromes. *Journal of Family Practice* 1999; **48**(12): 980–90.

110. Häuser W, Bernardy K, Uceyler N, Sommer C. Treatment of fibromyalgia syndrome with antidepressants: a meta-analysis. *Journal of the American Medical Association* 2009; **301**(2): 198–209.

111. Ford AC, Talley NJ, Schoenfeld PS, Quigley EMM, Moayyedi P. Efficacy of antidepressants and psychological therapies in irritable bowel syndrome: systematic review and meta-analysis. *Gut* 2009; **58**(3): 367–78.

112. Kroenke K. Efficacy of treatment for somatoform disorders: a review of randomized controlled trials. *Psychosomatic Medicine* 2007; **69**(9): 881–8.

113. Creed F. How do SSRIs help patients with irritable bowel syndrome? *Gut* 2006; **55**(8): 1065–7.

114. Harris LR, Roberts L. Treatments for irritable bowel syndrome: patients' attitudes and acceptability. *BMC Complementary and Alternative Medicine* 2008; **8**: 65.

115. Kroenke K, Bair MJ, Damush TM, Wu JW, Hoke S, Sutherland J *et al.* Optimized antidepressant therapy and pain self-management in primary care patients with depression and musculoskeletal pain: a randomized controlled trial. *Journal of the American Medical Association* 2009; **301**(20): 2099–110.

116. Bjelland I, Dahl AA, Haug TT, Neckelmann D. The validity of the Hospital Anxiety and Depression Scale. An updated literature review.

Journal of Psychosomatic Research 2002; **52**(2): 69–77.

117. Greco T, Eckert G, Kroenke K. The outcome of physical symptoms with treatment of depression. *Journal of General Internal Medicine* 2004; **19**(8): 813–18.

118. Rosenstiel AK, Keefe FJ. The use of coping strategies in chronic low-back-pain patients – relationship to patient characteristics and current adjustment. *Pain* 1983; **17**(1): 33–44.

119. Jensen MP, Keefe FJ, Lefebvre JC, Romano JM, Turner JA. One- and two-item measures of pain beliefs and coping strategies. *Pain* 2003; **104**(3): 453–69.

120. O'Connor AB, Dworkin RH. Treatment of neuropathic pain: An overview of recent guidelines. *American Journal of Medicine* 2009; **122**(10): S22–S32.

121. Volz HP, Möller HJ, Reimann I, Stoll KD. Opipramol for the treatment of somatoform disorders results from a placebo-controlled trial. *European Neuropsychopharmacology* 2000; **10**(3): 211–17.

122. Volz HP, Murck H, Kasper S, Moller HJ. St John's wort extract (LI 160) in somatoform disorders: results of a placebo-controlled trial. *Psychopharmacology* 2002; **164**(3): 294–300.

123. Kroenke K, Messina N, Benattia I, Graepel J, Musgnung J. Venlafaxine extended release in the short-term treatment of depressed and anxious primary care patients with multisomatoform disorder. *Journal of Clinical Psychiatry* 2006; **67**(1): 72–80.

124. Moja PL, Cusi C, Sterzi RR, Canepari C. Selective serotonin re-uptake inhibitors (SSRIs) for preventing migraine and tension-type headaches. *Cochrane Database of Systematic Reviews* 2005; **3**: CD002919.

125. Rains JC, Penzien DB, McCrory DC, Gray RN. Behavioral headache treatment: History, review of the empirical literature, and methodological critique. *Headache* 2005; **45**: S92–S109.

126. Fallon BA, Petova E, Skritskaya N, Sanchez-Lacay A, Schneier F, Vermes D *et al.* A double-masked, placebo-controlled study of fluoxetine for hypochondriasis. *Journal of Clinical Psychopharmacology* 2008; **28**(6): 638–45.

127. Greeven A, van Balkom AJ, Visser S, Merkelbach JW, van Rood YR, van Dyck R *et al.* Cognitive behavior therapy and paroxetine in the treatment of hypochondriasis: a randomized controlled trial. *American Journal of Psychiatry* 2007; **164**(1): 91–9.

128. Greeven A, van Balkom AJLM, van der Leeden R, Merkelbach JW, van den Heuvel OA, Spinhoven P. Cognitive behavioral therapy versus paroxetine in the treatment of hypochondriasis: An 18-month naturalistic follow-up. *Journal of Behavior Therapy and Experimental Psychiatry* 2009; **40**(3): 487–96.

129. Ipser JC, Sander C, Stein DJ. Pharmaco-therapy and psychotherapy for body dysmorphic disorder. *Cochrane Database of Systematic Reviews* 2009; **1**: CD005332.

130. Häuser W, Petzke F, Sommer C. Comparative efficacy and harms of duloxetine, milnacipran, and pregabalin in fibromyalgia syndrome. *Journal of Pain* 2010; **11**(6): 505–21.

131. Perahia DGS, Quail D, Desaiah D, Montejo AL, Schatzberg AF. Switching to duloxetine in selective serotonin reuptake inhibitor non- and partial-responders: effects on painful physical symptoms of depression. *Journal of Psychiatric Research* 2009; **43**(5): 512–18.

132. Kennedy T, Jones R, Darnley S, Seed P, Wessely S, Chalder T *et al.* Cognitive behaviour therapy in addition to antispasmodic treatment for irritable bowel syndrome in primary care: randomised controlled trial. *British Medical Journal* 2005; **331**(7514): 435.

133. Häuser W, Thieme K, Turk DC. Guidelines on the management of fibromyalgia syndrome – a systematic review. *European Journal of Pain* 2010; **14**(1): 5–10.

134. Arnold LM, Clauw D, Wang F, Ahl J, Gaynor PJ, Wohlreich MM. Flexible dosed duloxetine in the treatment of fibromyalgia: a randomized, double-blind, placebo-controlled

trial. *Journal of Rheumatology* 2010; 37(12): 2578–86.

135. Arnold B, Brinkschmidt T, Casser HR, Gralow I, Irnich D, Klimczyk K *et al.* [Multimodal pain therapy – principles and indications.] (article in German) *Schmerz* 2009; 23(2): 112–20.

136. Zastrow A, Faude V, Seyboth F, Niehoff D, Herzog W, Löwe B. Outcome of simultaneous psychosomatic/internal-medicine inpatient care – a naturalistic follow-up study. *Psychosomatic Medicine and Psychotherapy* 2009; 5(3): 229–47.

137. Chang L, Mayer EA, Johnson T, FitzGerald LZ, Naliboff B. Differences in somatic perception in female patients with irritable bowel syndrome with and without fibromyalgia. *Pain* 2000; 84(2–3): 297–307.

138. Arnold B, Häuser W, Bernardy K, Brueckle W, Friedel E, Köllner V *et al.* [Multicomponent therapy for treatment of fibromyalgia syndrome.] (article in German) *Schmerz* 2008; 22(3): 334–8.

Chapter

9

Training

Per Fink, Kurt Fritzsche, Wolfgang Söllner
and Astrid Larisch

Introduction

This chapter describes the training of doctors in different settings to improve their skills in managing patients with medically unexplained symptoms or somatoform disorders (henceforth referred to as bodily distress syndromes). The first section gives an overview of training at different levels with examples of the training developed in Denmark. The second describes the extensive training developed in Germany. In both Denmark and Germany, specialist centres have been set up to help this group of patients, but it has proved necessary, in addition, to establish training for non-specialists, in both primary and secondary care.

Teaching primary care physicians and other non-psychiatrists to diagnose and manage bodily distress syndromes

Teaching about the diagnosis and treatment of bodily distress syndromes happens at different levels (see Box 9.1).

Box 9.1 The range of teaching required to improve the care of patients with bodily distress

- Undergraduate training for medical students and other health professional students including psychologists
- Postgraduate teaching of non-psychiatric medical doctors and other healthcare professionals: there is an important difference between primary care physicians who themselves have treatment responsibility for their patients presenting with bodily distress syndromes, and most other medical specialists who do not have responsibility for treating the patients but for diagnosing the disorders and preventing inappropriate treatment. There may also be a particular training need for doctors in occupational and social medicine.
- Education of general psychiatrists
- Education of specialised consultation-liaison psychiatrists/psychosomaticists and health psychologists
- Education of specialists in functional syndromes and functional disorders (e.g. in university clinics)
- Education of non-health professionals, e.g. social workers
- Education of other healthcare professionals

Medically Unexplained Symptoms, Somatisation and Bodily Distress, ed. Francis Creed, Peter Henningsen and Per Fink. Published by Cambridge University Press. © Cambridge University Press 2011.

Education of medical, psychological and other students

Given the high prevalence of bodily distress in clinical practice, it is important that there is much more intensive teaching of bodily distress and health anxiety to medical students. This could improve the general basic knowledge about bodily distress among all doctors. The teaching may take the form of lectures as part of psychiatry or another specialty. Alternatively, teaching could take place in the setting of joint clinics or patient demonstrations between specialists in bodily distress and specialists such as rheumatologists and orthopaedic surgeons. In this way the students would learn that bodily distress syndromes are differential diagnoses that they always have to bear in mind, and they could acquire the necessary skills to make the diagnosis accurately and treat the disorder.

During the past decade, recognition of the importance of doctors' communication skills has increased, so today most medical schools worldwide train medical students in basic communication skills. Because bodily distress is a problem in most medical specialties, specific skills in communication with patients with bodily distress and health anxiety ought to be included in the communication training at a basic level. This may not always be the case, however. Furthermore, assessing the patients' illness beliefs and addressing them is not a part of basic communication skills training. These skills are best obtained by hands-on exercises, e.g. by a modified version of. The Extended Reattribution and Management (TERM) model (see below; [1]).

The TERM model: an educational programme for GPs and non-psychiatrists

Background

Up to a quarter of patients who consult their general practitioner (GP) do so with bodily distress. The underlying bodily distress syndromes often go undiagnosed and untreated, which may result in repeated examinations and treatment attempts that can inflict iatrogenic harm on the patient.

The relevant bodily symptoms vary in severity and the spectrum ranges from mild sensations or symptoms that are part of normal life to severe and disabling symptoms. Due to this broad spectrum of severity and the high proportion of patients presenting with bodily distress, most patients will be treated by their GP. This is also important as, at least in countries with a family doctor system, the GP may, by early intervention, be able to prevent mild or moderate bodily distress developing into a more severe or chronic condition.

Educational models

Various models for treatment in primary care have been developed to treat patients with psychological problems. In the early eighties, D. Goldberg and L. Gask from Manchester developed 'The Reattribution Model' as a method for training GPs in the treatment of patients with 'somatised depression and anxiety', i.e. patients with depression or anxiety disorder who present to their GP with somatic symptoms. The reattribution model has been tested in several studies, which indicate that it may improve GPs' communication skills. Several other brief intervention models for different types of problems have been developed for use by GPs in everyday practice [2;3].

However, none of these models target bodily distress in patients with no or few obvious emotional problems or mental disorder. The TERM model was specifically developed for treatment of the bodily distress syndromes seen in primary care (Box 9.2). It is named the TERM treatment model (The Extended Reattribution and Management Model) because it makes use of the earlier programmes and additionally includes classification and treatment of bodily distress. The main aim is to offer GPs an advanced course in assessment and treatment of patients with bodily distress syndromes in a form that is acceptable to and practicable for a broad section of primary care doctors. This means that the course caters in particular for the training needs of doctors who are inexperienced in this field, but all participants will be able to benefit from the training irrespective of their qualifications or experience.

Box 9.2 The TERM model

(A) Understanding
  (1) Take a full symptom history (seek clarification, identify accompanying symptoms, describe a typical symptom day)
  (2) Explore emotional clues
  (3) Inquire directly about symptoms of anxiety and depression
  (4) Explore life events, stress and other external factors (social, work-related and family)
  (5) Explore functional level (physical, social and family)
  (6) Explore the patient's health beliefs
  (7) Explore the patient's expectations of treatment and examinations
  (8) Make a brief, focused physical examination and, if indicated, non-clinical examination

(B) The physician's expertise and acknowledgement of illness
  (9) Feedback the results of the physical examination
  (10) Acknowledge the reality of the symptoms
  (11) Make clear that there is no (or that there is indeed) indication for further examination or non-psychiatric treatment

(C) Negotiating a New Model of Understanding (Reframing)
  Negotiate with the patient a new model of understanding of his/her illness in the light of the patients' illness perceptions and health beliefs which are thus modified
  (12) Primarily for the non-psychiatric specialist – clarify possible and impossible causal explanations

  Mild cases
  (13) Qualified normalisation
  (14) Reaction to stress, strain or nervousness
    (a) Palpitations when startled
    (b) Increased sensitivity when in low spirits
    (c) Muscle tensions when anxious or nervous
  (15) Demonstrate/present other associations
    (a) Practical (hyperventilation, muscular tension)
    (b) Establish the association between physical discomfort, emotional reactions and life events
    (c) Here and now (nervous about consulting the physician)

> **Box 9.2** (*cont.*)
>
> Severe cases
>
> (16) Known phenomenon with a name; 'bodily distress syndrome' or 'functional disorder'
> (17) Basically the cause is unknown, but possible biological cause is that 'Some are bodily more sensitive than others'
> (18) How one reacts to symptoms is important for how you cope in the future
>
> (D) Management of chronic conditions
> (E) Summary and planning of course
> Sum up agreements made during the consultation
> Agree on objectives, contents and form of the future course
>
> (19) Mild and transient cases ➔ terminate the treatment
> (20) Subacute cases ➔ agree with the patient a serious of scheduled therapy sessions of fixed duration
> (21) Chronic ➔ consider status consultation; agree on regular scheduled appointments
> (22) Consider referral to psychiatrist, psychologist or specialist service

Aim

The programme aims to transmit knowledge about bodily distress and the underlying disorders, train GPs in general interview techniques and specific treatment techniques for bodily distress, and initiate a change of attitude towards bodily distress. The programme intends to be acceptable to, and usable by, all GPs in everyday clinical practice, irrespective of prior qualifications.

The development

To ensure the clinical usefulness of the programme, it was developed in a close collaboration between psychiatric specialists and GPs. There were intensive discussions about the limitations imposed by the brief time available for GP training and for the consultation with patients in primary care. These limits were thoroughly discussed and defined when developing the course. First, it was assumed that most GPs would be unable to spend more than two days on a residential course and three to four evening sessions during one month. Second, it was presumed that the GPs would be compensated for the loss of earnings due to course participation. Finally, the model was designed to allow its use in everyday clinical practice without exceeding the time and financial constraints of primary care.

Prototocols have been developed for the academic content and the training methods and they are thoroughly described in *Psychosomatics* [1]. The programme is also available (in Danish) on the Aarhus University Hospital's website: www.functionaldisorders.dk. It is currently under revision, and the revised version will later be available in English.

Mode of delivery

The programme consists of a two-day residential course (two eight-hour days), followed by three two-hour evening meetings at one to two week intervals and a booster meeting after three months. The residential course consists of four modules of three hours in a fixed structure with: (i) a brief introduction to the exercises, including a short video demonstration;

Table 9.1 Main rules for interviewing in the TERM model

Dos	Don'ts
• Socratic questioning	• Use closed questions (questions that can be answered by yes/no)
– Be neutral and sincerely curious	• Offer a advice
– Use open questions	• Offer premature corrections
– Use encouragement (facilitating)	• Get involved in arguments and confrontations
– Keep the focus	• Try to persuade the patient to your view as ideas generated by the patients themselves are much more convincing
• Make frequent summaries	
• Use empathy / emotional feedback	
• Roll with resistance (rope-a-dope)	
• Support and empowerment – let the patients find their own suggested solutions and support the patients' feelings of power	

(ii) practical exercises in groups of two (either two GPs or one GP/one actor – sessions with an actor are video recorded); (iii) review of the recorded videos in groups of eight; and (iv) a plenary presentation of a theory.

The training is based on micro skills training principles and a multifaceted approach to the learning process. The practical training sessions consist of role playing (doctor/patient) and feedback. The doctor has seven minutes for the interview of the patient (see Table 9.1), and in each session the doctor's learning is restricted to a specific part of the overall model and a very limited range of specific interview techniques. Case histories are given to the patients, and the doctor is provided with written instructions on the specific learning objective for each session and examples of how the relevant questions can be framed. Every session ends with the patient giving positive feedback to the doctor. During the course, everyone will play both doctor and patient several times and be video recorded with an actor.

A course ideally accommodates 24 GPs. For the weekly evening booster meetings, they meet in groups of eight with two supervisors (a GP and a psychiatrist). The supervisors have been trained in a three-day residential course. The participants bring video recordings from their consultations with their real patients for review. Beforehand, the patients give consent that the recordings may be used for teaching purposes, and the recordings are erased afterwards. The review groups are subject to patient confidentiality.

Evaluation of effectiveness

Two cluster-randomised controlled trials were set up in 2000 to test the effect of the programme: one in Vejle County, Denmark, including 38 GPs and 2880 patients, who consulted their GP during the study period; the other in Aarhus County, including 38 GPs and 1785 patients. Half of the GPs were trained in the treatment model; the other half formed the control group. The patients in both groups were followed up after one and two years.

Main results

- The trained GPs changed their attitudes towards patients with bodily distress, and they were more confident and felt more comfortable and satisfied with the treatment of patients with bodily distress syndromes after the course, compared with the non-trained GPs [4].
- The trained GPs discussed more psychosocial issues with the patients after their training [5].
- The patients were significantly more satisfied if they consulted a trained GP, compared with a non-trained GP [6;7].
- Patients with somatoform disorders had less physical disability at two-year follow-up if treated by a trained GP, but in patients with 'medically unexplained' symptoms according to their GP, there was no significant improvement [5;8;9].
- Healthcare use for patients with somatoform disorders during the two-year follow-up period was one-third lower in the intervention group compared with the controls, but the difference was not statistically significant at a 5% level [5].
- The GPs attending the course were, in most respects, representative of all GPs in Aarhus county [5;8].

After the scientific trial period and current status

The TERM model has been implemented successfully in parts of Denmark after the positive results of the randomised controlled trials described above. There has been an explicit demand from GPs and other health professionals for more courses. The demand has not arisen because the GPs are persuaded by the scientific evidence, but because the word has spread among GPs that the TERM course is very beneficial.

More than 300 doctors have been trained in the model to date (about 20% of all GPs in Aarhus and Vejle counties). We have continuously tested the doctors' satisfaction with the model, and it has been extremely high. Of 205 participating doctors, 183 have evaluated the course (at nine courses), and the ratings are displayed in Figure 9.1.

In 2007, the TERM course was made compulsory for all doctors specialising in primary medicine in two out of the five regions in Denmark; and around 60 doctors have been trained each year since. Additionally, in one of the regions, all GPs in primary care, three sets of 15 doctors per year, undergo a brief one-day course in the model. At the present time, there are discussions about making the course compulsory for all new GPs nationwide. A slightly modified version of the training has been used in the teaching of other specialised doctors, e.g. rheumatologists and social medicine specialists.

Other parts of the healthcare system use the TERM model in education about management of patients with bodily distress. Some of the doctors who have attended the course have requested an extension of the course as they want to acquire skills in treatment of patients with chronic bodily distress syndromes, not only those with more short-lived problems, and we are currently developing an advanced course for the further treatment of these patients in primary care.

Training of general non-psychiatric specialists

Bodily distress syndromes are common in all clinical settings. It is paramount that all clinical medical specialists are familiar with these syndromes in order to make the differential diagnosis and guide the patients to receive the correct treatment. An early diagnosis may prevent iatrogenic harm and persistent symptoms with repeated help-seeking. It is

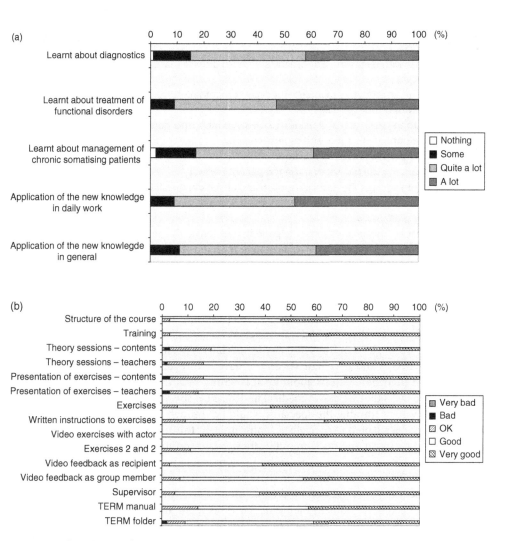

Figure 9.1 a,b Evaluation of nine TERM courses 2000–2007/N = 183/205

hoped that the intervention might prevent patients being referred to different special-ists throughout the healthcare system with multiple investigations and fruitless treatment attempts. Unlike GPs, medical specialists are not necessarily expected to treat bodily dis-tress syndromes themselves, but they should play an important role in initiating the treat-ment and motivating the patients for the treatment. Usually, the reason for referral to a specialist is suspicion of disease of a particular organ system. For further management, it is of pivotal importance that the specialist clearly explains to the patient that the exam-ination and clinical tests have revealed no signs of the disease in question and that the patient thus does not have that disease and that there is no need for further investigations. To meet the patient's expectations, it is absolutely necessary for the specialist to know about the patient's illness beliefs and expectations regarding examinations and treatment.

> **Box 9.3** The medical-surgical specialist's role in the management of patients with bodily distress
> - Rule out – within reason – any organically based disease that can be treated surgically or medically
> - Inform – in an empathic manner – the patient that there is/is no evidence of organic disease within your speciality
> - Explain to the patient that there is no indication for further somatic assessment
> - Treat the patient in a sober and professional way
> - Make the diagnosis of bodily distress
> - Avoid harming the patient or make the patient more ill
> - Attempt to address the patient's spoken and unspoken questions and expectations
> - Coordinate the patients future management with the patient's GP and other potential health professionals
> - Give clear and distinct responses to patient questions
> - Consider referral to psychiatric evaluation or specialist clinic, if available

The patient may have dysfunctional illness perceptions, which the doctor can only discover if they ask about this directly. The non-psychiatric specialist has a unique opportunity to correct such misunderstandings due to the specialist's position as a body-system expert; a position that GPs and psychiatrists do not have. However, some patients may be quite unyielding in their perceptions about what is wrong with them and therefore difficult to reassure. The tasks that we ask of medical and surgical specialists are listed in Box 9.3.

The best way of training the specialist would be through training programmes such as the TERM model adapted to specialists. Unfortunately, this may seldom be realistic. Due to the increased focus on doctors' communication, more and more doctors go through communication skills training, and a less ambitious aim would be to include specific communication techniques for bodily distress in these programmes. Although good communication skills are a necessary precondition for the treatment of bodily distress, they are not sufficient. Doctors also need basic skills in the particular assessment and management of bodily distress. This can be achieved by including these skills in the specialist training programmes of various specialists. In Denmark, for instance, workshops on bodily distress have been included in the curriculum of some specialist training programmes such as orthopaedic surgery, dermatology and neurology.

Education of general psychiatrists

General psychiatrists rarely see patients with bodily distress in psychiatric wards or outpatient clinics. For various reasons, the general psychiatrist may be inclined to dismiss or neglect bodily distress syndromes as not belonging to their specialty [10;11]. Instead, they focus on the 'severe' mental illnesses such as severe depression and psychoses. However, bodily symptoms are very prevalent in patients with various emotional disorders, and in schizophrenia and other psychoses, psychotic somatic delusions are quite common. Bodily symptoms are the most common reason for presenting to the healthcare system in depression [12]. Furthermore, bodily distress syndromes co-occur commonly with emotional mental disorders and vice versa. Therefore, general psychiatrists must be able to make this differential diagnosis.

At most general hospitals worldwide, there is no specialised consultation-liaison psychiatric or psychosomatic service, and therefore the general psychiatrists have the responsibility of providing a service to general hospitals. In this setting, the psychiatrists are often confronted with patients with bodily distress syndromes and the question of differential diagnosis between a medical condition and a functional disorder arises. If the psychiatric consultants do not have sufficient competencies in establishing the diagnosis of a bodily distress syndrome, it may have untoward consequences for the patients. Not only may they not be offered a potentially effective treatment, but they may also be exposed to iatrogenic harm due to the doctors' continuous efforts to exclude a medical disorder as the cause of the complaints. A typical conclusion of the non-experienced psychiatrist could be that 'there is no evidence of a formal mental disorder', which means that no signs of depression or anxiety or other emotional symptoms have been found. Because of their uncertainty regarding functional disorders and medical conditions in general, general psychiatrists may be even more inclined to stress organic explanations than their non-psychiatric colleagues. This is one of the reasons why positive diagnostic criteria for the bodily distress syndromes are important, as shown in Chapter 2, rather than it being just a diagnosis of exclusion.

Many general psychiatrists are private practitioners and are not employed at psychiatric hospitals, and they will quite often see patients with bodily distress referred from primary care. In fact, psychiatric generalists and health psychologists practising outside psychiatric hospitals should be managing the majority of patients with bodily distress who are too severely ill to be treated by their GPs, unless the GPs have the competencies and sufficient training. They could set up collaborative care with GPs. Some are working as consultants for the social security system and the like, and they therefore need courses and training in the diagnosis and treatment of bodily distress syndromes.

The training of general psychiatrists has many similarities with the training of GPs, but also some differences. The psychiatrists are in general well trained in communication skills, in establishing a psychosocial history and in assessment of emotional mental disorders, and therefore it is not necessary, as it is in the GP training, to include these particular components in the training. On the other hand, psychiatrists need to have the necessary theoretical knowledge about bodily distress syndromes to be able to assess a patient and diagnose this, when appropriate, including considering the relevant differential diagnoses. In cases of a bodily distress syndrome, the patient will often not understand the reason for seeing a psychiatrist since the patient has bodily and not emotional distress. The psychiatrists need to learn to address this dissonance and learn how to motivate the patient for therapy if indicated [13]. They have to learn (and be trained in) how to present the diagnosis of bodily distress syndromes to the patient and to inform the patient about the nature, the prognosis and the treatment of the disorder.

When patients are assessed by an unskilled psychiatrist, they often gain the impression that nothing is wrong with them – the same as they have been told by the non-psychiatric doctors. They are also often – erroneously – told by the general psychiatrist that they can not be treated if they do not have emotional symptoms. The necessary training of psychiatrists is best delivered by psychiatrists and other specialists in bodily distress, working in specialised university units for bodily distress, just as it is in all other diseases and specialties.

Training of the specialist in psychosomatics and consultation-liaison psychiatry

Consultation-liaison psychiatrists will often encounter patients with bodily distress because of the high prevalence of the disorder in general hospitals and the need for physicians or surgeons to refer such patients for psychiatric assessment and treatment. Greater responsibility is therefore placed on the psychosomatic and consultation-liaison psychiatry services as they are the only (sub)specialty that has patients with bodily distress syndromes as one of its target patient groups. In Denmark it is intended that psychosomatic medicine and consultation-liaison psychiatry services should be present in all general hospitals, where they should treat most of the patients with bodily distress syndromes at the specialist level. Currently, subspecialised units that only treat bodily distress syndromes are very rare, even at university hospitals. The education programmes in consultation-liaison psychiatry and psychosomatics should therefore include intensive training in the treatment and assessment of bodily distress. Unfortunately, this is not always the case.

Later in this chapter, one of the most comprehensive training programmes for the revlevant specialists is described: the German programme for training as a specialist in psychosomatic medicine.

Education of specialists in bodily distress syndromes

Specialised clinics for bodily distress syndromes are sparse worldwide, and therefore there is no widespread curriculum for training doctors and other healthcare professionals in the treatment of bodily distress. However, some pain clinics and clinics for other types of functional somatic syndromes, such as chronic fatigue syndrome, are in fact highly specialised in particular forms of treatment, such as physical methods of treating pain or particular exercise programmes for chronic fatigue. These are not relevant to other groups of people with bodily distress syndromes. Some countries have training programmes in pain for, for example, physicians and health psychologists, but these do not include bodily distress syndromes.

Specialised training programmes for doctors who will treat bodily distress disorders should include training in the relevant clinical skills drawn from both psychiatry and general medicine. This should include training in assessment and treatment of these disorders and in the relevant methods of research. Additionally, the programme should include training in how to cooperate in multidisciplinary teams including with physicians from various specialties, and in teaching and training in collaborative care. It is necessary that the specialists are well grounded in the broad field of general medicine to be able to assess the patients and to communicate with colleagues of other specialties. Finally, because the field lies between general psychiatry and general medicine, the administration and the leading of such units may be an extraordinary challenge to the hospital administration and to the relevant clinical directors of medical, psychiatric and psychological specialties.

As the basic skills needed by specialists in bodily distress are, in essence, the same skills as learned in psychiatry, usually it would be psychiatrists who subspecialise in this field. However, in Germany, there is a separate psychosomatic specialty within which non-psychiatrists such as internists or neurologists are also trained.

Consultation-liaison psychiatrists and specialists in psychosomatic medicine will posses many of the characteristics needed for the management of bodily distress (see below), but in many of the programmes, the training in bodily distress is very sparse as the focus is on other conditions [14], and a board certification in psychosomatic medicine or consultation-liaison psychiatry is by no means a guarantee that the doctors are qualified in assessment and treatment of bodily distress and functional somatic syndromes at the necessary highly specialised level.

Education of other healthcare professionals

Psychologists, nurses, physiotherapists and others will also need education in bodily distress. The programmes ought to be tailored for the specific groups, and ideally the groups should be taught, at least partly, by someone from their own profession.

Training psychologists in this special area is a particular challenge. These staff are often experts in psychological forms of treatment such as cognitive behavioural therapy, but their lack of additional general medical training can lead to problems. Assessment of patients with bodily distress involves assessment of the patients' medical history based on medical records and discharge letters, with which psychologists are not familiar. Understanding the process of differential diagnosis and excluding, where relevant, medical disorders, is a process with which psychologists need to collaborate closely with a suitably trained psychiatrist or medical colleague. In addition, the patients' illness beliefs are usually a very central issue in the treatment of bodily distress. It may be difficult, though, for a psychologist to work with their patient's illness beliefs if they do not have the necessary knowledge, or authority, to challenge those illness beliefs, when appropriate. Often this can be compensated for, at least in the less severe cases, by close cooperation between a doctor and the psychologist. Also, the focus of the therapy may be changed from the patient's illness beliefs to their behaviour, and the psychologist may focus more on the difficulties faced by the patient who may mistrust the doctor and fail to be reassured by negative investigations.

In health anxiety, the focus is much more on the cognitive and emotional disturbances, and psychologists will usually have no problem in assessing and treating these patients, although close collaboration with a doctor regarding questions about medical issues may be important. Education of practising psychologists is also important to prevent them inadvertently giving credence, or even support to, maladaptive illness beliefs – that something organic may be wrong and that more investigations are needed. This is also a risk when an unqualified or inexperienced psychiatrist assesses or treats the patient.

Education of non-healthcare professionals, e.g. social workers

Bodily distress syndromes often cause severe impairment resulting in sick leave and risk of exclusion from the labour market, and these patients account for a substantial portion of those taking early retirement pensions. Social security systems and the labour market often find it difficult to cope with patients who do not show obvious signs of illness and whose illness is based on subjective health complaints that are not supported by clinical tests or clinical findings. Often the patients are met with a negative attitude – as no positive signs of disease can be found, it must 'all be in their minds' and they just need to 'pull themselves together'. The social security system may put extreme pressure on these patients and force them into work, work ability testing or training programmes. In many cases, this stress may sabotage the treatment.

Therefore, social workers and others need to understand that the bodily distress disorders are a set of disorders that must be taken seriously, treated like any other medical or psychiatric disorder, and that undue stress may inflict severe suffering on the patients. To ensure cooperation between the social security system and the healthcare system, a common language and understanding of the problem is necessary. However, it is a precondition that the attitude to the patients is positive. If more intensive training is desired, a downscaled and modified version of the TERM model or similar may be the best solution.

Training in the specialty of psychosomatic medicine in Germany

The German Board for Psychosomatic Medicine has formulated curricula in psychosomatic medicine for individual medical professional associations (internal medicine, gynaecology and obstetrics, dermatology etc.). Such a programme has been obligatory in general medicine, internal medicine and gynaecology since 2005 [15].

Germany offers three levels of psychosocial medical services. The first is Psychosomatic Basic Care, for which each medical specialist (from general medicine to urology) receives training and in turn can be reimbursed for psychosocial care of patients by the health insurance company. The next level consists of more advanced training in psychosomatic and psychotherapeutic skills, which is open to all specialties (e.g. general medicine, internal medicine, gynaecology, dermatology etc.). This requires an additional three years of training on top of the usual residency training requirements for the chosen domain. Finally, there is a third level: a specialist in psychiatry and psychosomatic medicine, both requiring five years of training. The latter is unique to Germany.

Training in Psychosomatic Basic Care

Psychosomatic Basic Care is rooted in psychosomatic medicine and primarily influenced by psychoanalysts and internists who emulated Balint's approach (1964) stressing the integration of psychosomatic and holistic perspectives in medical practice model [16]. More recently, primary care physicians have become interested in psychosomatic medicine. The inclusion of Psychosomatic Basic Care into primary care routine in 1987 was a milestone in improving psychosocial care. This led to a growing interest in psychosomatic care by primary care physicians. In 1992, Psychosomatic Basic Care was defined as an educational standard for all clinical disciplines. Since 1994, there have been standard requirements for the training. According to these regulations, physicians must have completed an 80-hour training course in psychosocial primary care to be allowed to bill for these services. More than 60 000 of the 360 000 German GPs have attended courses in Psychosomatic Basic Care.

Basic and advanced training to improve the psychosocial skills of primary care physicians is offered by the Professional Board of Physicians in each German state, and by private institutions, licensed by the Board. Targeted skills include:

1. Identifying stressful emotional and mental conflicts using an extended psychosomatic interview
2. Promoting a helping alliance between the doctor, patient, and family members. This also includes identifying possible barriers on the doctor's, patient's, or family's part, and stressing core skills of empathy and sensitivity.
3. Improving patient skills in problem-solving: providing information on self-help groups; supporting management of adverse life events (e.g. severe illness, loss, separation or divorce); and avoiding unneeded medication, diagnostic procedures, or surgery.
4. Motivating and referring patients for psychotherapy. Additional skills in this area include collaboration around consultations and case management with psychotherapists and other psychosocial services.

Eighty hours of postgraduate training is required for certification. The training is divided into three parts: (i) an initial 20 hours on principles of psychosomatic medicine; (ii) a 30-hour

Box 9.4 Theoretical basis, and guidelines for training in Psychosomatic Basic Care

Theoretical basis for diagnosis and therapy
- Psychodynamic theory
- Cognitive behavioural approaches to initiating changes in thinking and learning
- Psychoeducation about stress, fear, and pain
- Systems theory, in particular, recognising and understanding dynamic processes in partner and family relationships; the complex effects of difficult treatment courses on the therapeutic system
- Principles of psychopharmacotherapy
- Differentiating among neuroses, psychoses and organic brain diseases

Guidelines for training:
- A combination of basic required courses with electives leading to greater flexibility in the courses of study, and permitting a concentration on fields of special interest
- Teaching methods that include lectures with practice-relevant introduction of the topic, live interviews with patients or video-demonstrations, small-group projects including 10–15 participants, and patient-oriented self-awareness (as in the Balint group)

block of exercises in psychosocial interventions; and (3) 30 hours' participation in a comprehensive Balint group. The training usually lasts 12 months, with sessions being spread out over the year. The Balint group provides an opportunity for participants to reflect on what they have learned and to progressively use the learning in actual medical practice.

Whenever possible, the Psychosomatic Basic Care courses are arranged regionally, encouraging a sense of continuity to the group work. There are also electives in specialty-related areas. Finally, participation in continuous quality circles (peer audit) is recommended, providing participants with the opportunities to further reflect on their individual behaviours and to assess whether improvements in patient-care outcomes might be achievable. The theoretical framework of Psychosomatic Basic Care is based on the biopsychosocial model as articulated by George Engel and promoted in Germany by Thure von Uexküll [17]. Special emphasis is placed on achieving and promoting health as stated in the concept of salutogenesis [18]. Box 9.4 summarises theories that form the basis for diagnosis and therapy.

Improving the psychosomatic competence in diagnosing and treating bodily distress syndromes

As part of the 'Quality Assurance in Psychosocial Primary Care' project [19], we demonstrated that psychosocially distressed patients who receive psychosocial interventions during a visit with their GP fared better in all outcome parameters (achieving a psychosomatic understanding, satisfaction with treatment and treatment success) than patients who were not offered this treatment opportunity [20]. We also found that psychosocially distressed patients without psychological attribution to their illness were offered less psychosocial treatment and responded less to routine medical care than patients presenting with emotional symptoms. The former group of patients may therefore need special psychosocial assessment and interventions in order to improve the outcome of their treatment.

Collaborative groups of GPs and psychotherapists were therefore established to develop and provide more specific treatments for patients with bodily distress. The treatment manual developed by these groups utilises training and interventions based on the reattribution model and the TERM model adapted to the German primary care setting [21;22]. The approach also includes treating bodily distress from a psychodynamic viewpoint, especially with regard to outpatient psychotherapy and specialised psychosomatic clinics [23]. The modified reattribution model includes three levels of intervention:

- *First level* – Patients' health beliefs and their treatment expectations are explored in order to reach consensus between the physician and the patient vis-à-vis an altered understanding of the symptoms. The following questions can be explored:
  - What do you feel caused your symptoms?
  - Why do you feel it started at this time?
  - How serious do you feel your illness is?
  - Which type of therapy would be the most beneficial to you?

  Patients with bodily distress syndromes benefit from regularly scheduled consultations, independent of the severity of their symptoms. The effectiveness of this approach with regard to holding down healthcare costs and improving the patient's general physical well-being has been demonstrated [24;25].

  For some patients, the interventions must be limited to this first step as these patients are unwilling or unable to delve deeper. One should avoid assuming a direct correlation between reported or assumed psychosocial problems and physical symptoms. Rather, the possibility of such associations should be discussed on a case-by-case basis, when and if the patient appears receptive. The pacing of treatment requires patience from the therapist. It is often the case that the problem cannot be realistically solved, only managed.

- *Second level* – The goal of the second level is to develop an alternative disease model by introducing the concept of psychophysiological associations. Below are two examples of relating the appearance of physical problems with current psychic stress.
  - When one is anxious or frightened, the body produces more adrenaline. That is why the heart beats faster in fearful situations.
  - When people feel pressured or emotionally distraught, their pain threshold is lowered. For example, joint pains may become unbearable when one is under stress.

  Cognitive processing mechanisms that accompany perception of the problem, such as the fear of having a serious disease, are vocalised and explained using a vicious-cycle model. Participation in relaxation training (progressive muscle relaxation, autogenous training) supports an understanding of the psychophysiological processes.

- *Third level* – When patients are already motivated, correlations between personality, the patient's life story, his or her current relationships, and the appearance of the problem can be addressed in an expanded social and medical history. Emphasis is placed on slowly replacing protective and avoidant behaviours in the social arena. The overemphasis of physical reactions protects the patient from addressing or confronting situations that are perceived as being overwhelming. This protective mechanism should be made to appear as something positive, not negative, so that the protective or avoidance behaviour is understood as being a consequence of environmental stress. By including partners or other significant persons from the patient's social environment, an understanding can be developed, and symptoms can be influenced within the framework of this social system [26].

Collaboration with mental-health specialists

If depression, severe anxiety disorder or suicidal risk are part of the clinical picture, then the physician should explain this to the patient and assist him or her to begin appropriate medication and psychotherapeutic treatment. Under these circumstances, collaboration between the psychotherapist and the primary care physician is important. Should the patient decline this treatment, there is still the possibility of carrying out a joint consultation with the psychotherapist at the GP's office, or even having the GP provide treatment in close collaboration with the specialist [27]. If the patient is at risk of harming him or herself, then psychiatric referral and inpatient hospitalisation should be considered.

To summarise, the Psychosomatic Basic Care model does not replace treatment by a mental health specialist, but rather the interventions concentrate on the symptoms, behaviour, and the accompanying cognition and affects. Limited objectives include decreasing unnecessary testing, avoiding harmful treatment and/or inducing a change in the symptom behaviour. It might also be possible to identify accompanying conflicts, without, however, necessarily working these through. Problem-solving skills are always related to the patient's actual, current situation.

New training models

To compare the effects of psychosocial interventions based on the modified reattribution model for patients with bodily distress syndromes in general practice with those of routine Psychosomatic Basic Care alone, we conducted a cluster-randomised clinical trial [28]. Effects of additional training in reattribution techniques compared with non-specific Psychosomatic Basic Care were small and limited to physical symptoms and healthcare utilisation.

Other projects of training primary-care physicians have been developed in some tertiary care centres. In Marburg, Rief and coworkers [29] established a one-day training course for GPs with the aim of better recognition and management of medically unexplained symptoms. Training included information about somatoform disorder, screening instruments, management guidelines and how to communicate with patients who have medically unexplained symptoms.

In Nuremberg, Söllner and co-workers in 2008 established training of basic psychosomatic care for hospital physicians. This training is similar to the training for GPs developed by the Freiburg group which is described in more detail elsewhere in this chapter [31]. Participants undertake 30 hours of communication skills training led by specialists of psychosomatic medicine experienced in consultation liaison services. In addition, they are offered 20 hours of lectures with a focus on 'medically unexplained' symptoms, as well as participation in 15 Balint group sessions lasting two hours each. Since 2004, 200 physicians (120 female and 78 male, mostly specialists in internal medicine and gynaecology and obstetrics) have taken part in this programme. Three months after attending the course, participants rated their competencies regarding recognition of bodily distress syndromes and managing a difficult interaction with patients suffering from 'medically unexplained' symptoms as significantly improved since baseline (and using five-point Likert scales).

Advanced training in psychotherapy and psychosomatics for physicians with any specialisation

This is the oldest model of an integrated psychotherapeutic and psychosomatic training for physicians from all disciplines e.g. general practitioners, internists, gynaecologists. It has been in existence for 60 years and since 1992 it is mandatory for psychiatrists. It includes 125 hours of theoretical and practical training, 100 hours of self-experience, 32 hours of relaxation techniques, 40 hours of Balint group and 120 hours of psychotherapeutic sessions under regular supervision. In daily practice, short-term psychotherapeutic interventions (three to five sessions) are the most common interventions [32].

Specialisation in psychosomatic medicine

A stand-alone medical specialisation in psychosomatic medicine was established by the German board of physicians in 1992. Training consists of three years in psychosomatic medicine (usually in a department of psychosomatic medicine; one year can be performed in a certified psychosomatic medicine practice), one year in internal medicine (half of the year may be performed in any other clinical specialty), and one year in psychiatry.

Training in psychosomatic medicine focuses on the assessment and treatment of patients with both somatic and psychiatric/behavioural disorders, e.g.:

- 'medically unexplained' symptoms (somatisation disorder, somatoform disorders)
- chronic pain syndromes
- somatic and psychiatric comorbidity (e.g. cardiovascular disease and diabetes plus depression or anxiety disorder)
- somatic disorder and problems of coping with illness, including adjustment disorder (any chronic disabling diseases such as cancer or multiple sclerosis)
- behavioural disorders with severe organic consequences (e.g. eating disorders).

In psychosomatic medicine departments, diagnostic assessment and treatment of such patients is taught in different settings: consultation-liaison services, outpatient clinics, inpatient psychosomatic wards (at least two years of residency) and day hospitals. Following a biopsychosocial approach, training in psychosomatic medicine takes biological as well as psychological and social aspects of illness and disease into account. Besides pharmacotherapy, special attention is given to the training in psychotherapeutic methods (either psychodynamic or cognitive behavioural, or both).

The psychotherapeutic training is intensive and includes 240 hours of theoretical training, 150 hours of individual self experience, 140 hours of self-experience in a small group setting, 70 hours of Balint group sessions, and 1500 hours of psychotherapeutic practise under supervision (with a 1:4 ratio between supervision and psychotherapeutic sessions). This intensive psychotherapeutic training is specific for the psychosomatic medicine specialist and greatly exceeds the degree of advanced psychotherapeutic training for other medical specialists including psychiatrists. Training of psychosomaticists in psychotherapeutic methods pays special attention to the treatment of the patient groups listed above and focuses on multimodal, short-term and more structured psychotherapeutic methods, including psycho-education, relaxation and imagery methods, supportive-expressive therapy, psychotherapy including relatives, and inclusion of body-centred methods in psychotherapy. Thus, this psychotherapeutic training exceeds the often narrow boundaries of psychotherapeutic schools (psychoanalytic or behavioural).

Outlook

A continuous curriculum of psychosocial medicine should be integrated into other aspects of medical school training. Topics to emphasise are the doctor–patient relationship, diagnostics, biopsychosocial systemic approaches and communication skills. Psychosomatic basic care is already part of the guidelines for postgraduate education in all clinical specialties. To ensure the adequacy and appropriateness of psychosomatic basic care, more quality measures should be developed to maintain existing quality standards for structure, process and outcome criteria. Also, appropriate remuneration is required for psychosocial services.

Although the development of curricula in biopsychosocial medicine is fairly advanced, there is still a need to educate more primary-care physicians to be teachers. Some general practitioners and other specialists are already involved in teaching and curriculum development. The German Board for Psychosomatic Medicine has developed curricula for individual specialist medical professional associations (internal medicine, gynaecology and obstetrics, dermatology etc.). Such a programme has been obligatory in general medicine, internal medicine and gynaecology since 2005 [15].

Training curricula in consultation-liaison psychiatry and psychosomatic medicine

The European guidelines for training in consultation-liaison psychiatry and psychosomatics identify as a specific area of knowledge, assessment and management of bodily distress syndromes [33]. There are other specific skills listed including the use of particular interview techniques relevant to these patients and explaining to them the causation of their disorder and its treatment when there are physical and psychological contributory factors present. It is likely, however, that the amount of training in relation to bodily distress syndromes varies considerably between centres, depending on the particular interest or emphasis of the local consultation-liaison psychiatry or psychosomatic medicine unit.

The American Board of Medical Specialties now recognises psychosomatic medicine as a subspecialty of psychiatry. The knowledge and skills required for certification in psychosomatic medicine include bodily distress as a topic [34]. The same is true of the competencies listed in the very recent consensus statement of the European Association of Consultation-Liaison Psychiatry and Psychosomatics and Academy of Psychosomatic Medicine [35]. In the USA there are, however, no specialised training programmes for the treatment of bodily distress in psychiatry or in psychosomatic medicine. This is so for many other countries worldwide.

Conclusion

This chapter has outlined the specific training of doctors aimed at improving their skills in managing patients with bodily distress syndromes. Such training is only available in a limited number of centres in Europe and this must clearly increase if the management of patients with these is disorders is to improve. The training must be made available to general practitioners, medical specialists and psychiatrists, as doctors in all of these areas of medicine are faced with patients with bodily distress syndromes. The evidence presented in Chapter 3 suggests that most doctors have not received sufficient training in this area of medicine to make them feel competent and confident in managing these disorders.

References

1. Fink P, Rosendal M, Toft T. Assessment and treatment of functional disorders in general practice: The extended reattribution and management model – an advanced educational program for nonpsychiatric doctors. *Psychosomatics* 2002; **43**: 93–131.

2. Rollnick S, Mason P, Butler C. *Health Behavior Change a Guide for Practitioners*,

1st edn. Edinburgh: Churchill Livingstone, 1999.

3. Catalan J, Gath DH, Anastasiades P, Bond SA, Day A, Hall L. Evaluation of a brief psychological treatment for emotional disorders in primary care. *Psychological Medicine* 1991; **21**: 1013–18.

4. Rosendal M, Bro F, Sokolowski I, Fink P, Toft T, Olesen F. A randomised controlled trial of brief training in assessment and treatment of somatisation: effects on GPs' attitudes. *Journal of Family Practice* 2005; **22**: 419–27.

5. Toft T. *Managing Patients with Functional Somatic Symptoms in General Practice.* Denmark: Faculty of Health Sciences, University of Aarhus; 2005.

6. Frostholm L. *Illness Perceptions in Primary Care Patients.* Denmark: Research Clinic for Functional Disorders and Psychosomatics, Aarhus University Hospital and Faculty of Health Sciences, University of Aarhus; 2005.

7. Frostholm L, Fink P, Ørnbøl E, Christensen KS, Toft T, Olesen F *et al.* The uncertain consultation and patient satisfaction: the impact of patients' illness perceptions and a randomized controlled trial on the training of physicians' communication skills. *Psychosomatic Medicine* 2005; **67**: 897–905.

8. Toft T, Rosendal M, Ornbol E, Olesen F, Frostholm L, Fink P. Training general practitioners in the treatment of functional somatic symptoms: effects on patient health in a cluster-randomised controlled trial (The Functional Illness in Primary Care Study). *Psychotherapy and Psychosomatics* 2010; **79**: 227–37.

9. Rosendal M, Olesen F, Fink P, Toft T, Sokolowski I, Bro F. A randomized controlled trial of brief training in the assessment and treatment of somatization in primary care: effects on patient outcome. *General Hospital Psychiatry* 2007; **29**: 364–73.

10. Creed F. Should general psychiatry ignore somatization and hypochondriasis? *World Psychiatry* 2006; **5**: 146–50.

11. Bass C, Peveler R, House A. Somatoform disorders: severe psychiatric illnesses neglected by psychiatrists. *British Journal of Psychiatry* 2001; **179**: 11–14.

12. World Health Organization. *Schedules for Clinical Assessment Neuropsychiatry.* Geneva: World Health Organization, Division of Mental Health; 1991.

13. Creed F, Guthrie E. Techniques for interviewing the somatising patient. *British Journal of Psychiatry* 1993; **162**: 467–71.

14. de Jonge P, Huyse FJ, Herzog T, Malt U, Opmeer BC, Kuiper B *et al.* Referral pattern of neurological patients to psychiatric consultation-liaison services in 33 European hospitals. *General Hospital Psychiatry* 2001; **23**(3): 152–7.

15. Neises M, Dietz S. *Psychosomatische Grundversorgung in der Frauenheilkunde.* [Psychosocial primary case in gynaecology.] Stuttgart: Schattauer; 1999.

16. Balint M. *The Doctor, His Patients and the Illness.* London: Pitman Medical Publishing; 1964.

17. Uexküll Th v, Wesiack W. Integierte Medizin als Gesamtkonzept der Heilkunde: ein bio-psycho-soziales Modell. In: Adler RH, Herzog W, Joraschky P, Köhle K, Langewitz W, Söllner W, Wesiack W (eds). *Psychosomatische Medizin,* 7th Edition. München: Urban & Fischer (Elsevier); 2011: 3–40.

18. Antonovski A. The salutogenic model as a theory to guide health promotion. *Health Promotion International* 1996; **2**: 11–18.

19. Fritzsche K, Sandholzer H, Brucks U, Härter M, Höger C, Wirsching M. Psychotherapeutische und psychosoziale Behandlungsmaß nahmen in der Hausarztpraxis [Psychotherapeutic and psychosocial treatment measures in the family practice.] *Psychotherapie Psychosomatik Medizinische Psychologie* 1999; **44**: 214–19.

20. Fritzsche K, Sandholzer H, Brucks U, Cierpka M, Deter HC, Härter M *et al.* Psychosocial care by general practitioners – where are the problems? Results of a demonstration project on quality management in psychosocial primary care. *International Journal of Psychiatry in Medicine* 1999; **29**: 395–409.

21. Fritzsche K, Larisch A. Treating patients with functional somatic symptoms. A treatment guide for use in general practice.

Scandinavian Journal of Primary Health Care 2003; **21**: 132–5.

22. Goldberg D, Gask L, O'Dowd T. The treatment of somatization: teaching techniques of reattribution. *Journal of Psychosomatic Research* 1989; **33**: 689–95.

23. Rudolf G, Henningsen P. Somatoforme Störungen: Theoretisches Verständnis und therapeutische Praxis [Somatoform disorders: Theoretical understanding and therapentic practice]. Stuttgart; Schattauer; 1998.

24. Dickinson WP, Dickinson LM, deGruy FV, Main DS, Candib LM, Rost K. A randomized clinical trial of a care recommendation letter intervention for somatization in primary care. *Annals of Family Medicine* 2003; **1**: 228–35.

25. Smith GR Jr, Rost K, Kashner TM. A trial of the effect of a standardized psychiatric consultation on health outcomes and costs in somatizing patients. *Archives of General Psychiatry* 1995; **52**: 238–43.

26. Cierpka M, Reich G, Kraul A. Psychosomatic illness in the family. In: L'Abate L, ed. *Family Psychopathology: The Relation Roots of Dysfunctional Behavior*. New York: Guildford Press; 1999.

27. Fritzsche K, Campagnolo I. Die kooperation zwischen Hausaerzten und Psychotherapeuten. Ein Beispiel für Psychosomatische Vernetzung [Collaboration between general practitioner and psychotherapist. An example of psychosomatic networking]. *Zeitschrift für Allgemeinmedizin* 1998; **4**: 318–20.

28. Larisch A, Schweickhardt A, Wirsching M, Fritzsche K. Psychosocial interventions for somatizing patients by the general practitioner: a randomized controlled trial. *Journal of Psychosomatic Research* 2004; **57**: 507–14.

29. Rief W, Martin A, Rauh E, Zech T, Bender A. Evaluation of general

practitioners' training: how to manage patients with unexplained physical symptoms. *Psychosomatics* 2006; **47**(4): 304–11.

30. Söllner W. Personal communication 2010.

31. Fritzsche K, Stein B, Larisch A, Weidner K, Diefenbacher A, Burian R et al. First curriculum for care of patients with mental and psychosomatic disorders in the context of a consultation-liaison service. *Psychotherapie Psychosomatik Medizinische Psychologie* 2009; **59**: 246–7.

32. Fritzsche K, Schmitt MF, Nübling M, Wirsching M. Arztliche Psychotherapie in der Haus- und Facharztpraxis: Eine empirische Untersuchung in Sudbaden [Medical psychotherapy in the house and speciality care practice: an empirical investigation in South Baden]. *Zeitschrift für Psychosomatische Medizin* **56**: 348–55. (in press).

33. Söllner W, Creed F. H and EACLPP Workgroup on Training. European guidelines for training in consultation-liaison psychiatry and psychosomatics: Report of the EACLPP Workgroup on training in consultation-liaison psychiatry and psychosomatics. *Journal of Psychosomatic Research* 2007; **62**(4): 501–9.

34. Angelino A, Lyketsos CG. Training in psychosomatic medicine: A psychiatric subspecialty recognized in the United States by the American Board of Medical Specialties. *Journal of Psychosomatic Research* (in press).

35. Leentjens AFG, Rundell JR, Wollcot DL, Guthrie E, Kathol R, Diefenbacher A. Psychosomatic medicine and consultation-liaison psychiatry: scope of practice, processes, and competencies for psychiatrists or psychosomatic medecine specialists. A consensus statement of the European Association of Consultation-Liaison Psychiatry (EACLPP) and the Academy of Psychosomatic Medicine (APM). *Psychosomatics* 2011; **52**(1): 19–25.

Achieving optimal treatment organisation in different countries

Suggestions for service development applicable across different healthcare systems

Francis Creed, Peter Henningsen and Richard Byng

Introduction

The early chapters of this book indicate that bodily distress syndromes are common and may be very disabling and expensive to health services. The data also indicate a wide range of severity of these disorders, which becomes important when considering the need for treatment. In general, a very high number of somatic symptoms is associated with marked disability and high costs.

Although it is incomplete, there is sound evidence that many of these patients can improve considerably with psychological or other forms of treatment, and that when this is successful there is often a reduction of healthcare costs. However, there is also evidence that most patients with bodily distress syndromes do not currently receive the treatment they need. There are also a few examples of new services and good practice, which we have highlighted.

Throughout this book there is reference to the barriers that need to be overcome if we are to improve treatment; these are specifically discussed in Chapter 5. The barriers are principally in four areas:

- Our dualistic system of medicine is ill-suited to problems that require the integration of medical and psychological forms of treatment.
- Many doctors lack the necessary skills to manage these problems appropriately and most do not have adequate time to do so.
- The negative attitudes towards psychological illnesses in our society affect adversely the way that patients, doctors and social agencies approach these problems.
- The situation is made worse by confused terminology and lack of understanding about these disorders, which can contribute to difficulties in patient–doctor encounters.

This chapter presents suggestions as to how the current situation can be improved. In view of the heterogeneity of healthcare systems in different countries, there is no single solution to these problems that will be applicable everywhere, so this chapter provides some overall principles in addition to specific examples. The next section provides important information for those preparing a case of need for local healthcare planners.

Medically Unexplained Symptoms, Somatisation and Bodily Distress, ed. Francis Creed, Peter Henningsen and Per Fink. Published by Cambridge University Press. © Cambridge University Press 2011.

Making the case of need

In Chapter 4, unmet need was defined as a recognised, treatable disorder that is not receiving adequate treatment and where the individuals, as a consequence, suffer impairment or disability because of untreated disorder.

At present, many doctors would not recognise bodily distress syndromes as a 'recognised, (set of) treatable disorder(s)'. The evidence presented in this book is intended to make the case that the bodily distress syndromes are indeed a well-recognised set of disorders that are treatable. We are optimistic that the current attention being paid to the revised classification of 'somatoform disorders' in relation to the *Diagnostic and Statistical Manual of Mental Disorders* (DSM)-V and International Classification of Diseases (ICD)-11 will highlight the current problems and produce a more satisfactory classification of these disorders. Even here, there is a problem of dualism as inclusion of these diagnoses in DSM-V implies that they come under the heading of 'mental disorders', whereas we have tried to make plain throughout the book that these disorders occur at the interface between 'medical' and 'psychiatric' disorders.

Throughout this book we have used, where possible, the term 'bodily distress syndromes' as an umbrella term to encompass what have been described previously in three ways: medically unexplained symptoms, somatoform disorders and functional somatic syndromes. The first two of these terms are particularly unsatisfactory and we propose a unitary phrase to enable doctors and healthcare planners to recognise a set of treatable disorders but without implying a single aetiology for all of them. The term 'bodily distress syndromes' includes patients who have well-recognised physical illnesses but also, concurrently have numerous somatic symptoms [1]. These people have been excluded from the previous terminology but they benefit from treatment in the same way as those with 'medically unexplained' symptoms, which are the hallmark of the previous diagnostic classification.

In discussion with patients, it is important to use whatever language or phrase allows the patient to understand the concept rather than stick rigidly to a particular 'diagnosis'. Patients vary in their own ideas about causation of symptoms and the label should be seen as a means to an end – less focus on symptoms and greater focus on improving functional ability.

General principles in defining the unmet need associated with bodily distress syndromes

Universal factors

The first step in making the case of need depends on understanding the local and national context in which the failure of current service provision occurs [2]. Although services vary greatly between different countries, there does seem to be a widespread problem that patients attending both primary and secondary medical care are being investigated for possible organic disease rather than being offered specific, effective treatment for multiple somatic symptoms. There seem to be three exceptions to this general rule. The first concerns symptomatic treatment for patients with functional somatic syndromes, such as irritable bowel syndrome and fibromyalgia, where drug treatment may be effective [3]. The second exception is the system of psychosomatic medicine in German-speaking countries, where patients may receive combined medical and psychological treatments without being labelled as 'psychiatric' patients (see Chapter 4). Third, there are specialist services, such as those described in Denmark and other countries where patients can receive the appropriate treatment for complicated, or multiorgan, bodily distress syndromes.

Even in these situations, where treatment is better than most others, there are problems. Far too often, doctors treating functional somatic syndromes continue with first-line symptomatic treatment when the patient actually needs psychological treatment or antidepressants for multiple somatic symptoms which have not been recognised [3]. Doctors working in psychosomatic medicine still report that patients avoid treatment in such departments because of the stigma associated with the psychological aspects of this service. Most of the specialist services have been developed for a single functional somatic syndrome, such as chronic fatigue syndrome, and are therefore not available to the vast majority of patients who need such treatments.

In summary, therefore, the arguments put forward in this book regarding unmet needs with respect to bodily distress syndromes probably hold across all healthcare systems. They can be used, therefore, to bring to the attention of healthcare planners the need to improve services.

Financial considerations

Although doctors tend to feel that the need for better treatment can be justified adequately by the obvious suffering endured by patients, a financial argument is also required. The principal argument is that this group of patients is currently very expensive to the healthcare system but this high expenditure leads to little or no health gain. This is because the money is spent on medical consultations, expensive investigations for possible organic disease and relatively ineffective symptomatic medications. Healthcare planners need to be persuaded that some of the costs currently incurred could be better spent on specific treatment that should lead to health gain. There is also a high societal cost through time missed from work and, sometimes, dependence on carers. A recent estimate for England suggested that this cost amounted to £14 billion annually [4]. These societal costs are independent of the healthcare budget, but should be of concern to politicians and economists; they should be included in the overall cost of these disorders.

We have seen that the diagnosis of 'symptoms and signs and ill-defined conditions', in which bodily distress syndromes will be included, is the fifth most expensive diagnostic category in the Netherlands and one of the most expensive categories of outpatients in UK. It is the fifth most common reason for doctor visits in the USA, where the phenomenon of multiple somatic symptoms is estimated to cost US$256 billion a year in medical costs alone. Bodily distress syndromes are among the most common presentations in primary care and can account for up to half of new patients attending specialist medical clinics, where the chance of expensive investigations is highest, but the chance of commencing effective treatment is least.

Local healthcare planning arrangements

Any proposal for a service development to improve the care of patients with bodily distress syndromes requires an understanding of the complex and confusing network of individuals and organisations involved in the planning process [2]. General practitioners (GPs) seem to be the group of doctors who are most concerned with the unmet need of this group of patients, presumably because they have sometimes to manage even severe disorders without any appropriate support from secondary care. In some countries GPs play an increasingly important role in commissioning health services, so this can be helpful. It is also becoming increasingly important that patient representatives and, where appropriate, self-help organisations, are involved in the planning process. This means that the case of need should not assume medical knowledge and should be framed in terms appropriate to the perspective of the individuals who will be involved in the planning process.

It is important that any potential service development has clear aims and objectives that are both achievable and measurable. The outcomes must be consistent with the broader aims of local health commissioning. It is best to provide a range of options for service development, including the 'do nothing' option. We have briefly described the disadvantages of the last option.

One of the greatest difficulties is trying to establish the importance of improving services for bodily distress syndromes in the eyes of the local healthcare planners. They have to rate the importance of developing such services against other services (e.g. for heart disease or diabetes) where patients have needs that are not currently met. Healthcare planners think in terms of priorities, so local knowledge of the way that priorities are determined is necessary if one is to be successful in gaining a high priority for improving services for bodily distress syndromes. A particular difficulty occurs when a service for bodily distress syndromes is proposed as it is not a high priority for either psychiatry or general medicine. Both these specialties have their own priorities and bodily distress can easily fall between them. It needs a particular 'champion' to push for bodily distress as a priority.

Any case of need must be realistic about the initial start-up costs. This includes the costs of training staff of all relevant disciplines as an appropriate skill mix is required. Costs of administrative changes need to be realistic. Wide consultation with all professional groups is necessary. One should also be able to demonstrate potential cost savings, although these may be delayed until the service has become established.

Components of a service to improve management of bodily distress syndromes

There are several major building blocks to developing a service for patients with bodily distress syndromes. The principal ones are changing aspects of the health services as a whole to make them less dualistic, training clinical staff in primary and secondary care, and modifying negative attitudes among healthcare planners/professionals, social agencies and the general public towards this group of disorders by disseminating helpful information about the recognition and treatability of these disorders. It is not clear whether tackling one of these areas alone is useful unless the other areas are also tackled. For example, training GPs may not be useful in itself unless the policy of medical specialists regarding investigation of patients with bodily distress syndromes can be changed also. Similarly, establishing a specialist clinic for patients with severe bodily distress syndromes will not have the impact that it should unless it is coupled with the training of primary and secondary healthcare professionals.

Since it is rarely possible to transform a whole medical system, more limited changes may be helpful. For example, developing a clinic for chronic fatigue is helpful to patients with this diagnosis if there has been, previously, no relevant service. Although this does not help patients who have bodily distress syndromes other than chronic fatigue, it may lead other medical specialists to recognise the advantages of a multidisciplinary clinic for patients with different types of bodily distress syndrome. This can lead to further service developments.

Alternatively, if one or more members of a consultation-liaison psychiatry team develop special expertise in, and devote dedicated time to, treating patients with bodily distress syndromes, this will help a limited number of patients. It may also lead to a change of attitudes among physicians who can begin to understand which patients with a bodily distress syndrome can be treated successfully. This is often accompanied by positive attitude change and greater support for developing a relevant service.

An example of a systems approach to medically unexplained symptoms is described below. This indicates the extent of change which needs to be considered if all aspects of the service relevant to patients with bodily distress syndromes are to be improved. The following sections briefly describe some more limited changes that involve only part of the healthcare system.

Developing a multidisciplinary team to treat severe bodily distress syndromes

Although many initiatives have started with training GPs, a local specialist multidisciplinary team should also be established, with primary responsibilities including treating severe bodily distress syndromes and supporting local GPs. As noted in Chapters 4 and 8, there are advantages if this team is located in the general hospital, as is the Danish specialist team in Aarhus. If the main push for its development comes from primary care, however, it could be a community-based team of specialists. Wherever it is sited, the members of this team must be involved closely in the training of GPs, medical specialists and other staff in order to improve their skills in treating this group of patients.

Such a specialist team needs to develop collaborative working relationships with all the other parts of the health services involved in the care of these patients. It also needs to develop clear referral guidelines for patients entering their own treatment programme. The latter are likely to be restricted to those with the more severe and persistent bodily distress syndromes. The team will therefore need to be active in helping GPs and medical specialists to manage those patients who have mild disorders which are not treated by the specialist team.

Training of GPs

The training of GPs to improve their skills in managing patients with bodily distress syndromes has been described in detail in Chapter 9. Such training is usually guided by members of the local specialist team who treat severe bodily distress syndromes. Following the initial training, there are two important aspects of care which need to be considered. First, GPs must arrange their time so that they can engage in longer consultations at prespecified times for the care of patients with moderately severe bodily distress syndromes. Such consultations are needed for patients requiring additional attention to avoid unnecessary medical referral, and also for those who have been discharged from specialist investigation. Second, it is important that the local specialist service provides ongoing support for the GPs. This is best provided in the form of collaborative care in conjunction with the GP, as there is evidence to show that this is beneficial to patients with moderately severe bodily distress syndromes. Other aspects of working with GPs are similar to those described below in respect of other medical specialists.

Training of medical specialists

One of the barriers to developing better treatment described in Chapter 5 is the fact that many doctors may inappropriately veer towards investigating physical illnesses and fail to recognise bodily distress syndromes. This is most likely in specialist medical clinics, which have ready access to investigations for possible organic disease. Some of these (e.g. magnetic resonance imaging and computed tomography) are expensive and their use in some conditions, such as headache, is questionable. Because of the general atmosphere of fear of litigation, many doctors have developed a low threshold for referring patients for extensive investigations 'to be sure', without thinking of the possible consequences for patients with bodily distress syndromes. Such investigations may well be clinically indicated, but much of the time the clinical indication is very questionable.

Part of the training of specialist physicians, therefore, concerns managing risk. This is best dealt with in conjunction with commissioners (see the section on a total systems approach below) as it is too threatening for individual clinicians to tackle this important issue alone. Having said that, there are some moves to try to reduce the extent of investigations performed for patients who have functional somatic syndromes. For example, the UK National Institute for Health and Clinical Excellence (NICE) guidelines for chronic fatigue syndrome and irritable bowel syndrome list recommended investigations, but they also list investigations that should *not* be performed unless they are clinically indicated [5;6]. Working with specialist physicians to ensure that such guidelines are followed locally is one way to reduce the use of investigations without detriment to patient care.

Other aspects of training specialist physicians have been described in Chapter 9. This topic is also described below in terms of persuading medical specialists to endorse the same type of management as employed by the GP with patients who have bodily distress syndromes. This includes alerting the patient to the likelihood of a negative investigation and the implications this has for understanding the likely cause of the patient's symptoms. It has been shown, for example, that a patient explanatory leaflet and brief discussion prior to a diagnostic exercise stress test can significantly reduce subsequent anxiety about heart disease [7] (see pp. 74–75, Chapter 3). Instituting such a leaflet and discussion as part of the normal routine of diagnostic stress tests should help subsequent care by the GP. The greater use of specially devised explanatory leaflets for patients with functional somatic syndromes would be very helpful. It has been suggested that both patients and doctors would benefit from the use of an algorithm focusing on positive diagnosis and evidence-based treatment of irritable bowel syndrome [8].

Both GPs and specialist physicians should be trained to ask every patient about the extent of their health worry, their expectations of the consultation, and screening questions for anxiety and depression, as this information can reduce difficult doctor–patient encounters by half [9]. Another important area for discussion with medical specialists and GPs is the use of screening questionnaires for multiple somatic symptoms. A very high score on the Patient Health Questionnaire (PHQ)-15, for example, should alert the physician that the diagnosis of bodily distress syndrome is very likely and management of the medical problem should be modified accordingly. If it seems likely that the patient has complicated, or multiorgan bodily distress syndrome, then preparing the patient for referral for cognitive behavioural therapy is much more helpful than prescribing symptomatic treatment for the leading somatic symptom.

A systems approach to 'medically unexplained' symptoms in Plymouth, UK

In the UK, an attempt has recently been made to develop a total systems approach to improve the care of patients with 'medically unexplained' symptoms. Because the phrase 'medically unexplained' symptoms is used in the project description, we will use it here although, as we see below, it caused difficulty with patient representation on the steering group [10]. This project is described in detail here as it highlights a broad range of issues that are relevant to developing services to improving the care of patients with bodily distress syndromes. The project aimed to develop guidance for the management of 'medically unexplained' symptoms by GPs, secondary care and medical specialists, and to develop a commissioner-led approach to medically unexplained symptoms. It also aimed to pilot the development of 'care pathways' for medically unexplained symptoms at the Plymouth Referral Management Centre. This required the establishment of a system-wide steering group and involvement of a wide range of stakeholders. The desired outcomes of this project were:

- no increase in missed diagnoses
- improved functioning, mental health and reported satisfaction by patients with unexplained symptoms
- more fulfilled and relaxed practitioners
- neutral or reduced cost of care.

Key messages from the literature

The project involved a literature review, and the main messages from this review were summarised as follows:

- 'Medically unexplained' symptoms can be associated with significant distress and impaired functioning for patients, high stress levels for clinicians and high costs to the healthcare system (see Box 10.1).
- The relationship between clinician and patient is crucial: the patient needs to feel listened to and understood.
- 'Medically unexplained' symptoms fall within a range of severity from mild to severe. Each type requires a slightly different type of management.
- A consultation-liaison model is recommended but difficult to implement in practice.
- Reattribution is a well-researched method, but has mixed results.
  - The Danish group developed a training method, the 'TERM' model, based on modifications of the reattribution model, including training and 'scripts' for use by GPs [17]. This has proved more successful than the original reattribution model (see Chapter 9).
- Communication between components of the healthcare system is vital for consistency of approach, so there is value in tackling all components of the system concurrently – patient, clinician and system.
- NICE guidelines should be followed for specific syndromes, where available.

Plymouth healthcare system

A review of the local healthcare system indicated that there was no specific provision within the clinical psychology services for people with 'medically unexplained' symptoms, except for those with some specific functional disorders. Patients with 'medically unexplained' symptoms were encountered at all tiers of the healthcare system and the clinicians who treated these patients recognised the need for training and tools to aid them in working with these patients. Clinicians were generally amenable to the use of training and tools to help them

Box 10.1 Why do 'medically unexplained' symptoms present such a problem?

For patients:

- Patient dissatisfaction [11]
- Conflict between patients' and physicians' explanations/beliefs [12]
- Stress and anxiety for patient [13;14]
- Iatrogenic harm
- Beliefs of physical causes become ingrained over time

For clinicians:

- 'Heartsink' patients
- Stress and anxiety for practitioner [13]; [14]
- Patient dissatisfaction [15]
- Conflict between patients' and physicians' explanations/beliefs [12]
- Unnecessary/excessive use of tests, resources and consultants' time
- Pressure/stress on consultant when delivering negative results

For the system:

- Cost of repeated consultations
- Cost to secondary care services [16]
- Unnecessary/excessive use of tests, resources and consultants' time

in working with patients who have medically unexplained symptoms – particularly those newer to the National Health Service (NHS), who have not yet built up their own strategies. A number of gaps in Plymouth health system were identified:

- the lack of psychological assessment and therapy services for people with 'medically unexplained' symptoms
- little community or primary care capacity for managing patients with longer term 'medically unexplained' symptoms
- a lack of consultation-liaison psychiatry for 'medically unexplained' symptoms.

Local data were collected. These indicated a high number of patients seen in gynaecology, neurology, cardiology, general medicine and gastroenterology clinics.

Stakeholder event

This event was essential to publicise the issue of 'medically unexplained' symptoms and involve stakeholders in possible solutions to the difficulties of improving care for these patients. Twenty-seven practitioners from eight different professional groups attended and there was agreement that this is a common area of difficulty within the local health community, which needed to be addressed. A systems approach was a helpful way of viewing the issue, but GPs should essentially be at the centre of management.

A *psychological toolkit* would be useful for consultants in secondary care, as this area of clinical practice is not emphasised in their training, and a *patient information leaflet* would be useful to support consultations. It was also recognised that there was a need for more *multi-disciplinary working*, and *risk management* issues needed to be addressed, including the need to reduce clinician anxiety. It was decided to develop and pilot both general guidance and a range of specific guides supporting clinicians at all stages of the pathway of care for patients with 'medically unexplained' symptoms. Psychological training for consultants and specialist teams was also recognised as essential.

It was decided that the *referral template* (used by Sentinel Community Interest Company (CIC), the GP-led referral management service) for patients being referred from primary to secondary care needed to be altered to encourage open discussion of possible/probable medically unexplained symptoms; but without 'labelling' this as a disease. Full, correct completion of the referral form should become part of the culture of referral.

Whole systems governance arrangements (i.e. full support from the local commissioning and provider bodies) to support these changes were necessary in developing clinical guidelines, developing risk-management guidelines and ensuring ratification of guidance with the local regulatory bodies. It was hoped that these changes in clinical practice would lead to fewer investigations for possible organic disease, more primary care input and a greater focus on attaining improved functional status (quality of life) of patients with medically unexplained symptoms. Key changes in clinical behaviour required to achieve these objectives are listed in Box 10.2.

Process and problems: some of the barriers met by the project

Development of such a system-wide approach was not without problems, some of which are described here for illustration purposes.

Referral management centre

Although the initial focus of the project was the referral management centre (Sentinel CIC), which processes all referrals from primary to secondary care, this newly created company had competing priorities so the team focused on other parts of the Plymouth healthcare system. This also meant that data-gathering regarding bodily distress syndromes was not possible.

General practitioners

Engagement of GPs was challenging, but GPs were successfully involved with the project both on an individual and at a practice level. Their engagement might have been improved if the referral management centre had been able to offer higher visibility sponsorship of the project. Many of the GPs taking an interest had developed strategies for dealing with 'medically unexplained' symptoms, which were incorporated into the guidance.

Less experienced GPs were able to articulate their lack of skills in managing 'medically unexplained' symptoms as an educational need; greater provision of training and tools at the GPs training stage is needed. Some experienced GPs had developed their own strategies for management, many of which mimicked very closely those suggested by research. Engaging experienced GPs without an interest in this topic was more challenging.

Patient involvement

Although a patient representative was on the steering group, and was consulted at several stages throughout the process, many patients do not understand or agree with the term 'medically unexplained symptoms' as a description of their symptoms. Patients were consulted regarding the patient information leaflet and the term was removed. It is a sensitive issue for both patients and clinicians, and it highlights the need to recognise and focus on

> **Box 10.2** Summary of key changes required to clinical practice
>
> Changes to primary-care consultations (as means of micro-commissioning):
> - Empathise and acknowledge symptoms
> - In 'medically unexplained' symptoms cases at low risk of disease, investigation and referral may not be required – clinicians can 'share risk' by discussing with patient, specialist or colleagues (and documenting)
> - In suspected cases of 'medically unexplained' symptoms, when referring for investigation or specialist opinion, patient should be informed of likely 'negative' results in order to manage expectations
> - Inform specialists of likely 'medically unexplained' symptoms in Sentinel referral letters (rather than feeling need to justify referral by emphasising symptoms)
> - Offer and explore, but don't push, psychosocial explanation
> - Focus on improving functional ability
> - Recognise and treat comorbid anxiety and depression
>
> Changes to specialist consultations:
> - In cases of suspected medically unexplained symptoms, when referring for investigation, patient should be informed of likely 'negative' results in order to manage expectations
> - Once a low risk of disease has been established, further investigation may not be required – clinicians can 'share risk' by discussing with patient and/or colleagues (and documenting)
> - Discharge to primary care once investigations are completed with clear negative results
> - Respond to GP's provisional medically unexplained symptoms diagnosis and actively support it verbally to patient and in writing to the GP

the symptoms in a way that is acceptable to both parties. In this respect, the issue of patient involvement throws up ethical problems. Involvement of patients to assess acceptability of new services is seen as critical.

Mental health service input

The project did not focus on the role of mental health services for 'medically unexplained' symptoms. It was agreed that improved treatment for comorbid depression and anxiety among these patients who recognised a mental health component to their problems was important. However, there was no clear agreement about whether the recently developed 'Improving Access to Psychological Therapies' service should provide cognitive behavioural therapy specifically for patients with 'medically unexplained' symptoms as opposed to depression or anxiety. Capacity in the newly formed service was an issue, but there was also disagreement as to whether patients who still considered their problems to be physical would engage with an overtly framed mental health service. There is also no clear pathway for those particularly complex patients with comorbid 'medically unexplained' symptoms and personality disorder.

System issues

Redesigning a service for medically unexplained symptoms is difficult because such a wide range of services and individuals is involved. While it can be easier to focus on a distinct functional somatic syndrome, as this reduces the number of staff involved in redesigning the service, the impact on the wider system will be limited. As well as looking at several ENT pathways as exemplars, this project was able to make recommendations for pathway, governance and training issues across the system.

Proposed next steps for NHS Plymouth

This project was evaluated and the list of proposed next steps indicates the complexity of a whole-systems approach to improving the care of patients with bodily distress syndromes.

- *Policy development for management of 'medically unexplained' symptoms.* With regards to commissioning, this work has been taken up by local commissioners, but not given a high priority. The guidelines produced within the project for the management of 'medically unexplained' symptoms were well received. These need to be ratified by the necessary regulatory bodies so they become clinical policy for primary and secondary general medical and mental health provider services. It is also necessary to gain approval for the Positive Risk Management Guidance [18].

- *As an alternative to a 'medically unexplained' symptoms pathway into the new psychological therapy service, a 'medically unexplained' symptoms franchise model was proposed.* This model aims to offer a 'consultancy' service to all departments in secondary care, develop care pathways for different bodily distress syndromes and develop a consultation-liaison model with health psychology and liaison psychiatry for secondary and primary care clinicians. This has similarities to the models of care outlined earlier in the chapter – the service would have a combined physical and mental health function and would involve specialists working across the primary–secondary care interface. This approach would create a specific pathway for mid-level problems on an 'as and when' basis. It would not proactively divert patients away from unproductive primary or secondary care. Such a model, developed by a GP in Cumbria, has been shown to be acceptable to patients and reduce the number of subsequent appointments,

- *Develop and deliver training programme across health community.* In addition to training GPs in the management of 'medically unexplained' symptoms and risk, there is a need to develop the key skills and knowledge for key departments throughout the healthcare system.

- *Commissioning new services.* The possibilities for new services include a symptom management group, consultation-liaison psychiatry, specialist 'training' service aimed at increasing capacity of (mental) health professionals and specific interventions.

- *Patient information and involvement.* A patient-information leaflet has already been produced and it conforms to patient information guidelines [19]. It should be distributed in conjunction with training. More effective patient involvement is required in this area of clinical practice.

It is intended that the output of the project – a local framework for the management of medically unexplained symptoms [19] – is a useful resource for others involved in developing care for patients with these disorders.

Among the barriers to success were competing priorities of commissioning, including the fact that this topic is never first on anyone's agenda and it is easy to leave in the 'too difficult' box, compared with other more limited service developments. 'Medically unexplained' symptoms are once again being prioritised in Plymouth and it is hoped that many of the principles in the guidance will be put into action. The guidance has been used to influence commissioners in several areas in the UK. In the Devon Partnership Trust a 'symptom management pathway' has been developed. Patients identified from primary and secondary care with 'medically unexplained' symptoms are referred to a primary care-based clinic to see a specialist mental health practitioner and GP focusing on symptoms and function. This kind of pathway promises rewards not only of improved function but also of reduced NHS costs.

Conclusions

The Plymouth whole-systems *'medically unexplained' symptoms* project has succeeded in engaging shareholders across the system to produce:

- guidance for practitioners in the form of a whole-systems pathway
- positive risk management guidance to support clinicians by gaining whole-system governance approval
- an outline for integrating educational interventions for patients and clinicians into a whole-systems approach.

The project also described key clinical changes across the system. Using practice-based commissioning as a specific mechanism, in order to shift care away from investigation and hospitals towards primary care, a focus on improved functional status remains elusive. The experience described and the products developed should be of use to others across the UK and other countries developing services for patients with 'medically unexplained' symptoms. The service development in Plymouth has emphasised some of the important ingredients of successful integration of general medical and psychiatric services, which have been listed by Kathol and colleagues [20]:

- close professional relationships between collaborating mental health and general health professionals, and co-location of the two groups of staff with frequent and sustained interaction over time
- clearly identified leaders who 'champion' the service
- gradual development of the service over time with attention to implementation of all critical components
- use of case managers who operate under close supervision of experienced psychiatrists
- a triage system to identify and work with patients who have complicated medical-psychiatric problems
- consolidated general medical and psychiatric clinical records
- mental health staff prepared to adjust their working practices to fit the medical setting.

Kathol *et al.* also listed some of the difficulties in developing integrated general medical and mental health services [20]. One of these, mentioned by several organisations, was a fast pace of change. Since culture change is required in the relevant organisations to achieve successful integration, a gradual pace of change to this end appears important.

Key features of developing a service for bodily distress syndromes

Developing a steering group

In most countries there is very little 'top down' pressure from the respective department of health, or equivalent national body, to develop a service for bodily distress syndromes. In the absence of such guidance, it is necessary to try to influence national healthcare planners, but most people will be trying to work with local healthcare planners.

The first step to developing a service for bodily distress syndromes involves convening a group of doctors who are interested and enthusiastic about such a development. Since consultation-liaison psychiatrists are the only group of specialists who have this specific remit in their job description, it is likely that such a person might initiate a steering group. That person needs to involve at least one GP, who has influence within the local sphere of primary care. It is also preferable to have a medical specialist involved because of the necessity of influencing both primary and secondary care medical specialists if one is to bring about the changes that are needed.

Early involvement of the professions likely to be involved in developing the service is helpful. This will include psychologists, nurses, occupational therapists, physiotherapists and administrators, with other staff according to local service configuration. It is also necessary to bring on board those staff who can facilitate the service development by helping to modify existing general medical services. This involves the development of facilities for longer, private patient–doctor interactions, reducing investigations for organic disease (some of which may bring income to the hospital) and improving communication between primary and secondary health services.

It is also advisable to involve a local healthcare planner from an early stage. The description of the experience in Plymouth, UK, makes it clear that this is a complicated and difficult area of development. For this reason, to avoid much wasted time and effort, it is necessary to be guided by a healthcare planner, but it is crucial to try to persuade this planner to become a champion of the development. One would hope that the financial arguments, coupled with the degree of suffering and inability to work associated with bodily distress syndromes, would enable at least one senior member of the healthcare planning team to become involved.

The model to be developed

As mentioned previously, one may need to be flexible about the form of service to be developed. Because the development of a full service for bodily distress syndromes may not fall readily into one of the 'boxes' of the healthcare development schemes, which are usually specialty-specific, it may be necessary to 'sell' the model by comparing it with similar services. A multidisciplinary pain clinic is one such model and most healthcare planners will be aware of the need for such a clinic and have an idea about how they are run. Another key model is seen in the clinical services for chronic fatigue syndrome (see Appendix 10.1), which has been widely established in some countries, including the UK and Belgium. The drawbacks of limiting such a service to a single group of patients should be spelled out.

Although it is preferable to establish training of GPs and medical specialists and a specialist clinic for severe bodily distress syndromes simultaneously, this may not be practicable.

A step in this direction, however, can be made if a consultation-liaison psychiatrist devotes special time to this work and operates a collaborative care model with local, specially trained GPs. In this way, it may be possible to improve the care of some patients with bodily distress syndromes and thereby provide a model through which healthcare planners and other healthcare professionals to witness an alternative to the repeated normal investigations/no health gain model.

Local initiatives to demonstrate need

If possible, it is well worth collecting local data in the form of an audit to demonstrate the high proportion of new medical outpatients who have bodily distress syndromes and the number of investigations they receive. The latter can be costed and contrasted with the amount of specific treatment that they receive for their bodily distress. There is little doubt that locally collected data are more persuasive than national data, even though the latter are more extensive. Examples of local audits can be seen in two published papers [21;22].

Another worthwhile type of audit measures the extent to which local general and specialist medical practice conforms to guidelines, such as those produced for irritable bowel syndrome, chronic fatigue syndrome and for 'somatoform disorders', if these have been produced in your country. If your country does not have guidelines for bodily distress syndromes, it is best to encourage their development.

A consultation-liaison psychiatrist could devote a specified amount of time each week to assessing and treating patients with bodily distress syndromes. It is very likely that any such clinic would soon develop a substantial waiting list because demand will outstrip the supply of adequate treatment. There have been instances where this has persuaded commissioners to develop the service further. In Denmark, demand by GPs for training in the TERM model has been very helpful in making the case for more resources to be devoted to such training. Irrespective of patient outcomes, after the training, GPs have reported feeling more confident and more comfortable with patients who present with bodily distress. This is a very important step in changing attitudes.

Suggested ways of meeting the need

The service development in Plymouth has been described in detail and the services provided in Denmark and Germany have been described in earlier chapters of this book. Recent initiatives in Belgium have been outlined in Chapter 4. Some very helpful material has recently been provided by primary care commissioners in Birmingham, UK [18]. Guidelines for the care of patients with bodily distress syndromes have been developed in several countries. It is hoped that the European Association of Consultation-Liaison Psychiatry and Psychosomatics (EACLPP) will facilitate the development of services for patients with bodily distress syndromes in the following ways:

- ensuring that guidelines that are developed in European countries are widely circulated and, if appropriate, facilitating the modification of these guidelines for different healthcare systems
- facilitating the production of patient information leaflets that can be widely distributed
- seeking ways to engage with the general public and patient organisations in order to facilitate attitude change towards this group of disorders

- facilitating the transfer of training programmes between countries and enabling more consultation-liaison psychiatrists and other appropriate professional staff to become proficient in the training of GPs and medical specialists
- promoting the development of a 'psychological toolkit' for medical specialists to help them to improve their management of patients with these disorders
- circulating widely information concerning the risks involved in changing clinical practice and how these risks can best be managed.
- continuing to promote the importance of better care for patients with bodily distress syndromes through publicity, pressure on European or national bodies responsible for healthcare, encouragement of training and research.

Conclusion

This book has brought together a wealth of information about bodily distress syndromes in the hope that this will provide impetus to the development of services for these syndromes. It is up to local doctors and other healthcare professionals and planners and national health departments to take these developments further.

All those concerned with the production of this book are committed to pressing for improved services for patients with bodily distress syndromes. It is hoped that the production of this book will bring to the attention of the relevant healthcare planners, healthcare professionals, patient organisations, general public and politicians the enormous unmet need regarding these disorders and the importance to healthcare systems of recognising the cost-effectiveness of services to meet these needs.

Appendix 10.1
Description of services for chronic fatigue syndrome
Leeds and West Yorkshire Chronic Fatigue Syndrome/Myalgic Encephalopathy Service

For full details, see: www.manchestercfsme.nhs.uk/document_uploads/Co-ordinators_Resource/Operational_Policy_March_06.pdf

The mission statement of this service indicates that it is:

'a multidisciplinary service, which aims to help people who have a diagnosis of or are debilitated by Chronic Fatigue Syndrome or related problems and live in the West Yorkshire area. The service aims to provide specialist assessment, therapy interventions, and management advice from a range of disciplines. The service also aims to provide expert advice, education and support to health professionals, statutory and non-statutory organisations, service users and carers on the condition.'

In addition to a clinical team manager, administrative support and a medical secretary, the multidisciplinary team includes a part-time consultant and another doctor in liaison psychiatry, a clinical nurse specialist in cognitive behaviour therapy, another nurse, several occupational therapists and physiotherapists, and input from a clinical psychologist, a consultant in immunology and a dietician. This means that a range of treatments is available after the initial assessment to decide which treatments are required.

The treatment is organised into three levels according to the severity of the condition. For mild to moderate disorder, brief advice, workshops and a chronic fatigue syndrome programme are available. At the moderate to severe level, multidisciplinary assessment is required with individual work and assessment, and treatment by liaison psychiatry if necessary. At the very severe level, home rehabilitation and even inpatient management is available. Full details are available on the website (see above).

There are six adult chronic fatigue syndrome/myalgic encephalopathy services in the Manchester region. There is an extensive assessment scheme, which may be followed by one of six forms of treatment: activity and exercise; cognitive behavioural therapy; complementary approaches; relaxation techniques; and symptomatic control. There are a variety of different disciplines involved in the Manchester regional scheme. For details, including the guidelines for treatment of chronic fatigue syndrome, visit www.manchestercfsme.nhs.uk/services/.

References

1. Kroenke K, Zhong X, Theobald D, Wu JW, Tu WZ, Carpenter JS. Somatic symptoms in patients with cancer experiencing pain or depression prevalence, disability, and health care use. *Archives of Internal Medicine* 2010; **170**(18): 1686–94.

2. Peveler R, House A. Developing services in liaison psychiatry. In: Peveler R, Feldman E, Friedman T, eds. *Liaison Psychiatry. Planning Services for Specialist Settings.* London: Gaskell; 2000: 1–13.

3. Henningsen P, Zipfel S, Herzog W. Management of functional somatic syndromes. *The Lancet* 2007; **369**(9565): 946–55.

4. Bermingham SL, Cohen A, Hague J, Parsonage M. The cost of somatisation among the working-age population in England for the year 2008–2009. *Mental Health in Family Medicine* 2010; 7: 71–84.

5. National Institute for Health and Clinical Excellence. *Chronic Fatigue Syndrome/ Myalgic Encephalomyelitis: Diagnosis and Management of CFS/ME in Adults and Children.* London: NICE; 2007.

6. National Institute for Health and Clinical Excellence. *Irritable Bowel Syndrome in Adults. Diagnosis and Management of Irritable Bowel Syndrome in Primary Care.* London: NICE; 2008.

7. Petrie KJ, Muller JT, Schirmbeck F, Donkin L, Broadbent E, Ellis CJ et al. Effect of providing information about normal test results on patients' reassurance: randomised controlled trial. *British Medical Journal* 2007; **334**(7589): 352–4.

8. Quigley EM, Bytzer P, Jones R, Mearin F, Quigley EMM, Bytzer P et al. Irritable bowel syndrome: the burden and unmet needs in Europe. *Digestive and Liver Disease* 2006; **38**(10): 717–23.

9. Jackson JL, Kroenke K, Chamberlin J. Effects of physician awareness of symptom-related expectations and mental disorders – a controlled trial. *Archives of Family Medicine* 1999; **8**(2): 135–42.

10. NHS Plymouth. *Medically Unexplained Symptoms (MUS): A Whole Systems Approach in Plymouth.* NHS Plymouth, 2009.

11. Reid S, Wessely S, Crayford T, Hotopf M. Medically unexplained symptoms in frequent attenders of secondary health care: retrospective cohort study. *British Medical Journal* 2001; **322**(7289): 767–9.

12. Salmon P, Peters S, Stanley I. Patients' perceptions of medical explanations for somatisation disorders: qualitative analysis. *British Medical Journal* 1999; **318**(7180): 372–6.

13. Salmon P, Humphris GM, Ring A, Davies JC, Dowrick CF. Primary care consultations about medically unexplained symptoms: patient presentations and doctor responses that influence the probability of somatic intervention. *Psychosomatic Medicine* 2007; **69**(6): 571–7.

14. Engel CC, Liu X, McCarthy BD, Miller RF, Ursano R. Relationship of physical symptoms to posttraumatic stress disorder among veterans seeking care for Gulf War-related health concerns. *Psychosomatic Medicine* 2000; **62**(6): 739–45.

15. Page LA, Wessley S. Medically unexplained symptoms: exacerbating factors in the doctor–patient encounter. *Journal of the Royal Society of Medicine* 2003; **96**: 223–7.

16. Reid S, Wessely S, Crayford T, Hotopf M. Frequent attenders with medically unexplained symptoms: service use and costs in secondary care. *British Journal of Psychiatry* 2002; **180**: 248–53.

17. Fink P, Rosendal M, Toft T. Assessment and treatment of functional disorders in general practice: the extended reattribution and management model – an advanced educational program for nonpsychiatric doctors. *Psychosomatics* 2002; **43**(2): 93–131.

18. Chitnis A, Dowrick C, Byng R, Turner P, Shiers D. *Guidance for health professionals on medically unexplained symptoms (MUS).* 2011; Available at: www.wmrdc.org.uk/wmrdc/en/mental-health/primary-care/medically-unexplained-symptoms/ (Accessed, 3 April, 2011).

19. NHS Evidence – commissioning. *Medically unexplained symptaus (MUS): a whole systems approach in Plymouth.* Improving access to Psychological Therapies (IAPT); 2009. Available at: www.iapt.nhs.uk/silo/files/medically-unexplained-symptoms-mus-a-whole-systems-approach-in-plymouth.pdf (Accessed 3 April, 2011).

20. Kathol RG, Butler M, McAlpine DD, Kane RL. Barriers to physical and mental condition integrated service delivery. *Psychosomatic Medicine* 2010; **72**(6): 511–18.

21. Hamilton J, Campos R, Creed F. Anxiety, depression and management of medically unexplained symptoms in medical clinics. *Journal of the Royal College of Physicians of London* 1996; **30**(1): 18–20.

22. Mangwana S, Burlinson S, Creed F. Medically unexplained symptoms presenting at secondary care – a comparison of white Europeans and people of south Asian ethnicity. *International Journal of Psychiatry in Medicine* 2009; **39**(1): 33–44.

Index

Printed in the United States
By Bookmasters